Linda Clark on This Book and Its Author

- **Who Is Your Doctor and Why?** was one of the turning points of my life.

- I have leaned upon the knowledge supplied by Dr. Shadman in **Who Is Your Doctor and Why?** to choose and use these wonderful remedies, remedies which are safe, natural and do not have the side effects attributed to drugs.

- I would not be without these remedies, or the book by Dr. Shadman, to help me understand how homeopathy works and to apply it to my health.

  — Linda Clark (from her book **Get Well Naturally**, paperback edition published by Arco Publishing, New York, N.Y.)

WHO IS YOUR DOCTOR AND WHY?

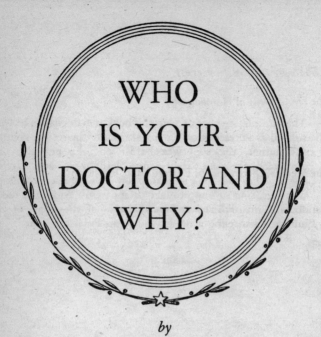

WHO IS YOUR DOCTOR AND WHY?

by

ALONZO JAY SHADMAN, M.D.
With comments by LINDA CLARK

KEATS PUBLISHING, INC.   NEW CANAAN, CONNECTICUT

The information contained in this book is in no way to be considered as a prescription for any ailment of the reader. Neither the author, the copyright holder nor the publisher has authorized the use of their names or the use of any material contained in this book in connection with the sale, promotion or advertising of any product or apparatus. Any such use is strictly unauthorized and in violation of the rights of the author, the copyright holder and Keats Publishing, Inc.

WHO IS YOUR DOCTOR AND WHY?

Copyright © 1958 by Alonzo Jay Shadman
Copyright © 1980 by Mrs. Norman Meyer
Pivot Health Edition published by arrangement with
Mrs. Norman Meyer
Special contents copyright © 1980 by Keats Publishing, Inc.

All Rights Reserved

No part of this book may be copied or reproduced in any form
without permission of the publishers

ISBN: 0-87983-227-4
Library of Congress Catalog Card Number: 80-82320

Printed in the United States of America

PIVOT HEALTH EDITIONS are published by
Keats Publishing, Inc.
36 Grove Street, New Canaan, Connecticut 06840

PREFACE

When Dr. Shadman's book first appeared in 1958, the ideas presented therein were skeptically received; his philosophy of HEALTH as a totality of man's natural state, and Homeopathy as a therapeutic system to aid simple physiological disorders, ran counter to the current orthodoxy of chemotherapy. A skilled surgeon himself, head of a 150 bed hospital in Boston, he incurred medical wrath with his charge of unnecessary operations and fee-splitting.

Yet the intervening years have proved Dr. Shadman's observations to be correct: on smoking, the harms of x-ray, the dangers of the sulpha drugs, to name a few. His views on diet have been strengthened by many sources, from Adelle Davis to Beatrice Trum Hunter. One of his most controversial statements, that more children died of vaccination than from smallpox, was corroborated (Lloyd Shearer's *Intelligence Report*, Oct. 3, 1971) by the United States Public Health Service, which is considering the abolition of routine smallpox vaccinations.

Dr. Shadman's warning of the dangers of putting fluorides into the public water supply has been solidly researched in the United States by such men as Dr. George Waldbott, Detroit allergist, Professor A. W. Burgstahler of the University of Kansas, Dr. Alfred Taylor of the Clayton Foundation; and in Europe by such men as Professor G. Frada of Palermo, Italy, and D. G. Steyn of South Africa. Recently, the political-economic pressures surrounding the fluoridation issue have been underscored by Ralph Nader and supported, in fact, by action against the fluoridation of public water supplies in Sweden, Switzerland, West Germany, and Italy.

A continuous demand for this book after Dr. Shadman's passing in 1960 has necessitated this printing.

A growing number of voices are joining the call for medical truth and urging an investigation of the medical-chemical complex. Once alone, Dr. Shadman would have been pleased with this company.

Time has shown Dr. Shadman to have been a perceptive prophet, dedicated to maintaining man's *natural* state — his miracle of health.

N.M.
Wellesley, Mass.

CONTENTS

WHO IS YOUR DOCTOR AND WHY?

CHAPTER I

Who Is Your Doctor and Why?

In 1953 bills for doctors and medicine cost 1,500,000 United States families one half or more of their entire income.

Of these families 500,000 spent all or more than all of their income on medical bills (thus burdening themselves with debt for years to come).

Drugs worth $14,000,000,000 (14 *billion* dollars) are purchased annually by the American public in its quest for health.

Millions of dollars are solicited and spent every year by research foundations with the avowed purpose of finding cures for the diseases which plague the nation.

These figures are staggering and their size alone might suggest that, at great financial sacrifice, we are at last becoming a healthy nation. Yet one further statistic quickly pops any such balloon of optimism: it is estimated that there are in our country today 45,000,000 chronic sick (over one quarter of the population), few of whom will ever be completely cured! The number is growing steadily and such major diseases as heart trouble and cancer, on which so much is spent, far from decreasing, are taking an ever greater toll of life.

Isn't this a horrible discrepancy? Doesn't the return on such tremendous expenditures seem pitiful in the light of the true condition? Aren't we justified in asking questions about the effectiveness of our research and the drugs so universally used? Shouldn't we try to find out just what kind of men we have appointed as guardians of our health?

In fact, with the knowledge of such an appalling state of affairs, isn't it imperative that we probe deeply and earnestly into our whole medical system and philosophy to determine whether or not we are wasting immeasurable effort and money because of possible widely-held misconceptions of the nature of disease and the means of cure?

It must be remembered that all living organisms have an innate power to recover from sickness without help. The *right* kind of help, of course, is always welcomed by nature, but do you know what doctor to get to provide the remedy which can really give nature the help it sometimes requires?

At least 90 per cent of all who become sick can eventually get well without a doctor. The remaining 10 per cent could use real medical help to good advantage. Therefore, the question arises: *What is real medical help and where are you going to find it?*

Today every community has its allopaths, osteopaths, chiropractors, naturopaths, eclectics, physiotherapists, hydrotherapists, electrotherapists, and a host of religious and semi-religious cults, claiming cure through faith to say nothing of voodooism, mesmerism and those who believe in the laying on of hands. All of these are engaged in the treatment of disease, and *no two methods agree on the treatment* in any given case.

You undoubtedly believe that your doctor can cure you when you are sick, regardless of what school, cult or pathy he follows, otherwise you would not employ him. If your car needs repairing and the repairman does a good job, the result is self-evident because the car would not repair itself. However, you may be giving credit to your doctor for having done a good job when nature cured you, possibly in spite of him!

In the meantime, your confidence in your doctor grows and is so firmly established eventually, that when serious sickness comes to you or your family he will be the one on whom you will rely. His actual ability, or lack of it, not your faith in him, will determine the outcome. If death ensues, whether in spite of him or because of him, your previously established confidence in him will absolve him of all blame, and death will be charged to the inscrutable Providence whose will must be done. If the patient lives, whether in spite of the doctor or not, your confidence will, therefore, in your opinion have been justified.

The mortality rate of the so-called cults is lower than that of Orthodox medicine principally because they do not risk the possible poisoning of their patients with strong drugs. Of the two kinds of medical doctors (M.D.'s) today, one kind is right, the other I believe to be absolutely wrong — and they are as far apart as the poles.

One kind will cure quickly, quietly, permanently and inexpensively, all in accordance with Nature's Law of Cure — Homœopathy, the new school.

The other kind, the old school — organized Orthodox — will use strong, often dangerous, expensive drugs that change and modify the symptoms, that have been known to kill within a few hours and only too often will change the original ailment into artificial ones which are difficult to cure. This is in accordance with a false conception of sickness.

This book will tell you how to choose your family doctor, if after reading it, you still feel that you need one.

*　　　*　　　*

I always wanted to be a doctor.

I had an unusual respect and great admiration for such men as our old family physician, Dr. Bailey of Titusville, Pennsylvania, where I was born. I wanted to be like him. I have never outlived the influence he had on me.

Of course my great ambition was only a dream — I feared I could never make it. I had a profound inferiority complex, although we had no name for it then. It was just bashfulness, modesty and lack of self-assurance.

One day while working for the Library Bureau in Boston, selling office systems, card indexes, etc., I had occasion to go into a drug store carrying my sample case, which was just like the bags the doctors carried, and the clerk came up and said, "Good morning, Doctor, what can I do for you?" Well, that did it! No more doubts assailed me. If I looked like a doctor to the clerk, then a doctor I would become.

This happened in May, and in the fall I was in medical school, just like that.

After graduation, I went to the Emerson Hospital in Forest Hills, Massachusetts, and learned surgery under Dr. Nathaniel W. Emerson. He was a clever surgeon and a fine Homœopathic doctor. He and I were like father and son. I learned much from him.

After his passing I took over the hospital. My new hospital had a capacity of one hundred and sixty-five beds. There were on the courtesy staff nearly five hundred (old-school) physicians, each one of whom was family physician to many. I was of the new school — Homœopathic.

There I had a most unusual opportunity to observe and study orthodox measures and to compare the results with new-school treatment. This position offered me a rare chance to discover for myself, from first-hand experience, those concepts and practices which were false and unreliable and those which were true and curative. Of the latter I found none in the old-school medical practice.

The knowledge which I thus acquired should belong to everyone, physician and layman alike.

I had seen the bad effects of many pre- and post-operative procedures and changed them for something better. As an instance: I was impressed by the fact that in emergency operations — where there was no time for cathartics, enemas and pre-drugging — the patient always seemed to get along better than those who were treated by routine measures. Thereafter I left out all the customary pre-drugging, cathartics, enemas, etc. The patients all did well. I stopped all *post*-operative druggings, as I had seen so many killed by drugs after an otherwise successful operation.

Before operating, we used to scrub our hands in strong solutions of various kinds, and I would go to bed nearly every night with the backs of my hands so sore, tender, and even bleeding, that the pressure of the bed clothing caused pain.

I stopped all that. We just scrubbed with soap and water and rinsed with alcohol. We stopped the soap poultices that were applied to the field of operation and just cleaned normally, dried and swabbed with 1½% iodine. After that everybody was happy. Patients did better. Doctors and nurses did not go around exuding the awful smell of chloride of lime, and there were actually much fewer cases of "wound infection."

Before I acquired my own hospital it was routine practice to syringe septic wounds with various substances supposed to be germicides. We used to buy these large glass syringes by the gross. The wounds were very slow in healing under this treatment.

I gave the matter a lot of thought and study and finally concluded that in washing out the wounds, more harm than good resulted, because the healing serum supplied by Nature was washed away too.

As soon as I got the opportunity to put my ideas into practice, wounds healed very quickly without disinfectants, and so I was finally convinced that there were no known germicides — except Nature's own. We bought no more syringes after that.

I watched the effects of homœopathic remedies on my patients and compared them with the results of drugging. In fact, many doctors, when asked by the nurses, "What are your orders for the patient?", replied, "Do whatever Dr. Shadman does." And so, under such an opportunity I gradually became aware of a great many truths in medicine and surgery that apparently escaped others.

At the time when I entered medical school I feared germs as much as anyone. All my life I had heard about germs causing this disease, that disease, etc., and that good germicides were absolutely necessary to preserve life and health.

As I studied, observed and practiced, I began to feel that there was something wrong with the germ idea of sickness. I began to notice that people were not cured or even helped in any way by using germicides.

I saw cases of malaria cured by a dose or two of the homœopathic remedy in an almost infinitesimal dose, when large doses of quinine given to kill plasmodium (germs) failed. (A prominent Boston doctor once grew the malaria plasmodium in a strong solution of quinine.)

I saw cases of typhoid cured with unbelievably small doses of the indicated homœopathic remedy, when it was the style in Orthodox medicine to give the patient strong drugs — such as salol, for instance, thus hoping to kill the typhoid germ — only to have many patients die under such treatment.

I saw many cases of pneumonia cured with small doses of homœopathic medicine; so small that the pneumococci (the fancied cause of the disease) could not possibly be influenced in the slightest degree.

I personally have never lost a case of pneumonia in my entire half century of practice, and I never used anything but Homœopathic remedies. Its treatment by strong, old-school drugs caused an average mortality of 29% and often much higher. All this I saw and experienced with a mind alert to make comparisons of the two radically different forms of treatment.

I saw cases of cerebrospinal meningitis cured by the Homœopathic method and saw them die by the current Orthodox measures.

I saw many hundreds of cases of septic wounds clear up quickly under the treatment of just clean dressings, changed when necessary, where under Orthodox germicidal treatment it took a very long time indeed for a cure finally to obtain.

Considering all these facts, there was but one conclusion to which I could arrive and that was — germs are *not* the cause but the result of disease. That goes for virus too, as there is no such thing. What conclusion could any thinking, intelligent person draw?

Consequently my fear of germs, contagious infection, left me, left me free of fear, left me with a clear mind to investigate and discover *the real cause* of man's many illnesses.

It took many years of study and actual experience to jolt erroneous ideas from my head. Today, instead of fearing germs, I *fear the morbid conditions which feed them.*

At that time I believed in vaccination to prevent smallpox. No one ever told me that vaccinated people get smallpox, but only in a worse form, and many died who would have lived through it had they not been vaccinated. Later on when I saw epidemics of smallpox and discovered by personal experience that this measure did not protect one, doubts began to creep into my mind and so today I thoroughly condemn such so-called "immunizing" practices as not only useless but dangerous. More evidence will be presented later.

Because I had accidentally discovered before entering medical school that there were two distinct schools of thought in medicine, I was more or less prepared to accept the teachings I was to receive there. Many another student was not so prepared; consequently he could not take kindly or with credence some of the philosophy of disease, cause and its cure as taught in the Homœopathic school. It violated all his preconceived ideas.

I had always believed that disease was a thing, a definite entity, something that had to be killed by strong medicines, and that if a little medicine was good, a lot was better. That seemed to be the concept of most people and most doctors. They also thought, as I did, that if a medicine was expensive it must be good, which of course is not true. The individual old-school doctor relies less and less on his drugs the longer he practices, and eventually becomes a therapeutic nihilist helpless in cases which require curative medicine.

I soon found by clinical evidence that medicine applied according to the methods of the new school cured quickly, gently and permanently all curable ills, leaving no after or "side effects," and at practically no cost for the medicine. The law of cure which guides to proper prescribing is permanent.

The new-school doctor became a better and better physician the longer he practiced. He learned the *Materia Medica* and was able to remember it because it never changes.

The unfortunate old-school doctors, with many of whom I was later to be closely associated, were uncertain because the drug salesmen recommended a drug for a certain disease today, only to condemn it on his next trip. So what could they do? I used to feel sorry for them. I would try to advise them and did succeed in converting quite a number. One of them said, "Oh! if I had only known about it twenty years ago. Twenty years of absolutely wasted time, I am happy now for the first time since I began to practice. Now I know how to cure sickness."

Of course such incidents always pleased me. I had seen so many patients killed by the strong drugs given by their family doctors — nice fellows and good friends of mine — but somehow or other they didn't dare throw away everything that they had been taught (even sometimes knowing they were wrong) for something they had been led to believe in their schooling was a humbug.

As the years went by we outgrew my original hospital and had to build a much larger one. Continued success, both professional and financial, followed. Many of my old-school associates, even if they wouldn't right-about-face and learn the new-school method, used me as surgeon and consultant for their patients, and soon every bed was filled and remained so until I sold my hospital to the Massachusetts Memorial Hospital forty years later. After nearly a half century (at the time of sale) of very active practice of surgery (20,000 cases) and medicine, I grew tired of the commercial trend of the profession and decided to sell.

Several years earlier there had sprung up in the profession the unethical and pernicious request for splitting of surgical fees with the doctors who supplied the cases. I would not cooperate in this practice, and it caused embarrassing situations. It was the determining factor in my decision to sell and get out of surgery. It was too easy for the family doctor to exploit his patient. The fee-splitting surgeon wasn't too particular about diagnosis. What he was after was the fee. The patient seldom realized he was "taken for a ride." No, he usually felt he had a wonderful family doctor, one who knew just when to be broad-minded enough to call in an expert. Sometimes the family doctor didn't care much about diagnosis either, it was money he was after too. Let me cite a couple of cases which will serve as an example of how the "fee-splitting racket" was worked.

I came to the hospital late one afternoon and saw three men and a little boy standing in the lobby. The men were arguing; I listened. The father of the little boy was saying, "Do you think my little boy is in danger, Doctor — does he really need an operation?"

The family doctor said, "Why do you suppose I brought him to the hospital and called in the Professor?"

The Professor, a surgeon, then said, "If your little boy isn't operated on very soon, he will die of peritonitis."

The poor father said, with tears in his eyes, "O.K., Doctor, if you say so."

Then the great Professor said, "It will cost you two hundred dollars, paid in advance," to which the father replied, "But, Doctor, I can't pay you now — I haven't any money."

"Well," said the doctor, "in that case we will put the boy to bed and watch him till morning; in the meantime you try and raise the money."

One hundred dollars was for the surgeon and one hundred dollars for the family doctor. I was so indignant that I took a hand in the matter. The next morning I saw the boy and sent him home — there was no need for an operation. Both doctors were thereafter denied the privileges of the hospital. Who is your doctor and why?

A very prominent doctor from a nearby town brought in an emergency Cæsarean case. After the operation the doctor handed me fifty dollars, saying, "These people are strangers to me but I managed to get fifty dollars for your fee; it is better than nothing."

In a few days the mother of the patient came to see me and said, "Dr. Shadman, I will have to move my daughter into a ward as your surgical fee of two hundred and fifty dollars took most of our money and we cannot afford a private room any longer." Up until that moment I had had a great deal of respect for that doctor. I said nothing to the woman but phoned the family doctor immediately and told him that henceforth he would not be welcomed at the hospital. I never saw him again!

Then, a few years back, everyone wanted to be a "specialist," mostly in surgery. My hospital was an open staff, community hospital — as all hospitals should be. Any physician in good standing and of good moral character was permitted to use it for his patients.

Many young doctors representing themselves as competent surgeons sought permission to operate there. It was more expedient for me to take their word for it and then observe the quality of the work performed than to depend on unreliable references.

Many got no further than their first cases. Some of them came in and studied and worked under me and later became good surgeons. One fellow on being denied further privileges complained, "A fellow has to fill a graveyard before he becomes a good surgeon." How would you like him for a family doctor or surgeon?

A large percentage of my surgery was referred to me by other doctors. More than fifty percent were sent home as they needed no operation, but they did need curative medicine. This did not always please the doctors who sent them to me.

During the epidemic following World War I, I saw hundreds die of influenza under old-school drugging — 25 to 60%. Under new-school medicine only 1% plus died.

With the advent of the "miracle drug" sulfa, the slaughter really began. Close personal friends of mine were killed by it. Everyone seemed to want to be treated with the "miracle drug."

I saw the deadliness of this treatment in its concentrated form, one might say, which the public never sees. Deaths occurring here and there all over the country caused no public concern.

One good old school friend of mine came to see me and said, "Alonzo, I've got a cold coming on and want a private room."

"All right, Ed," I replied, "Take Room 212, I'll get you a remedy and you'll be O.K. in a couple of days."

He seemed a little embarrassed but he said, "I have made arrangements with my brother (who was also a doctor) to give me the new 'miracle drug,' they claim it will cure a cold over night."

"Don't do it," I said. He did, however, and in two days he was dead. If that wasn't legalized murder, what do you call it? Thousands met the same fate. No one told the public what caused these deaths. The whole world *now* knows what happened to people under the administration of the "miracle drug" sulfa. How many of your relatives or friends died of it?

No matter what the diagnosis, if the "miracle drug" was given and the patient managed to struggle through, it was the "miracle drug" that did it. If one died, it must have been the Will of Providence.

Today, ten years later, the "miracle drug," (except around the fringes) has lost its glory — gone the way of so many which preceded it and many which will follow.

I did all in my small power to prevent the use of this deadly drug, but as a reward reaped only ridicule.

No *good* homœopath ever fell for the "miracle drug." Homœopaths had their remedies, their philosophy, their guiding principle, all as reliable as the law of gravity and as unchanging as the Universe.

With the passing of the "miracle drug," there ended what was known in the profession as Chemotherapy (i.e. treatment by chemicals). It lasted only about ten years. Today is the Antibiotic Age, and if anything, it is more deadly than its predecessor.

Chemotherapy could kill its victims sometimes in three hours, sometimes delayed for three years. Antibiotics modify sickness and often create (as so-called side-effects) many other ailments which the profession bunches together as Virus X. These ailments run the gamut of human suffering and either they become chronic, or the patient dies of drug poisoning.

Natural ailments yield readily to curative remedies. Artificial ailments are difficult to cure even with Homœopathy. At best they can only be palliated with sleeping pills, painkillers, cathartics and hundreds of newly-concocted drugs which further change and modify, but never cure. Already as of July, 1957, the people have spent an estimated two hundred million dollars for the so-called tranquilizers.

The information which may be obtained from reading this book should and will dispel the deadly fear of sickness which assails most people. It will do much more than that. It will assure you that sickness is unnatural and should seldom occur. *Sickness is not inevitable. Health is natural.* This book will reveal how easy it can be to remain well. It will give you courage and faith in Nature and her remedies; the result will be that you will seldom have occasion to call a doctor.

I know of many families who have not had a doctor for years, because of advice given them that is contained in this book. Before that, their apprehension and fear of sickness cost them hundreds of dollars each year for doctors and drugs.

CHAPTER 2

The Practice of Medicine

The origin of medicine is lost among the legends and fables of the earliest ages. Mythology has man learning the art of healing directly from the gods. Certainly we may assume that the earliest inhabitants of the earth must have made observations which helped them to combat the diseases that afflicted them as well as the injuries they suffered by accident and in war.

Today, even among the most primitive tribes, we find evidence of some degree of medical and surgical practices. Like these tribesmen, early man, when his sorry efforts at cure failed, resorted to charms and incantations. In the religion of Egypt, we find a blend of superstition and the art of healing. The first Egyptian physicians were priests. There have come down to us, today, records and descriptions of the solemn processions in which these physician-priests marched through the temples and palaces of Thebes and Memphis bearing the symbolic bed of the Goddess of Love and Beauty.

The Jewish priests continued to be their only physicians until about 200 B.C. The Law of Moses directed them in their duties. These Jewish priest-physicians were probably the first to isolate persons suffering from certain diseases, such as leprosy.

Like the Egyptians, the Greeks of a later civilization considered disease a direct sign of their gods' displeasure, and the people looked to the temple priests, who were the divinely favored agents and representatives of these deities, to avert the pestilences the gods had visited upon them. The priests believed there were thirty-six spirits or demons of the air, who divided various parts of the body among themselves. Each part had its name, and by invoking the spirit to whom the afflicted parts belonged, the priests would attempt to cure the patient.

Later, medicine was divided into numerous branches or specialties.

According to Herodotus, "Each physician applies himself to one disease and only one." All places abounded in physicians at that time. Some were for the eyes, others for the head, others for the teeth, some for the abdomen, and others only for internal disorders. After many centuries, the cycle is complete and specialism is again in style. However, specialism is now again on the wane.

Everywhere we hear of the so-called psychosomatic[1] medicine. It has finally dawned on Orthodox medicine that not only has the specialist failed in his own field, but that it is actually unreasonable to divide a man arbitrarily into his component parts and to try to treat the various parts separately.

A few thinkers here and there have finally concluded that man, when ill, should be treated as a whole — but how to do it successfully is something else, something beyond their lore. For this they will eventually have to turn to Homœopathy for advice and instruction.

The most celebrated Greek physician of the fabulous ages was Æsculapius, whose fame won him, after his death, a place among the gods. But even while he lived he was highly revered by the people, and the first medical schools and hospitals the Greeks founded were known as the Temples of Æsculapius.

About a hundred of these hospitals were scattered throughout the Roman Empire. Here came the sick, the lame, and the blind seeking cures. These patients were admitted to the temples only after they underwent a process of purification. The oracle had to be consulted, too, and the patient would await the answer in the temple. And then would come days of abstinence, prayer, fasting and sacrifices. Even keen-minded old Socrates, with his dying words, asked that his sacrifice be not forgotten: "I owe a cock to Æsculapius; do not forget to pay it."

The priests told new patients about the cases they had treated successfully, much as doctors do today. It was here, in these Temples of Aesculapius, that the first records of treatments were made and transmitted to posterity on plates of metal, wood or stone.

The Greek priests knew how to select healthful sites. This, together with the effects of change of scenery, the benefits derived from the long journeys to the temples, the new hope the patients felt, and the con-

---

[1] Medicine for the entire man: *psyche* (mind), *soma* (body).

fidence which the priests inspired in the minds of their patients, all contributed to the frequent successes the priests had and, consequently, to their fame. They also enjoyed the advantage of that peculiar psychology which makes men observe faithfully certain rules of hygiene as prescribed religious observance and scorn and neglect those advised only on the basis of common sense and science!

The priests did not rely solely on oratory and oracles to influence their patients. They also used opium, blood-letting, purgation, emetics and friction, mineral waters and sea bathing. Materia Medica was limited to a small number of substances whose powers were not really understood. Anatomy and physiology were practically unknown.

Aesculapius had many followers who carried on long after his death, handing down from father to son the secrets of the art. Medical lore in those days was kept within the family and among the favored few.

Hippocrates, who was born in 460 B.C., was the most ancient medical authority to have his ideas, in a large measure, carried over to our times. His theories on the causes of disease were, of course, not entirely accurate; but they were, in general, based upon careful observation.

All he knew of anatomy was what he had learned by dissecting cats, dogs and other animals. Only once in his life did he see a human skeleton. He refers much to blood and bile, supposing there were but two fluids contained in the body. He emphasized the good and bad effects of sleep, stressed the importance of exercise and rest, and was very careful in prescribing diets.

Even Hippocrates could not slough off priestly influence. In his writings we find much importance placed on the courses and changing of the winds, the seasons, the rising and setting of the stars and certain constellations, the times of the equinoxes and solstices.

Hippocrates was followed by Serapion, who, in about 287 B.C. founded what he called Empiricism, which will be described later. This sect, depending on personal opinion alone, pitted itself against the dogmatists who advocated the value of theory.

During this era of activity in Greece and Egypt, the science and practice of medicine remained entirely unknown in Italy for six hundred years. (They got along as well or better than those who relied on the medical profession.) The usual efforts of the ignorant were undoubtedly made to mitigate suffering, but there was no one class of men who took care of the sick, and people put their faith in their priests and oracles. Not until about 234 B.C. was the religion of the Greeks and so-called science of medicine introduced to Rome.

It was shortly thereafter that Archagatus of Peloponessus settled there to practice medicine and surgery. The Romans considered surgery incompatible with kindness and humanitarianism although later they were to surpass anything the Greeks had accomplished in surgery. At any rate, they did not take kindly to anything emanating from Greece, and we find the Roman censor favoring the expulsion of any Greek found practicing medicine in Rome.

A hundred years or so later we come upon Asclepiades, who openly opposed the theories of Hippocrates. By his general condemnation of the practices of his own contemporaries and the disparaging manner in which he referred to all medical practitioners of the past, he attracted a large share of attention to himself.

"His arts," reports Pliny, "were such as every fashionable physician employs" — soothing the patient and avoiding everything that might give pain until nature cures or the patient sinks under the disease.

It was Asclepiades who originated the doctrine of the self-limitation of disease and asserted that the principal cure for a fever is the disease itself. He, himself, escaped disease and lived to an advanced age before being killed by a fall.

In the year 4 A.D., Celsus was born. He was the only distinguished medical writer in Rome for the period of two hundred and fifty years from Asclepiades to Galen. Celsus agreed to some extent with Hippocrates but rejected the often revived and equally exploded doctrine of critical days. It was while he was engaged in writing in an elegant manner his principal work, a long treatise on the state of the medical profession at that time, that the cities of Herculaneum and Pompeii were destroyed by the eruption of Vesuvius in 79 A.D.

Years passed before the birth of Galen in 131 A.D. He was evidently superior to all of his contemporaries. So successfully did he expose the deficiency of their knowledge and the futility of their reasoning that he triumphed over his opponents and attained a very high rank in medicine.

He swayed the opinion of physicians and the public alike on all points in the field of medicine never before known and was the propounder of the theory of opposites — *"contraria contrariis curantur"* — (opposites are cured by opposites) — in the prescribing of medicine. If a man couldn't sleep he was given a sleeping potion, dope; if he was sleepy, a stimulant was given.

Galen discovered that the arteries contained blood and not air, as proclaimed by predecessors. This was the most important discovery in physiology thus far made. He wrote a great deal, and while he had no correct ideas as to the cause or treatment of disease, his writings influenced the medical world for the next thirteen hundred years. Nobody dared to advance any ideas or theories contrary to those of Galen.

Then, in 1493, in Switzerland, was born Paracelsus, who was to upset the entire philosophy of Galen and boldly advance a theory of chemical therapy (reminiscent of the present "miracle" chemicals for which so much is claimed but so little forthcoming). Paracelsus' claims for his chemicals were just as fantastic as those of our "miracle" and "wonder" drugs today. He claimed that his remedies would even give immortal life; but, alas, he himself died at the early age of forty-seven, blasting the hopes his claims had raised in the hearts of the people.

The authorities stopped the use of his chemical drugs because of their deadliness. Although he displayed so many unfavorable traits of character — insolence, conceit, insincerity and vanity, as well as immorality — he rendered important service to our race by breaking down the despotism of the schools and sects of his time. He wandered from place to place teaching fragments of truth, seldom changing his clothes, generally intoxicated, going to bed only infrequently. He excited the envy of some, the emulation of others, and inspired the industry of all.

The next great step in the progress of medicine was to be made by Michael Servetus, who was born in 1509. He was proceeding rapidly with his research and had completely established the fact of the passage of the blood through the lungs, when he happened to be passing through Geneva. There, John Calvin, the Christian reformer, had him arrested, charged him with heresy, and had him burned at the stake with his books to kindle the flames. Thus a brilliant man's life was sacrificed to the bigotry and stupidity of medicine and religion.

It was not until seventy-five years later that Harvey, through the work already done by Servetus, was enabled to discover the general circulation of the blood. For this, he too was cruelly "crucified" by his professional contemporaries, though his life was spared. He lived to see his discovery accepted by the world.

At this late date, the universities which possessed the sole power of authorizing physicians to practice medicine were ecclesiastical institutions. They taught very little and persecuted all who attempted to learn anything not found in the writings of Galen. For example, hot irons or hot oils and pitch were applied to wounds to stop the flow of blood. It was generally considered better practice to let a limb drop off through gangrene than to perform an amputation. Compression by pitch plasters was used for this purpose. Ambrose Pare saw the dire results of such practice and invented the mode of arresting bleeding by tying the arteries and healing wounds by mild dressings.

These discoveries, although of greater benefit to humanity than all of the improvements made by routine followers of Galen for a thousand years, were not permitted to be published, and Pare had to recant, even as did Galileo his important discovery in Astronomy.

Then followed Sydenham and Boerhaave, both great men, thinkers and philosophers, who brought many reforms to both the theory and practice of medicine. They, in their time, had no bigoted *religious* persecution to fear. However, they used absolutely no *guiding principle* or *natural law* for guidance in the selection or prescribing of remedies.

Disease was still more or less a mystery. Physiology was practically unknown and anatomy had not yet been explored to any great extent. Under all these limitations, therefore, it may be reasonable to suppose that the time was perhaps not ripe for men to have learned how to apply medicine properly.

Such is not the case, however, because there existed, coeval with the human race, the natural law which could direct the use of remedies for almost any disease but which, up until the eighteenth century, remained undiscovered. Why? Not because of man's general stupidity or ignorance, for he had made remarkable advance up to that time in chemistry, mechanics, physics, painting, poetry, etc. No, it was not ignorance. It was bigotry. It was the kind of bigotry that manifests itself especially in the fields of organized religion.

Bigotry in religion we may excuse; but in medicine we cannot do so if medicine is to be a science. If it is not a science, it is nothing. Yet, today, bigotry is responsible for the failure of Orthodox medicine to cure sickness. Orthodox medicine has always refused to accept any philosophy, discovery or tenet emanating from anyone outside its own constituted authority.

It was roused to fury when *cinchona bark,* from which quinine is made, was introduced by the Jesuit priests as a cure for Malaria. It had been discovered and used by the Indians of South America. It may not be generally known, but Oliver Cromwell was allowed to die of malaria rather than be given this hated specific. To this day, Orthodox medicine does not know how to use quinine properly for the cure of malaria.

It must be remembered also that during all this time there were many individual doctors who considered themselves units in a great and glorious profession. They were educated, refined gentlemen who did their utmost to cure sickness. When their patients recovered, they were happy, and when they died, they were sorrowful and sympathetic toward the relatives and friends of the departed.

They did the best they could. They could do no better than those at the head of the medical orthodoxy would allow them to do. The latter would seldom depart from established methods and measures lest they admit their lack of knowledge, which to them would be suicidal.

It will be difficult to convince most of you that Orthodox medicine is not as yet in its entirety the grand and noble profession that you think it is. That there are many grand and noble men in the profession, I admit. There are individuals of lofty mind and character in every school, cult and pathy. Their numbers are so few, however, that they have very little influence in correcting the abuses which abound. Each one of you will fight tooth and nail for your own family or personal doctor. Whatever *he* does will be accepted by you, even as in the past. When the physicians of George Washington bled him to death, they were not criticized — not then, not in their lifetime — not until later generations of people were born, lived and died. Finally, only when the event could be analyzed in the glaring light of history, was there just criticism of a most absurd, cruel act.

By consulting the third volume of the *Medical and Physical Journal* published in London in the year 1800 by T. Bradley, M.D., R. Battey, M.D., and A. A. Noehden, M.D., there will be found on page 409 a description or report of the last illness of Washington, and the treatment given him. At present it is interesting as an example of too much doctoring, to say the least. It is as follows:

"Some time on the night of Friday, the 10th inst., having been exposed to a rain on the preceding day, General Washington was attacked with an inflammatory affection of the upper part of the windpipe, called in technical language cynache trachealis (Tonsillitis, or as Orthodox doctors would call it today, Strep Throat). The disease commenced with a violent ague, accompanied with some pain in the upper and fore part of the throat, a sense of stricture in the same part, a cough, and a difficult rather than a painful deglutition,[2] which was soon succeeded by fever and a quick and laborious respiration. The necessity of bloodletting suggesting itself to the General, he procured a bleeder in the neighborhood, who took from his arm in the night twelve or fourteen ounces of blood.

"He could not by any means be prevailed on by the family to send for his attending physician till the following morning, who arrived at Mount Vernon at about 11 o'clock on Saturday. Discovering the case to be highly alarming, and foreseeing the fatal tendency of the disease, two consulting physicians were immediately sent for, who arrived, one at 3:30 and the other at 4 o'clock in the afternoon. In the meantime employed two pretty copious bleedings, a blister was applied to the part affected, two doses of Calomel were given, and an injection administered, which operated on the lower intestine, but all without perceptible advantage, the respiration becoming still more difficult and distressing. Upon the arrival of the first of the consulting physicians, it was agreed, as there were yet no signs of accumulation in the bronchial vessels of the lungs, to try the result of another bleeding, when about thirty-two ounces were drawn without the smallest apparent alleviation of the disease.

"Vapors of vinegar and water were frequently inhaled; ten grains of Calomel were given, succeeded by repeated doses of Tartar emetic, amounting to five or six grains, with no effect other than a copious discharge from the bowels. The powers of life seemed now manifestly yielding to the force of the disorder. Blisters were applied to the extremities, together with a cataplasm[3] of vinegar and bran, to the throat. Speaking, which was painful from the beginning, now became impracticable. Respiration grew more and more contracted and imperfect till 11:30 on Saturday night, retaining the full possession of his intellect, when he expired without a struggle.

"He was fully impressed at the beginning of his complaint, as well as through every succeeding stage of it, that its conclusion would be

[2] The act, process and power of swallowing.
[3] A soothing poultice.

mortal; submitting to the several exertions made for his recovery rather as a duty than from any expectation of their efficiency. He considered the operations of death upon his system co-eval with disease; and several hours before his death, after repeated efforts to be understood, succeeded in expressing a desire that he might be permitted to die without further interruption.

"During the short period of his illness he economized his time in the arrangements of such few concerns as required his attention with the utmost serenity, and anticipated his approaching dissolution with every demonstration of that equanimity for which his whole life has been so uniformly and singularly conspicuous."

JAMES CLARK, *Attending Physician*
ELISHA C. DICK, *Consulting Physician*

Homœopathy would have selected Aconite for President Washington which would have cured him as it has hundreds of similar cases, or at the very least it would not have stood in the way of recovery. George Washington died over 150 years ago. Such mistreatment cannot happen today — or can it?

Recently a patient came to my office to get help for a condition that had been diagnosed as asthma. This patient was about forty years of age, the mother of two grown daughters. It was revealed that about six years ago she developed a cold and someone advised her to get a doctor. This was the first sickness she had had for years. The doctor came and, after looking her over, said, "It is a good thing that you called me because I think you are about to go into T.B."

The patient was naturally frightened. He then said, "You must come to my office and have a chest X-ray."

She did as she was told, and he took and developed the picture and held it up to the light and said, "See! It is just as I said. T.B. has already begun," and he pointed out various shadows, etc.

Consequently, for the next six years she was under his domination and expenses which took every cent she had or could earn. Finally the doctor told her, "Now you have asthma, for which there is no cure and you will have to learn to live with it."

Then he said, "I have just got a wonderful new drug which will give you great relief, but it is very expensive. It will cost you $15 a shot!"

That was the last straw. It was at this stage that I was consulted.

I immediately stopped all the drugging that she was receiving and gave her a curative remedy. She got relief immediately and just ten days later, she reported that she felt fine, had slept well, and felt like a new person.

The unwillingness of orthodox medical men generally to open their minds to new discoveries, the failure to study and accept what others have found beneficial is *criminal bigotry*.

The handful of men who were responsible for the spread of Homœopathy throughout the world were all graduates of Orthodox medical schools. They were the intelligent and courageous ones — the ones fitted by nature to follow the wonderful science of medicine. When they investigated, they recognized the truth, and their honest, open and intelligent minds directed its adoption and practice. All men are not fitted for the noble profession.

A most natural question now comes up, a question that I have been asked hundreds of times. That question is, "What is Homœopathy?" That is a fair question and one that should be answered in such a way that people can get a full understanding of just what it is.

CHAPTER 3

Hahnemann and Homoeopathy

Just one hundred and fifty years ago, for the first time in history the method for applying true, curative medicine was discovered. From that time on there have been two schools of medicine — the old and the new, the Allopathic (Orthodox) and the Homœopathic.

The graduates of both these schools are entitled to use the title of M.D. and legally permitted to practice medicine if and when they qualify with the State Board of Registration.

The word *Homœopathy* (from the Greek "homoios," meaning *like,* and "pathos," meaning *suffering* or *sickness*) is used to describe the practice of curative medicine, where medicines are prescribed according to a permanent law of Nature, the Law of Similars: Let Likes be treated by Likes.

The natural law through which the choice of remedies must be prescribed has always existed. This law is unchanging; it is not man-made. Hippocrates just missed it as long ago as the fourth century B.C. when, speaking of the drug Hellebore and its effect upon insanity, he said that "like cures like," but he went no further.

It remained for a man who took his medical degree some two thousand years later to discover this Law of Cure. A study of the historical background of this man's time explains much of his reform work in medicine. It is interesting that present-day changes in medical ideas were foreshadowed, a century ago, by him.

This great man's name was Samuel Hahnemann. Hahnemann was born in Saxony in 1755. Many talents and strong drives went into his make-up, including the "glorious gospel of discontent"[1] with all that was senseless, useless, harmful, inept — which practically sums up the med-

[1] "Discontent is the Mother of Ambition." — Shadman

icine of his day. He was a great linguist, a master of many languages, including Arabic, at a very early age.

At twelve years of age he was already teaching the rudiments of Greek. His knowledge was voluminous, as was his memory. More than once in his early years he was in charge of, or closely associated with, large and important libraries (Hermanstadt and Dresden); and his erudition was commensurate with his opportunities.

At Leipzig, "the Saxon Athens," in 1812, in order to obtain permission to lecture, he had to deliver a "speech of qualification" from the Upper Chair. This he delivered in Latin; it was entitled "Dissertatio historico-medica de Heleborismo veterum." In this speech, we are told, he was able to quote verbatim and give the location of the passages from manifold German, French, English, Italian, Latin, Greek, Hebrew and Arabic medical writers, and he could examine their views — either in disagreement or in extension. He quoted from fifty more or less known doctors, philosophers and naturalists.

In chemistry his methods of chemical analysis and some of his discoveries are still in daily use — among them his "mercurius solubilis," the black oxide, and in Crell's Annals (1793) Hahnemann was already mentioned as "the famous analytical chemist."

In the reformed treatment of the insane, Hahnemann was among the great pioneers. Already, in 1792 (in Pinel's time), he had devised humane treatment. He never allowed any insane person to be given painful bodily chastisement. There could be no punishment for involuntary actions; these patients deserved pity and were always made worse and not better by such cruelty. He even went further than Pinel in advising psycho-therapeutical measures.

He was a prodigious worker and was only one year short of ninety when he died. In the course of his long life (according to Ameke) he published 116 large works and about 120 pamphlets. He was always "filling gaps in his education," as he expresses it, as when he studied botany, or "took small journeys to learn mining science and metallurgy." He was not only a chemist but a good musician and an astronomer, and he was versed in every branch of knowledge connected with medicine. Ameke says, "When Hahnemann came out with his new system of medicine he was universally spoken of with respect and even reverence, but with regret for his folly. But, after a year or so, he was denounced as an ignoramus and a scoundrel."

His great work was in the field of therapeutics.[2] He was, above all, a born physician and reformer. His great idea of *Similia* was first communicated in 1796 in an essay on *The New Principle for Ascertaining the Curative Powers of Drugs,* and some examinations of the previous principles.

His three classical works are (1) his *Organon of Medicine*: wherein he justifies his position and teaches how, and what to prescribe, and why; (2) his *Materia Medica Pura,* which embodies exhaustively the answers of the healthy human body to the assaults of morbific agents or drugs; that is to say, the exact symptoms produced when drugs are tested on the healthy, in order to apply them, with assurance, for the healing of the sick of "like" symptoms; (3) his *Chronic Diseases* — almost too much, in the past, for even his keenest disciples and followers — is assuming new importance in the light of discoveries of today.

Those who study these works discover with amazement that Hahnemann in his views of disease expressed the all-importance of *vital resistance to adverse environment,* that disease can only be cured by stimulating the vital force of the patient, which is a modern concept, abreast always (when it is not ahead) of science. What Hahnemann has to give us is exactly what medicine the world over is now waking up to demand. One feels that Hahnemann is, at long last, coming into his kingdom.

The medicine of Hahnemann's day was based on the assumption that sickness was caused by humours that had to be expelled from the body by every method that could be devised, expelled not only by the natural organs of excretion, which were taxed to the limit, but also by artificial and unnatural methods of excretion.

Exutories, cauteries, setons, moxas, fontanels, meaningless names to our generation, are of interest only to the historian of medicine. We can have no conception of what a torture chamber was the medicine of Hahnemann's day, when all these barbarities were designed to provide "new organs of excretion."

The Cautery: Iron at white heat, or some chemical agent, was employed to dig deeply these "new organs" into which dried peas were introduced and compressed by means of a bandage. These wounds were given their daily supply of peas.

The Seton: The flesh was pinched up and an incision made, by means

---

[2] Applying curative medicine to sick people.

of which a skein of cotton on silk was inserted. When the wound was dressed, the skein was drawn out, and the part saturated with discharge cut off. The seton was applied to the back of the neck to drain foul humours from head, eye, etc.; to the region of the heart to "clean and polish it up," or to other parts of the body to draw some organic derangement from the liver, lung, or joint, or for a dropsy.

The Moxa: This was a cone of some combustible material applied to the skin, when its apex was set on fire. "Here," we are told, "as the flame advances, the heat becomes more intense; the skin crackles and shrivels — turns brown — and is scorched till nearly black."

Prolonged blisterings with cantharides at times led to the loss of a limb; wounds were powdered with arsenic, often with fatal results. One would think, in reading of these things, that the devil was responsible for medicine in the days of Hahnemann.

To an unmerciful extent, purgation, emesis, sweatings and salivation were also resorted to, while "issues" were not only established, but maintained for years. Above all, bloodletting was to an incredible degree in favor. Leopold of Austria, Count Cavour (the "saviour of Italy"), and the English Princess Charlotte were among its illustrious victims; while Raphael, Lord Byron, Mirabeau and a host of celebrities were, we are told, seriously injured by bleedings. Goethe in his 82nd year having had a serious hemorrhage, was bled to the extent of two more pounds. You have read how our own George Washington was bled to death.

Hahnemann protested against these brutal and unnatural methods, which weakened the patients to the verge of incurability.

Granier, a French doctor, who wrote in 1858, contrasting Homœopathy with the medicine that obtained even in his day, says; "If it be not true that diseases can escape by cauteries, it is at least certain that they can enter the system by this means. It is really a new organ of absorption."

Hahnemann denounced in particular the prevalent idea that venesection draws off only the bad blood, that continual purging evacuates only the depraved humours, and that a vesicating agent can select, collect and remove only injurious humours.

Against such practices — and against Broussais, who carried the custom of the times to a ridiculous length, earning for himself the nickname of "the medical Robespierre" of whom it was said "he had shed more French blood than Napoleon," Hahnemann fulminated his thunder. It must have required not a little courage to break away from what was deemed on all hands to be essential, and to treat acute inflammatory conditions with his small doses of Aconite (which obtained the name of "the Homœopathic lancet") and to confess, as he did in 1833, that for forty years he had not "drawn a single drop of blood, opened one seton, used pain-producing processes, *etc.* . . . had never weakened patients by sudorifices, or scoured them out with emetics and laxatives, thus destroying their organs of digestion." Thus you can see the medical climate of Hahnemann's time.

"While surrounded by anxiously watching adversaries, ready to pounce at the slightest mistake . . .", his followers, seeing his accomplishments and joyfully following in his steps, were unmoved even when haled into the Courts and prosecuted for not practising phlebotomy (bloodletting). The great Hufeland, who had previously been just to Hahnemann amid all the injustice and persecution Hahnemann suffered, said in 1830 that "anyone who neglected to draw blood when a man was in danger of suffocating in his own blood (this was the idea regarding inflammatory fevers) was a murderer by omission."

In regard to the necessity for bleeding in acute fevers, Hahnemann wrote, "Anyone who has felt the tranquil pulse of a man an hour before the rigor that precedes an attack of acute pleurisy, will not be able to restrain his amazement if told two hours later, after the hot stage has commenced, that the enormous plethora present urgently requires repeated venesections. He will naturally enquire by what magic power could the pounds of blood that must be drawn off have been conjured into the blood vessels of this man which but two hours previously he had felt beating in such a tranquil manner. Not a single dram more of blood can now be circulating in those vessels than when he was in good health, not yet two hours ago."

Hahnemann contends here that "the sole true *Causa Morbi* is a morbid, dynamical, inflammatory irritation of the circulatory system, as is proved by the rapid and permanent cure of general inflammatory fever by one or two inconceivably minute doses of *Aconite* juice, which removed such irritation homoeopathically."

One must admire Hahnemann's enormous courage — the courage of strong conviction — which, if it did not procure sudden, universal recognition for his system of medicine, at least civilized, and that speedily, medicine in general, not only by putting to shame its degrading· barbarities, but by proving that they were wholly unnecessary.

That this was so, we have curious evidence. In 1852 we find Professor Allison of Edinburgh broaching the famous theory that inflammatory diseases, which hitherto had been treated by bloodletting and debilitating methods, now no longer required those methods, but an utterly opposite mode of treatment, because the *diseases* had *"changed their type"*[3] and were no longer what they used to be. He confessed that he was led to adopt the new treatment — or rather to abandon the old — chiefly from the report of physicians who had "witnessed the practice of Homœopathic hospitals on the Continent."

Mark Twain — himself once a Mississippi pilot — in nautical phraseology pays his tribute to Homœopathy for the purifying work it has accomplished in medicine. He says:

So recent is this change from a three or four thousand year twilight to the flash and glare of open day that I have walked in both, and yet I am not old. Nothing today is as it was when I was an urchin; but when I was an urchin, nothing was much different from what it had *always* been in this world. Take a single detail for example — medicine. Galen could have come into my sickroom at any time during my first seven years — I mean any day when it wasn't fishing weather, and there wasn't any choice but school or sickness — and he could have sat down there and stood my doctor's watch without asking a question. He would have smelt around among the wilderness of cups and bottles and phials on the table and the shelves, and missed not a stench that used to gladden him two thousand years before, nor discovered one that was of later date. He would have examined me, and run across only one disappointment — I was already salivated;[4] I would have him there; for I was always salivated, calomel (mercury) was so cheap. He would get out his lancet then; but I would have him again; our family doctor did not allow blood to accumulate in the system. However, he would take a dipper and ladle, and freight me up with the old familiar doses that had come down from Adam to his time and mine; and he would go out with a wheelbarrow and gather weeds and offal, and build some more, while those others were getting in their work. And if our revered doctor came and found him there, he would be dumb with awe, and would get down and worship him. Whereas if Galen should appear among us today, he could not stand any-

---

[3] It reminds me of the present-day claims of the adherents to the Germ Theory that when germicides and antibiotics and chemical drugs currently in vogue fail, it is because the germs have changed their type.

[4] A well-known physiological action of mercury is to produce an immense amount of saliva, and so they had a slogan in those days, "In salivation there is salvation."

body's watch; he would inspire no awe; he would be told he was a back number, and it would surprise him to see that counted against him, instead of in his favour. He wouldn't know our medicines; he wouldn't know our practices; and the first time he tried to introduce his own, we would hang him.

And after giving many examples of ancient practice, with its crude ideas, its horrible mixtures, etc., he concludes by declaring:

When you reflect that your own father had to take such medicine as the above, and that you would be taking them today yourself but for the introduction of Homœopathy, which forced the old school doctor to stir around and learn something of a rational nature about his business, you may honestly feel grateful that Homoeopathy survived the attempts of the Allopaths to destroy it, even though you may never employ any physician but an Allopath while you live.

At this point it may be interesting to quote Professor Chapman of Philadelphia, now deceased, in describing the woeful effects of mercury: "Who is it that can stop the career of mercury at will, after it has taken the reins in its own destructive and ungovernable hands! He, who, for an ordinary cause, resigns the fate of his patient to mercury, is a vile enemy to the sick; and if he is tolerably popular, will in one successful season have paved the way for the business of life; for he has enough to do for ever afterward to stop the mercurial breach of the constitutions of his dilapidated patients. He has thrown himself in fearful proximity to death and has now to fight at arms length as long as the patient maintains a miserable existence, and this dreadful poison is the most common — yes, the daily remedy of allopathy (Orthodox medicine) for almost every disorder, whether mild or severe, acute or chronic. This is the substance with which unfortunate mortals are drugged, from the time they come into the world until their wretched, too often premature departure.

"Calomel (mercury) and opium were the common remedies in traditional practice for a large number of diseases. Glancing at the standard works on the practice of medicine will confirm the fact that there is scarcely a single malady, either acute or chronic, for which one or both of these drugs is not recommended as an all important, if not indispensable, means of cure."

That was yesteryear in allopathic medical practice. Yet no one was ever cured by such treatment. Many were killed; many more made chronically ill for life.

Today the same irrational, nonsensical, dangerous procedure continues; except, in place of mercury and opium, we have the so-called "miracle" and "wonder drugs" being prescribed for almost every conceivable ailment.

Hahnemann found himself in conflict, too, with the system, or rather, want of system, in the prescription of medicines in his day. Here all was imagination, tradition, hoary authority. Of science, there was none. "The life and health of human beings were made dependent on the opinions of a few, and whatever entered their precious brains went to swell the materia medica."

"The god-like science, practical medicine," had become a "degrading commerce in prescriptions — a trade that mixes the disciples of Hippocrates with the riff-raff of medical rogues, in such a way that one is indistinguishable from the other."

Polypharmacy[5] flourished to an unbelievable extent. We are told that the largest number of ingredients recorded in one prescription was four hundred. The famous "Venice Treacle" contained sixty-five ingredients; and I have seen a world-famed prescription called "Mithridate," of fifty ingredients, which was actually in the Pharmacopœia of 1785, at the time when Hahnemann was beginning his fight for purity and simplicity in medicine. "Nature," says Hahnemann, "likes simplicity and can perform much with one remedy while you perform little with many. Imitate nature."

As early as 1797 he wrote, "May I be allowed to confess that for several years I have never prescribed more than one medicine at a time, and I have never repeated the dose until the effect of the previous one has been exhausted." He says that thus he has successfully cured patients, and has "seen things he would not otherwise have seen."

The chemists who perceived that the hope of their gains must vanish with the advent of Homœopathy, fought the iconoclast; got laws enacted to restrain him from preparing and dispensing his medicines, and drove him from city to city. No wonder that Hahnemann thundered: "Away with this excessive mixing of medicine, this prescription tomfoolry! Down with the apothecaries' privileges! Let the doctor have freedom to make his own medicine and administer it to his patients. We cannot be shown the correct way by a deluding tradition."

Hahnemann wrote that in his day, in order to decide on something positive in regard to the instruments of cure "the powers of the different

[5] Prescription containing many drugs.

medicines were inferred from their physical, chemical and other irrelevant qualities; also from their odour, taste and external aspect, but chiefly from impure experiences at the sick bed, where, in the tumult of morbid symptoms, only mixtures of medicines were prescribed for imperfectly described cases of disease."

Can one wonder that in his earlier days Hahnemann revolted, not only against the senseless cruelty, but the utter uncertainty of lawless medicine. He says: "My sense of duty would not allow me to treat the unknown pathological state of my suffering brethren with these unknown medicines. If they are not exactly suitable (and how could the physician know that, since their specific effects had not been demonstrated) they might with their strong potency easily change life into death, or induce new and chronic maladies, often more difficult to eradicate than the original disease.

"The thought of becoming in this way a murderer or a malefactor towards the life of my fellow human beings was most terrible to me; so terrible and disturbing that I wholly gave up my practice in the first years of my married life, and occupied myself solely with chemistry and writing."

Then, in the anguish of impotence when one of his own children was ill and suffering terribly from the treatment she underwent, he set his soul to discover, as he expressed it, "if God had not indeed given some law, whereby the diseases of mankind would be cured."

"Where," he cried in that hour of agony, "can I obtain certain and sure help in our present knowledge? — based as it is on vague observations, hypothetical opinions, and the arbitrary views of disease in our pathologies."

In this labyrinth, he said, a man can only remain complacent who is ready to accept assertions in regard to the healing powers of medicines because they are printed in a hundred books.

He knew from experience what little help was to be got from the methods of Sydenham and others — Boerhaave, Stoll, Quarin, Cullen.

"Can it be," he asked, "that the nature of this science (as great men have said) is incapable of certainty? . . . Shameful, blasphemous thought! . . . that Infinite Wisdom should be unable to create the means of assuaging the sufferings of His creatures. Surely there must be a reliable way of regarding disease from the right angle, and for determining the specific, safe and reliable use of medicines."

Mankind is the only earthbound animal created by God who was ordained to learn how to use the whole world as his rightful habitat. In
his efforts to learn how to adapt himself to adverse environment, mistakes
were bound to occur, thus causing sicknesses. Therefore it is natural to
expect that there should be a reliable guide to the choice of proper remedies
for the sickness thus arising.

It was useless, as Hahnemann had discovered, to "seek the means of
healing in arbitrary opinions — false conclusions" — or on the authority
of "highly celebrated men of delusions. Let me seek it," he cried, "where
it may be near at hand, and where all have passed it by, because it did
not seem artificial or learned enough, and was uncrowned with laurel for
its system, its pedantry, or its high-falutin' abstractions."

To the patient seeker of Truth and Law comes sooner or later revelation
— and so with Hahnemann. The Law that he sought came to him as a
flash of inspiration, as we shall see, and, once it was grasped, the rest
followed, surely and faultlessly, so that no one, in all those hundred years,
has been able to add to, or to take from, our legacy from Hahnemann.
Once his eyes were opened, it was merely a question of devoting a long
life to the elucidation of the Law and establishing it as a practical basis
of therapeutics.

It was in 1790, when translating Cullen's *Materia Medica,* and dis-
agreeing with the author's dictum that Peruvian bark owed its anti-
pyretic [6] power to its tonic effect on the stomach, that Hahnemann made
his first pure experiment with cinchona bark upon himself, and thereby
discovered its powers of exciting the familiar symptoms of intermittent
fever.

Hahnemann seems to have realized instantly the enormous importance
of the discovery, which subsequent observations and experience with
other drugs never failed to confirm. "With this first trial," he says, "broke
upon me the dawn that has since brightened into the most brilliant day
of the medical art, *that it was only by their power to make the healthy
human being ill, that medicines can cure morbid states;* and, even so,
only such morbid states whose symptoms the selected drug can itself
produce in the healthy."

An episode with belladonna in a scarlet fever epidemic was also illuminating in this connection to one who knew the extraordinary similarity
between the symptoms of scarlet fever and those of belladonna poison-

[6] Preventive or alleviative of fever.

ing: the burning skin, the dry sore throat, the red rash, the dilated pupils, and the delirium.

In a family of which several members were attacked by scarlet fever, one, a child whom he was treating with belladonna for some other ailment, remained immune. He thereupon gave this "providential remedy" to other children, who remained well, even when subjected to the greatest risk of infection. Here Hahnemann made his first successful experiments in homoeo-prophylaxis (Homœopathic prevention):

From his day on, belladonna has been used by Homœopaths all over the world to protect from or to modify and cure scarlet fever. Besides the minimal mortality, it has been the unfailing observation that cases so treated do not exhibit the sequelae which are often the serious feature of attacks of scarlet fever.

Expressions of agreement from contemporaries as to the value of belladonna in scarlet fever are to be found in Hufeland's Journal for May, 1812, etc., and Hufeland (the one big figure in medicine in Hahnemann's day) himself published in 1825 a work entitled "The Prophylactic Effect of Belladonna," ascribing this efficacious remedy for scarlet fever to Hahnemann. In 1838 the Prussian Government ordered the doctors of that country to use belladonna in small doses against the epidemics of scarlet fever which were then prevalent.

Hahnemann realized that if the Law of Similars was ever to be practical it was imperative to test, or "prove," medicines as to their powers of vitiating human health, in order to have them at hand for curative purposes.

Here began a lifetime of proving medicines, on himself first, then presently on a large circle of disciples and friends. "At first," he says, "I was the only one who made the proving of medicinal powers the most important of all his duties; since then I have been assisted in this by a number of young men who have made experiments on themselves, and whose observations I have carefully reviewed."

With what extreme care these experiments were conducted, checked, and registered, we are told. The drugs were put up in milk-sugar powders. The prover never knew what drug he was taking and had no idea when the proving began (so he would have no preconceived ideas).

Provers had to bring their day-books to Hahnemann, who questioned the provers regarding observed symptoms in order to get the verbal expression of their sensations and sufferings as accurately as possible, as

well as the exact conditions under which the symptoms occurred. Their
mode of life and diet was strictly regulated during a proving, so that
alterations in health should be absolutely due to *drug action*.

Hahnemann says, "Medicines should be distinguished from each other
with scrupulous exactness with regard to their powers and true effects
upon the healthy body. For upon the accuracy of this proving depend life
and death, sickness and health of human beings."

In regard to *Materia Medica,* he lays it down that "a true materia medica
will consist of a collection of genuine, pure and undeceptive effects of
simple drugs" . . . and that such a materia medica "should exclude every
supposition — every mere assertion and fiction; its entire contents should
be the pure language of Nature, uttered in response to careful and faithful
enquiry."

By his provings, Hahnemann introduced an entirely novel and scientific method of studying drug-action. He demonstrated the effect of drugs
on the living human being — surely a method far superior to the study of
their toxic effect on animals! Even if the drugs did affect animals in precisely the same way that they affected all other animals and humans —
which is not the case — what animal would visibly respond to the suicidal
impulses of *Aurum,* the terror of death of *Aconite* and *Arsenicum,* the
terrors of anticipation (even to diarrhea) of *Argentum Nit.* and *Gelsemium,* the indignation and the effect on health of the bottled-up sense of
injury of *Staphisagria,* the fear of knives for the impulses they suggest of
Nux and *Arsenicum,* the shamelessness in mania and delirium of
Hyoscyamus, the indifference to loved ones of *Sepia* and *Phosphorus?*
These, and such symptoms, have led to the most brilliant curative work,
and they can only be found by provings on sensitive men and women.

Hahnemann insisted that what a drug can cause, *that* and *that only,* it
can cure, whether in the mental or the physical sphere; that its curative
powers depend entirely on vital reaction to drug-stimulus; that the stimulus must only be sufficient to evoke reaction in organs rendered hypersensitive by disease; that reaction must be respected and allowed to run
its course before a repetition of the stimulus (should it be called for).

Dominant medicine seems to think that the dose should be the largest
tolerated, and that its repetition is a mere matter of opinion, or of individual practice, or of experience drawn from many experiments (at
the expense of many patients), or of authority, when someone whose
name is prominent lays down the law. It has yet to grasp the idea, which

we owe to Hahnemann, that there is a law in all these things.

Illustrations and corroborations come from all sides. The Arndt-Schultz Law shows that the same poison, to the same cells, may be lethal, inhibitive or stimulating, according to the largeness or the smallness of the dose; while Professor Bier endorses Hahnemann as to the infinite sensitiveness of diseased parts to the vital stimulus.

Hahnemann showed that: "Homœopathy is absolutely inconceivable without the most precise individualization." The *names* of *disease should never influence* the physician who has to judge and cure diseases, not by names, but by the *signs* and *symptoms* of *each individual patient*. Since diseases can only express their need for relief by symptoms, the *totality of the symptoms* observed in each *individual* case of disease can be the only indication to guide in the choice of the remedy.

Hahnemann "knew no disease, only sick persons."

He taught that all parts of the body are intimately connected to form an invisible whole in feelings and functions; that all curative measures should be planned with reference to the whole system, in order to cure the general disease by means of internal remedies. (Even an eruption on the lip, he says, "cannot be accounted for without assuming a previous and simultaneous diseased state of the body.") Read Corinthians I, Chapter 12, Verses 25 and 26.

A sick organism, whether it be man or beast, is very sensitive. It can easily and quickly be relieved by the proper remedy, or made much worse or even killed by improper substances given as remedies. Nature is constantly supplying new cells for worn out ones. Injuries begin to mend almost immediately, as Nature is always on the alert for such conditions. The same applies to sickness of all kinds. Too often, however, the symptoms which are manifested to the doctor, such as fever, for instance, are wrongly conceived to be the disease itself, and strong drugs are forced into the patient, which instead of helping, aggravate and often kill.

I believe, barring an accident, that very few people would die of acute natural diseases even without medicine. If, however, they could have the benefit of the proper Homœopathic remedy, the cure would be much quicker and more permanent.

In looking upon a sick person, you are viewing something that you have never seen before, nor will ever see again. You may see again something similar, but never in your lifetime will you see anything quite identical. That is the secret to proper and perfect medical prescribing.

There are as many variations in sickness as there are persons — no two are alike, although the diagnosis may be the same. Nature, if given the chance, will cure most cases of illness. It may take some time, however, if it is left unaided. It is really harder to get sick than to remain well, provided a person lives in a sensible manner and obeys the laws of health.

Nature needs a boost now and then, and that is where the Homœopathic remedy comes in. It always *helps,* it never interferes. Homœopathy will remove predisposition to health disturbance, tendencies, etc.

Years ago a baby was born at my hospital. She was a blue-eyed blonde. At birth she had a gland in the left side of the neck about the size of a walnut, and a lump on the right breast about the size of a hazel nut. The allopath would have removed them by surgery. What caused these growths in the first place? Some constitutional taint, or predisposition or inheritance. Would surgical removal of the growths have removed their cause? Certainly not! A careful study of the child, parents, and grand-parents was made. A properly selected constitutional remedy was given and the lumps disappeared as if by magic. The little girl, now ten years old, is the brightest, healthiest, happiest and most beautiful child one could wish to see. She can eat anything, never has a cold or symptoms of any kind. It was not the lumps prescribed for, it was the constitution of the baby which was deranged enough to have allowed the occurrence of the lumps. The diagnosis would probably have been cervical and mammary adenitis. No one will ever know how this little child would have fared if she had been subjected to surgery.

There is always some danger connected with the most trivial operation, but in this particular case there would have been not only considerable danger from the operation itself, but the greatest danger would be in the withholding of the remedy that was needed to cure the constitutional, deep-lying causes of the condition with which she was born.

Such is the kind of case Homœopathy is curing every day, all over the world, and no other system thus far discovered can do it.

CHAPTER 4

The Decline of Homœopathy

I have often been asked: "If Homœopathy is as good as you say it is, why then is its practice so rapidly declining in the U.S.?"

It is, indeed, difficult to understand the stubborn bigotry that takes a stranglehold on the minds of men in a profession which has for its purpose the relieving of man's suffering. This is a mission so important that one would assume that every substance offering the slightest promise of having some hidden, curative virtue would be gladly and eagerly studied. Any measure that claimed to be of benefit to suffering mankind should be investigated, whatever its source.

The success of Homœopathy caused hatred, jealousy, and consternation in the hearts of those too prejudiced to use it themselves. The tearing down of Homœopathy has been going on for many years. In the van of its detractors have been the ignorant, the fearful, and those who would stand to lose if it were to succeed.

I would like you to read the following partial transcript of a trial that took place in Massachusetts in the last century. I think it will give you a pretty good idea of the treatment accorded Homœopathy by established orthodoxy.

STATEMENT OF THE TRIAL

In November, 1871, the following notice was received by each of the following gentlemen viz:—

William Bushnell, M.D.	George Russell, M.D.
Milton Fuller, M.D.	I. T. Talbot, M.D.
Samuel Gregg, M.D.	David Thayer, M.D.
H. L. H. Hoffendahl, M.D.	Benj. H. West, M.D.

All of Boston.   NORTHAMPTON, MASS., NOV. 4, 1871.

To................................M.D.

SIR, — Charges having been preferred against you by a Committee of the Massachusetts Medical Society of "Conduct unbecoming and unworthy an honorable physician and member of this Society," *to wit:* "by practising or professing to practise according to an exclusive theory or dogma, and by belonging to a Society whose purpose is at variance with the principles of, and tends to disorganize, the Massachusetts Medical Society."

You are hereby directed to appear before a Board of Trial at the Society's Rooms, No. 36 Temple Place, Perkins Building, on Tuesday, November 21, 1871, at 11 o'clock, A.M., to answer to the same, in accordance with by-laws and instructions of the Society.

SAMUEL A. FISK,
PRESIDENT OF THE MASSACHUSETTS MEDICAL SOCIETY.

At the time and place appointed the persons notified appeared before a board consisting of

Jeremiah Spofford, M.D., of Groveland.
Augustus Torrey, M.D., of Beverly.
George Hayward, M.D., of Boston.
Frederic Winsor, M.D., of Winchester.
Francis C. Greene, M.D., of Easthampton.

The charges were then presented, signed by

Luther Parks, M.D., of Boston
R. L. Hodgdon, M.D., of Arlington
Thos. L. Gage, M.D., of Worcester
Asa Millet, M.D., of Bridgewater
Benjamin B. Breed, M.D., of Lynn

The accused protested against being tried upon charges of so vague a character; against the manner in which the so-called board of trial was constituted; and also against the manner in which the trial had thus far been conducted.

The board refused to receive or consider these protests, when the trial was interrupted by a temporary injunction from the Supreme Court.

Arguments on the question of an injunction were made by counsel before the Supreme Court, and the injunction was removed, the Court declining, at this stage of proceedings, to decide upon the powers of the Society under its charter.

In April, 1873, the following notice was received by all the persons accused, except Samuel Gregg, M.D., removed by death.

BOSTON, April 1, 1873.

To.............................M.D.

SIR: — Specifications having been demanded of charges preferred against you by a Committee of the Massachusetts Medical Society of "Conduct unbecoming and unworthy an honorable physician and member of this Society," *to wit:* "by practising or professing to practise according to an exclusive theory or dogma, and by belonging to a Society whose purpose is at variance with the principles of, and tends to disorganize, the Massachusetts Medical Society," and you having been directed to appear before a Board of Trial at the Society's rooms, No. 36 Temple Place, Perkins Building, on Tuesday, November 21, 1871, at 11 o'clock, A.M., to answer to the same. In accordance with By-laws and instructions of the Society.

By DR. FISK,
PRESIDENT OF THE
MASSACHUSETTS MEDICAL SOCIETY.

The Committee now specify that the exclusive theory or dogma referred to in said charges is the theory or dogma known as Homœopathy, and the Society therein referred to, whose purpose is at variance with, and tends to disorganize the Massachusetts Medical Society, is the Massachusetts Homœopathic Medical Society.

The Committee file the following as further specifications:

CHARGE I. — That you are guilty of an attempt to disorganize and destroy the Massachusetts Medical Society.

SPECIFICATION 1. — That you have joined, and are a member, of a certain Society, known as the Massachusetts Homœopathic Medical Society, whose purposes are at variance, and which tends to disorganize, the Massachusetts Medical Society.

SPECIFICATION 2. — That you belong to, and are a member of, a certain Society called the Massachusetts Homœopathic Medical Society, which adopts as its principle in the treatment of disease a certain exclusive theory or dogma, known as Homœopathy.

CHARGE II. — That you are guilty of conduct unbecoming and un-worthy an honorable physician and member of the Massachusetts Medical Society.

SPECIFICATION 1. — In that you practise, or profess to practise, medicine according to a certain exclusive theory or dogma known as Homœopathy.

SPECIFICATION 2. — In that while a member of the Massachusetts Medical Society you have joined, and are a member of, a certain Society called the Massachusetts Homœopathic Medical Society, which adopts as its principle in the treatment of disease a certain exclusive theory or dogma known as Homœopathy, and whose purposes are at variance with, and which tends to disorganize, the Massachusetts Medical Society.

SPECIFICATION 3. — In that you are a member of a certain Society, called the Massachusetts Homœopathic Medical Society, which adopts as its principle in the treatment of disease a certain exclusive theory or dogma, known as Homœopathy, whose purposes are at variance with, and which tends to disorganize, the Massachusetts Medical Society.

You are further hereby reminded that to try the same, the Board of Trial *stands adjourned* to April 29th, 1873, at 11 A.M., at 36 Temple Place.

> GEO. C. SHATTUCK,
> PRESIDENT OF THE
> MASSACHUSETTS MEDICAL SOCIETY

At the time and place of adjournment the accused appeared. R. L. Hodgdon, M.D., of Arlington, was the only one of the prosecutors present. He presented the charges as amended and added to; and as documentary proof he exhibited the Act of Incorporation of the Massachusetts Homœopathic Medical Society and the section of its by-laws which state that "Any person who . . . acknowledges the truth of the maxim SIMILIA SIMILIBUS CURANTUR may become eligible to membership" of the Society.

He read extracts from the *Organon,* in which Hahnemann states that Homœopathy is the opposite of, and can have nothing to do with Allopathy.

He presented the section of a By-law of the Massachusetts Medical Society, passed in 1860, as follows:—

"No person shall hereafter be admitted a member of the Society who professes to cure diseases by Spiritualism, Homœopathy or Thompsonianism."

Also a resolution adopted by the Massachusetts Medical Society in 1871 to the effect, that the practice of Homœopathy is "conduct unbecoming and unworthy an honorable physician and member of this Society."

Also, the fact that the accused were known as practitioners of Homœopathy and members of the Massachusetts Homœopathic Medical Society.

Dr. I. T. Talbot appeared as counsel for Dr. William Bushnell, in behalf of whom and for the rest of the accused, he made the following demands of the Board of Trial:—

1. That the trial should not be held with closed doors, but that their friends should be allowed to be present.
   Demand refused.

2. That reporters for the press should be allowed to be present; that as this was a matter affecting the character of the accused, the public had a right to know the evidence produced and the manner of conducting this trial.
   Demand refused.

3. That the accused be allowed legal counsel, since it is proposed to dispossess them of rights, privileges and personal property.
   Demand refused.

4. That they be allowed to have an advocate, not a member of the Massachusetts Medical Society, present to advise them.
   Demand refused.

5. That, as they have reason to object to the record of the Secretary a phonographic reporter of the trial should be appointed by mutual consent, and sworn to the faithful performance of his duty.
   Demand refused.

6. That the accused may employ a phonographic reporter.
   Demand refused.

7. That an amanuensis, not a member of the Massachusetts Medical Society, be allowed to sit beside the accused and assist him in taking notes of the trial.
   Demand refused.

8. The right to peremptory challenge.
   Demand refused.

9. The right to challenge members of the Board of Trial for good and sufficient reasons.
Demand refused.

The accused then presented the following protest and asked the Board to receive it and put it on file.

EVIDENCE FOR THE DEFENSE

The following documentary evidence was introduced in the case of Dr. Bushnell, and was accepted by the Board of Trial as applying to all the cases:—

1. The Act of Incorporation of the Massachusetts Homœopathic Medical Society, showing that membership of the said Society was authorized by law.
2. That section of the By-laws of said Society relating to membership, as originally adopted.
3. That portion of the present By-laws of said Society relating to the objects of the Society and to membership.
4. The Act of Incorporation of the Massachusetts Homœopathic Hospital.
5. The Act of Incorporation of the Homœopathic Medical Dispensary.
6. The Act of Incorporation of the New England Homœopathic Medical College.
7. Correspondence with the Treasurer of the Massachusetts Medical Society, showing that the accused had faithfully paid their dues to the Society.

The following is a resumé of testimony introduced. It was proposed by the accused to give it under oath, but the chairman ruled that the word of any respectable physician would be accepted by the Board.

EVIDENCE OF GEORGE RUSSELL, M.D.

I am seventy-seven years old; have been in practice fifty-three years; began to investigate Homœopathy in 1846 or 1847, and have since continued such studies; I believe it is the best system of medicine, but should be very glad to find any better; have never sought to injure, destroy, or disorganize the Massachusetts Medical Society, but have sought to learn from it as much as possible. Think that if Homœopathy were investigated by the Society it would greatly benefit its members.

THE CHAIRMAN. Why, if you believe in Homœopathy, do you remain in the Massachusetts Medical Society?

DR. RUSSELL. Because I see no good reason why I should leave it. It is a Society designed to include all educated physicians of good character, and has nothing to do with medical opinions or belief.

DR. HODGDON. What is allopathy?

DR. RUSSELL. I suppose, from the derivation of the word, it means the opposite of homœopathy.

DR. HODGDON. Do you consider the Massachusetts Medical Society an allopathic society?

DR. RUSSELL. I do not, though some of its members may be allopaths. If the Society were such, I should leave it at once.

EVIDENCE OF DAVID THAYER, M.D.

I have been practising medicine for thirty years; I joined the Massachusetts Medical Society in the year 1845; and was one of the original corporators of the Massachusetts Homœopathic Medical Society, in 1856; its object is the improvement of the science of medicine in accordance with the principle *Similia Similibus Curantur;* Homœopathy is not yet perfect, and the object of the Society is to improve it; I have never known of an effort being made on the part of the members of the Massachusetts Homœopathic Medical Society to destroy or injure the Massachusetts Medical Society.

There is not, and never has been, required from the members of the Homœopathic Medical Society a pledge to practice in accordance with any particular theory.

THE CHAIRMAN. Do you consider it honorable, as a member of the Massachusetts Medical Society, to practice Homœopathy?

DR. THAYER. Perfectly so. The Society is chartered by law for physicians of every school. Education and character are, by that charter, the only requisites for membership. Medical opinions legally form no part of the qualifications of members.

DR. TALBOT. Do you consider it honorable, as a member of the Massachusetts Medical Society to give unmedicated sugar pellets, and pretend that they are homœopathic medicine?

DR. THAYER. I should consider it very dishonorable and downright dishonesty.

DR. TALBOT. If it were known that a physician was in the habit of practising such deception, should you think him sufficiently honorable to be worthy of a place on any board of trial?

DR. THAYER. No; I should think he deserved expulsion from any honorable society.

DR. TALBOT. Will you state the history of the Massachusetts Homœopathic Medical Society?

DR. THAYER. It was first established in 1840 by four or five physicians, and was called the Homœopathic Fraternity. Its meetings were informal and social in character, and were held at the houses of the members. As the members increased, the name was changed to the Massachusetts Homœopathic Medical Society, about 1850, and in 1856 it was chartered by the State without any change in the objects of the Society, which were to develop a branch of medicine not cultivated by the Massachusetts Medical Society. At present there are between one and two hundred members of the Homœopathic Society.

THE CHAIRMAN. Have you ever been prevented by the Massachusetts Medical Society from making any investigations in regard to Homœopathy?

DR. THAYER. No, I never have; and from many of the members who knew that I believed in, and practised, Homœopathy, I have received only the greatest courtesy and kindness; but there are members of this Society, who, at its meetings, and at other times and places, have gone out of their way to insult those members who believe in Homœopathy; and I consider that this prosecution is designed to prevent the investigation of Homœopathy by members of this Society.

EVIDENCE OF C. W. SWAN, M.D.
In answer to questions by Dr. Talbot.

I am Secretary of the Massachusetts Medical Society, and have been for several years. The society has about 1,200 members. Think it is as prosperous now as ever before. Have never known the accused to do anything to injure or destroy the society. So far as I know they have been peaceable members of the society.

R. L. Hodgdon, M.D., the prosecutor, refused to testify.

The accused offered to present the testimony of every member of the

Massachusetts Homœopathic Medical Society, if it were necessary to prove that the object and character of that Society was such as had been already stated by witnesses.

THE CHAIRMAN. Cumulative evidence on these points will not be necessary, and will not add to the strength of testimony.

The accused proposed at this point to present no further evidence.

WHO ARE THE MEN ON TRIAL?

Look at the character and standing of the accused, and the methods adopted by this singular tribunal.

DR. WILLIAM BUSHNELL: a man of singular purity of character and life, who after faithful study under approved teachers has conscientiously performed the duties of his profession, and whom the breath of slander has never touched.

DR. MILTON FULLER: a favorite student with the elder Dr. Townsend, a painstaking pupil in a school of acknowledged ability, who has for more than forty years devoted himself to his profession with universal acceptance, and finds himself now, for the first time in his life, charged with conduct unbecoming a gentleman and a physician.

DR. H. L. HOFFENDAHL: who graduated from Harvard University with the leading honors of his class, and who has brought the severe training and broad culture of the University into the service of the profession, and whose reputation is such as may well be envied.

DR. SAMUEL GREGG: who for neary half a century, day and night, devoted himself to the welfare of his patients, among whom were some of our foremost men in professional and mercantile life, glad to trust to his intuitive skill and education and sagacity their own lives and those of their families, but who in early professional life was compelled to join this Society, in order to have the benefit of consulting with its members, and at a time when he was so poor that even the ten dollars required for membership was a serious tax on his scanty resources. Here in his old age, after having done all that the Society could even ask of a member, after having honored the Society, as few men are privileged to do, by a life of rare usefulness and deserved success, after having believed and practised in accordance with the Homœopathic principles for more than thirty years, he was to be expelled and dishonored on the accusation of men belonging to a generation which was in its cradle when he was watching at the bedside of some of our noblest citizens, their trusted counsellor, to whose skill and care they acknowledged that they owed health and life.

DR. GEORGE RUSSELL: now nearly fourscore years of age, the good physician of three successive generations, whose professional success testifies for him, and whose uprightness, honesty, and integrity are unimpeachable.

DR. DAVID THAYER: whose professional skill has not only been rewarded with a large practise and the well-earned confidence of a wide and influential circle, but whose admitted ability and integrity have advanced him to many places of public trust.

DR. BENJ. H. WEST: whose character as a scholar, as a physician, and as a public man, needs no eulogy here.

These are the men whom you seek to brand as guilty of a crime worthy of expulsion, from whom you would take rights given them by the State; whom you would deprive of property which they themselves have helped to contribute to the Society and to science.

DR. THAYER'S DEFENCE

Dr. Thayer spoke especially in behalf of himself and Dr. Milton Fuller.

MR. CHAIRMAN AND GENTLEMEN OF THE BOARD OF TRIAL:—

In addressing myself to the defence which I find myself here to make, against certain charges brought by a Committee of the Massachusetts Medical Society, it seems proper that I should first rehearse those charges in your hearing. They are as follows, viz.:—

NORTHAMPTON, MASS., NOV. 4, 1871.

To DAVID THAYER, M.D.:

SIR — Charges having been preferred against you by a committee of the Massachusetts Medical Society of "Conduct unbecoming and unworthy an honorable physician and member of this Society," *to wit:* "by practising or professing to practise according to an exclusive theory or dogma, and by belonging to a Society whose purpose is at a variance with the principles of, and tends to disorganize, the Massachusetts Medical Society," —

You are hereby directed to appear before a Board of Trial at the Society's Rooms, No. 36 Temple Place, Perkins Building, on Tuesday,

November 21, 1871, at 11 o'clock, A.M., to answer to the same, in accordance with by-laws and instructions of the Society.

SAMUEL A. FISK,
PRESIDENT OF THE MASSACHUSETTS MEDICAL SOCIETY

I pass by the insult implied in the phrase *"professing to practise."* It is of a piece with many other things in this trial. It requires no notice, and is wholly unworthy of gentlemen representing our venerable Society and members of an honorable profession. The substance of the charge is that in practising on the homœopathic system and in joining the Homœopathic Society I have been guilty of conduct inconsistent with my duty as a member of the Massachusetts Medical Society.

What is the nature and object of that Society? Its charter provides in its preamble that those physicians who are educated and qualified to practise physic may be distinguished from those who ignorantly and wickedly administer medicines. The object of the Society is apparent from this preamble. That object is to bring educated physicians together for mutual support, consultation, and recognition. The Society proposes to marshal in its ranks all those physicians who have submitted to a thorough and sufficient education and preparation before assuming the responsibilities of the profession. The object of the Society is to distinguish such men from the presumptuous and ignorant quack who, without training or study, administers drugs of which he knows nothing, and the use of which in disease is fraught with danger to health and life. The Society prescribes no method or system of medicine, no rule of practise; neither does it forbid any. It endorses neither allopathy nor Homœopathy nor antipathy nor hydropathy. It neither denies nor affirms Cullen's theory of fever, nor Todd's. It does not make belief in Bigelow's notion of self-limited diseases a condition of membership; neither would it expel old Dr. Shattuck or Strong, or any of our old heroic practitioners, were they alive, because they did not accept Holmes' idea of a good physician; viz., to watch your patient carefully, but trouble and endanger him with as little medicine as possible. On all such points it is silent. It only demands that its members shall be men who have faithfully weighed and examined all systems; men of trained minds, competent to form a judgment on such questions, men of such education, skill, and experience as justify them in assuming the care of the sick. It runs no line between this system or that. The line that it intends to draw is one that shall separate education from ignorance, the man of careful and honest training from the charlatan and the quack. Inside of this line it leaves every one of its members entirely free to exercise the healing art according to his own best judgment. All systems and theories are free to all. They may and do practise, some on one principle and some on another, while many follow no principle or theory, but are guided entirely by experience — and no one objects or has any right to object. All may give large doses of medicine or small ones, or none at all. Many use all the means known to the art of healing — ponderable bodies and imponderable agencies, all the various uses of water — hot and cold — electricity and galvanism, Perkinsism and animal magnetism, and whatever else that is known or to be known.

All that our Society undertakes to secure is that its members shall be men sufficiently educated to be competent to decide between rival theories, and of such good judgment that their course shall honor the profession, and serve the public health. If I am not correct in this statement of the purposes of this Society, please, gentlemen, open its records and show me where it states what particular system it *does* sanction. Please to show us in the by-laws or charter of the Society any indorsement of any system of practise. You cannot do it, for it is not there. As Dr. Luther Parks, the Chairman of the Prosecuting Committee, said in the beginning of these trials, "We have no system; every one is entirely free to do as he pleases. In this room," said he, "the doctors used to contend with old Dr. Strong against his enormous doses; but no one could deny his right to do just as he pleased, and every one had the same right." Various and numerous have been the theories believed in, practised on and promulgated in this Society. Even Perkinsism was allowed and practised in this Society, within the last century. It went out of use, not by summoning its votaries before this tribunal: that might have prolonged its use. Perkinsism and Astrology might be used in the Massachusetts Medical Society today, and undisturbed, so long as it was unsuccessful, and the large fees did not find their way into the pockets of the astrologers and tractorators. The learned and witty Dr. O. W. Holmes ridicules the efficacy of nine-tenths of all the drugs which the founders of this Society used, and excepting one or two, he considers all drugs injurious, — is sure mankind would be healthier if drugs had never been discovered, and is not quite sure the same would not have been the case had physicians never appeared. You remember his saying:

"If all the medicines were thrown into the sea it would be all the better for mankind, but all the worse for the fishes." Is this treason to the Massachusetts Medical Society? If we are justly accused, what of Dr. Holmes? Does any one propose to arraign him as undermining the very foundations of this Society? Why not, if the theory on which we are accused be correct?

Now, gentlemen, if my representation of the Society be correct, why are we arraigned? Educated we certainly are to the Society's content; otherwise we should never have been admitted. Besides, we can point to as many years of faithful study and practise as you can. How, then, have we violated our duties since? Have we ludicrously failed in grappling with disease? Have we sported with the lives of our patients? Have we deluded the ignorant classes to their hurt, extorting fees and rendering nothing in return? Have we disgraced the Society by parading a notion of medicine that no sane man would countenance, which trifles with human life and brings contempt on the profession? Gentlemen, on all these points we are willing to measure ourselves with you. Your system has had possession of the Commonwealth for two centuries. Ours has been known here not quite forty years. Making fair allowance for time, we have as many families trusted to our care as you have. And our patients are not the careless, the ignorant, the needy, who must take what they can get, or the reckless, carried away by every new whim. No; we count among our patients the rich, who have tried every clime for health, every city for medical skill, every theory for efficient help; we have the foremost men at the bar, in the pulpit, on the exchange. In intelligence, social position, and world-wide culture, the men and women who trust their lives to us may be fairly measured with any who consult you. On this point we have done the Society no dishonor.

But, second, have we failed to help these friends? Have we been found wanting in severe disease? Forty years is sufficient time for trial. The evidence that they find us efficient helpers is that they continue to trust us.

Third: But is our method empiricism and quackery? Who is authorized to say that of a system which two generations of the best educated men in this country and in Europe continue to trust; which the foremost governments of Europe recognize; which has its hospitals, both city and national, all over the world; which dares to compare its success in curing disease with the best of you? If world-wide recognition, unequalled success in curing disease, and the confidence of the most enlightened classes here and in Europe do not lift a system into sufficient character to prevent its use disgracing this Society, please describe to us, gentlemen, what evidence of usefulness you do demand?

Again, gentlemen, other members of the Massachusetts Medical Society have organized themselves into other societies for the cultivation of medicine and for special purposes, just as the homœopathists have done. The Gynæcological Society, whose blatant and noisy members have done so much to disturb the harmony of this Society, has for its object the study of the diseases of women. Yet no one of them has been arraigned here. Why not? Is it because they have no principle or system? But we who have a system, and practise in accordance with it, are called to answer for it. The object of the Massachusetts Homœopathic Medical Society is the culture of medicine according to a law of nature, which law is recognized (ignorantly perhaps) even in the Massachusetts Medical Society.

This law is expressed by the formula of Hahnemann — *"Similia Similibus Curantur."* Hippocrates acknowledged the truth of this law, and Hufeland sent some patients, whom he could not cure, to consult Dr. Hahnemann. Why do you apply snow to a frozen part, and distant heat to a burn? These practises are traditional, and are used empirically by the members of the Massachusetts Medical Society, never thinking that this is Homœopathy of the rankest kind. There are many other instances in which you cure diseases homœopathically without once dreaming that you are guilty of trenching on the domain of Homœopathy. One of these is the use of purgatives in affections of the bowels, and thus hundreds are killed every year in this city by your heroic and dangerous doses. If the allopaths would follow out and profit by the experience of the homœopaths, and give their minute doses, the results would show them the superiority of the latter over the former. They have lately learned that minute doses of ipecacuanha will cure nausea and vomiting, while they have given the large doses of that drug for a century — first increasing vomiting and thereby curing it — on the homœopathic principle, to be sure; but so "ignorantly and wickedly" applied, that great mischief is often done thereby. But some wise observer among them has discovered that very minute doses of ipecacuanha will cure nausea and vomiting in a more prompt and satisfactory manner. This astonishing discovery is explained, they think, by the bold statement that ipecacuanha is a tonic! How cunningly they avoid the homœopathic law — *"Similia Similibus Curantur!"*

There are many other instances of the same nature which might be stated, showing that the members of the Massachusetts Medical Society for years have blundered along the road towards Homœopathy; but if told of it, the learned reply is, "Homœopathy is a humbug," and that is the end of it. The motto on the seal of the Massachusetts Homœopathic Medical Society is *Certiorem Medendi Usum Maluit.* This motto expresses the meaning and the aspirations of thousands of earnest homœopathists in this country — "to make the art of healing more certain."

If it be proved that the Massachusetts Homœopathic Medical Society has done something to benefit science and to aid in the cure of disease and to make medicine a more certain science, then I boldy assert that, instead of tending to disorganize the Massachusetts Medical Society, the tendency is rather to benefit and to aid that ancient corporation, and to put it on a higher plane of observation. Any member of the Massachusetts Medical Society, should he become so far enlightened as to perceive that there is truth in the direction of Homœopathy, could join the Massachusetts Homœopathic Medical Society by avowing a desire to learn Homœopathy.

But leaving general statements, I propose to show you in detail that Homœopathy is not what Dr. Luther Parks declared it to be — a fraud, an imposition, "like the little joker, sometimes here and sometimes there" — but that it is a useful and beneficient system of medicine, as true as any law known to physics. In order to make this clear I must state to you something which Homœopathy has done. In the report made to the Massachusetts Medical Society, twenty-three years ago, Dr. George Hayward, Dr. Oliver W. Holmes, and Dr. J. B. S. Jackson said that Homœopathy had done much good by teaching us that a great deal less medicine will do just as well, — (I quote from memory). Has any other special theory of medicine in your books or system of practise lived so long as Homœopathy has — more than three-quarters of a century? and is it not still fast gaining in favor with the best and most intelligent of the people? Homœopathy *has* done some good.

There are cures made every day by Homœopathy which would astonish the whole medical world if they were known and understood. In the cure of diarrhœa of adults in New England nothing can surpass the efficacy of this little white powder. It is sweet to the taste, inodorous, and I doubt if your chemistry can detect even a trace of medicine in it. It contains only one-millionth part of a grain of the drug in each grain, yet it cures with astonishing quickness — tute, cito, et jucunde. But even this medicine is too strong for the enteritis of infants, and if given will endanger life.

Dr. Jacob Bigelow says that syphilis is not a self-limited disease; by which he means to say that the patient will never spontaneously recover. If that is true, then I am able to demonstrate the efficacy of homœopathic medicine in that terrible disease. This little vial contains also a white, sweet, and inodorous powder — just one ten-thousandth part of it is medicine, the rest is sugar of milk. For the primary chancre I always give a small dose of this powder two or three times a day for one week. The sore will always look worse at the end of that time. I then give it only once or twice a day. When improvement is visible I give the medicine less frequently, and the patient is cured. Sometimes the young homœopathist will be impatient as the chancre looks worse, and will be tempted to make some local application, especially if he has been graduated at an allopathic college. But let him wait, and his faith and works will be rewarded. No application to the chancre itself should be made, further than to keep it clean; and this little white harmless powder will effect a cure without secondary symptoms. I am able to assure you, Mr. Chairman and gentlemen of the Board of Trial, that it is a very rare circumstance that one of my cases has ever developed secondary symptoms. This powder contains only one ten-thousandth part of the drug, while the other 9,999 parts are nothing but sugar of milk. This medicine has been ground four hours in a mortar. Dr. Jacob Bigelow says this disease is not self-curable. Then I ask you what cures these cases? If this homœopathic drug does not do it, please tell us what does? Or is Dr. Bigelow mistaken? Or am I mistaken? Very strange I should not know the disease after the study and practise of medicine more than a third of a century, and living in a city where it is very common.

One or two more illustrations and I will not tire you with a fourth. The disease known as gall-stone, you, Mr. Chairman, none of you, gentlemen, members of the Massachusetts Medical Society, can cure. Not one of you ever pretended to have attained to that knowledge; yet nothing is easier. The gallstone colic is easily recognized. Your only remedy is opiates, hypodermic injections, the inhalation of ether, or some other narcotic to allay the sufferings of the patient, and perhaps an aperient to hasten the discharge of the gallstone. This is the best you know — the best you can do. In the winter of 1854-55 the discovery was made that gallstone colic can be cured, radically cured. By the radical cure of gallstone colic is meant that change in the system which prevents the recurrence of the malady. The remedy I hold in my hand. It is in these small, round pellets of sugar. They have been slightly moistened by a solution containing only one-millionth part of the drug and 999,999 parts of alcohol and water. This bilious colic is caused by the lodgment of a calculus in the duct of the gall bladder too small for its easy passage, or by other biliary obstructions. It is apt to recur every two or three weeks, once a month, and sometimes after longer intervals. One of its strong characteristics is periodicity. The remedy which I have exhibited has periodicity for one of its characteristics as well as a special affinity for the gall bladder. It is now more than nineteen years since the value of this remedy came to my knowledge, and from that time to this it has not in a single instance failed to prevent the recurrence of the disease. I usually give six of these little pellets twice a day till ten doses are taken, then once a day till ten doses are taken, then every other day till ten doses are taken, etc., etc., till at length they are taken only once a month. In the last nineteen years I have treated hundreds of cases, from all parts of the continent, and without a single failure.

There are many other diseases, the remedies for which are equally reliable and well known to the accused. Can any of you gentlemen cure organic disease of the heart? Every member of our Society can. Are any of you able to tell us the remedy for rachitis infantum? We can tell you, for we have not failed once in more than twelve years. And we don't use any iron braces, nor any mechanical appliances whatever, only some of those little sugar pills, moistened with a solution of a drug, only one-millionth part of which is medicine, and 999,999 parts of which are alcohol and water — nothing else.

We are indicted for belonging to a Society which teaches these things, and for practising Homœopathy, by means of which cures are made of diseases which those unacquainted with Homœopathy would pronounce incurable. Is this "conduct unworthy and unbecoming an honorable physician"? And does it "tend to disorganize the Massachusetts Medical Society"?

If you don't believe these statements, we will obtain permission to refer you to the persons who have been cured of these (incurable?) diseases, who are only too grateful to Homœopathy not to be willing to tell you the truth. We may perhaps be permitted to refer you to the members of the Massachusetts Medical Society, who pronounced those cases incurable.

You charge us, gentlemen, with attempting to disorganize the Massachusetts Medical Society. Your only evidence is, that we have joined another society and practise Homœopathy. I invite you, gentlemen, to show us how either of these acts tends to disorganize the Massachusetts Medical Society. You have not offered one tittle of evidence. On the contrary, I offer you the evidence of any and all of the accused, or any other member of our Homœopathic Society. They have told you that they never heard a word uttered, or knew of a plan laid to weaken your Society. But, on the contrary, that we have always cherished its welfare and sought its usefulness, and we have annually paid our dues.

Now, gentlemen, let me ask you: Is there any by-law or rule in your Society which forbids its members from investigating Homœopathy? If not, suppose you take the lead and examine it. I have no doubt, if you will do so, you will all become homœopathists. For I can say, as has been often said, "I never knew a scientific man to fairly examine it who did not believe in it." Now, gentlemen, I make you this proposition, that at the next annual meeting of the Massachusetts Medical Society, in June next, you ask that a committee be appointed — one from each County in the State — or, if you prefer, one from each town and ward of the cities, to investigate the claims and pretensions of Homœopathy, with instructions to report at the next annual meeting. I pledge you, gentlemen, that we will aid you all in our power. Every facility shall be given you that can aid your inquiries.

DECISION OF THE BOARD OF TRIAL

The undersigned, having been appointed a Board of Trial for the purpose of trying William Bushnell, Milton Fuller, H. L. H. Hoffendahl, George Russell, I. T. Talbot, David Thayer, Benjamin H. West, upon the foregoing charges and specifications, met the several parties charged on the 29th day of April, A.D. 1873, and by adjournment on other days between the said 29th April and the date hereof, and heard the evidence adduced in support of said charges, and heard the said several defendants, all of whom were personally present, and their evidence, averments and arguments in answer to said charges and specifications, and the parties having been fully heard, and the evidence and arguments on each side fully considered, we do find and determine that the said charges and specifications are all fully proved against each of said accused persons, and they are severally guilty of the charges aforesaid, and we therefore adjudge and determine that the said William Bushnell, Milton Fuller, H. L. H. Hoffendahl, George Russell, I. T. Talbot, David Thayer, Benjamin H. West, be therefore expelled from their membership of the Massachusetts Medical Society, and report this our determination to the Massachusetts Medical Society at its annual meeting, for such action thereupon as to the Society may seem fit.

> (Signed) JEREMIAH SPOFFORD,
> AUGUSTUS TORREY,
> GEORGE HAYWARD,
> FREDERIC WINSOR,
> Being a majority of the Board of Trial.

Dated MAY 19, 1873   CHAS. W. SWAN,
A true copy.   *Secretary, Board of Trial*

*   *   *

Should not every member of the Massachusetts Medical Society blush with shame for any part — passive or active — that he may have had in this so-called trial, which produced not one scintilla of evidence of guilt on the part of the accused, yet ended with the verdict of "guilty"?

This trial was a farce and the final judgment pre-arranged.

What "wonderful" men to serve as family doctors!!!

The men who were forced to suffer the indignity of this trial were of the highest integrity — professionally, intellectually, and morally. They were doctors who had discovered how to really cure sickness.

Dr. I. T. Talbot later became Dean of Boston University Medical School.

The accusers of these men were bigoted orthodox doctors. It was their type of medical practice that aroused Holmes to such acid castigation. Theirs was a practice based on empiricism, the futility of which led Professor H. C. Wood, an orthodox physician of repute, in the preface of his *Treatise on Therapeutics, Materia Medica and Toxicology,* to say:

"Therapeutics developed in this manner (empiric) cannot, however, rest upon a secure foundation. What today is to be believed, is tomorrow, to be cast aside, certainly has been the law of advancement and seemingly must continue to be so. What has clinical therapeutics established permanently and indisputably? Scarcely anything beyond the primary facts that Quinia will arrest an intermittent fever, that salts will purge and that opium will quiet pain and lull to sleep. Yet with what a babble of discordant voices does it celebrate its thousands of years of experience."

Looking back, we find that hardly a single method of medical treatment in vogue at the time of this suit and used by each and every member of the Massachusetts Medical Society is used today. The years have proved that many of their methods were not only useless but more deadly than the diseases they were meant to cure. On the other hand, the same homœopathic remedies used by the doctors who stood trial are being used throughout the world by Homœopaths today exactly as they were used then and with the same excellent results.

They were doctors who for many years were Fellows of the Massachusetts Medical Society and were highly esteemed by their fellow members. They were evidently and obviously superior to the others because somewhere during their many years of practice, they acquired a conviction that they were not as successful in their orthodox method of practice as they would like to be.

One by one they were led to investigate a so-called new "cult" in medicine that had recently been introduced in America. It was called Homœopathy. Results of prescribing by this method were claimed to be superior to anything heretofore used. They found these claims to be true and they adopted and practiced Homœopathy to the great benefit and satisfaction of their patients. *

But think of it — only eight out of twelve hundred members of this medical society at that time were interested in becoming better doctors. All the others were very well aware of the fact that they knew no curative medicine nor any guiding principle. The situation today is no different than it was then.

The usual prevailing professional bigotry prevented most orthodox doctors from even daring to look into the matter; and they immediately became the enemy of any doctor who did have the courage and honesty to do it. It is not only a right, but an absolute duty of all physicians to investigate very carefully everything that may be of benefit to sick people.

The majority of the Members of the Massachusetts Medical Society not only would not investigate the new discovery in medical procedure that had interested their former respected fellow members, but sat supinely by, indifferent to the fate of these superior men — and yet all these men were the trusted, loved and respected family physicians to many, many people.

Those who adopted the new system, Homœopathy, and prescribed according to it, achieved curative results never before experienced. Its patrons included the illustrious names of:

Elizabeth Stuart Phelps	Henry Wadsworth Longfellow
Nathaniel Hawthorne	Wendell Phillips
Elizabeth Palmer Peabody	Thomas Wentworth Higginson
William Loyd Garrison	Julia Ward Howe
Thomas Starr King	Louisa May Alcott
A. Bronson Alcott	Theodore Parker
	Thomas Bailey Aldrich

The number of Homœopathic physicians in Boston over the past nearly one hundred years was as follows:

1861 — 16	1882 — 124
1870 — 57	1889 — 200
1874 — 74	1904 — 645

The peak was reached around 1904. Today there are not more than a dozen.

It was about the year 1900 that the AMA began its crusade against allegedly inferior medical schools. This activity was brought to my attention in 1904 or 1905 when President Merlin of Boston University asked me to come to his office in the medical school building. He told me that the AMA frowned on homœopathic teaching and had advised its discontinuance. It would be allowed as an elective course only to comply with the school charter.

Had I any comments to make on the situation? To me it seemed pretty arbitrary and high-handed, considering the fact that the buildings and other physical properties of the school came largely through the gifts from grateful patients who wished to establish an institution where such scientific, curative medicine could be taught to medical students. So I replied in plain English — perhaps too plain for some — "Why don't you tell the AMA to go to hell!"

He replied that the AMA had usurped authority to classify all medical schools, and if we did not comply with their demands the B. U. Medical School would be given a Class C rating and as such its graduates would have great difficulty taking and passing the State Board examinations to get a license to practice.

Then I said, "Why don't you fight them?"

His reply was that the B. U. Board of Trustees would not go for that. It wanted no controversy and no trouble. It *did* want a large school.

Who were these trustees? Just some individuals who evidently did not take the situation seriously — could not foresee the dire results which were sure to follow and which did follow as proved by subsequent events. Thus in my opinion was destroyed a fine medical school and its well-trained homœopathic teachers were replaced by orthodox doctors who knew nothing about curative medicine; therefore no curative medicine was taught. And so Boston University was then able to boast a Grade A medical school when, if you ask me, it ceased then and there to be a *real* medical school at all. Its birthright was sold for a "mess of pottage."

Of course the misinformed public was bamboozled into thinking that the great AMA was doing a wonderful thing in its efforts to produce the "best kind" of medical schools and therefore the "best kind" of doctors.

At present in this country, the only schooling available for pure homœopathic training is the Post Graduate School for Physicians conducted by the American Foundation for Homœopathy, Inc., Washington, D. C.

CHAPTER 5

The Stories of Two Doctors

An inquiring mind capable of freeing itself of preconceived ideas can bring a man great satisfaction. In this chapter you will read the stories of two doctors who, unlike so many others, refused to reject the evidence of the Homœopathic Law of Cure.

TWO DECADES IN MEDICINE
T. H. Hudson, M.D.
Kansas City, Missouri

Nearly twenty years ago I began the study of medicine in an eastern allopathic college. I never dreamed that there was a better place, more efficient teaching, or wiser instructors. And, indeed, this was for my purpose at that time sufficiently true. The institution was splendidly equipped, the faculty composed of earnest, thoughtful, brainy men. The thought that any mistake could have been made as to schools never once occurred to me. If it had, the teaching which I there received would have banished such thoughts from my untutored mind.

I remember especially one professor of splendid physique and magnificent presence, an orator and capable teacher, who used to stand six feet two before our class of three-hundred students, and in his magnetic way say: "Gentlemen, when you leave your *alma mater* go not after strange gods; chase no 'Will o' the Wisp' through the bogs and marshes of Homœopathy or eclecticism! All that is worth teaching in medicine we know; all that is worth knowing we teach." And so, under such teachers (the best of their kind), and from such an institution (as good as the best), I graduated.

For nearly one decade I practiced *regular medicine,* with as much success as my colleagues and neighbors, and I was satisfied. No "Will o' the Wisp" crossed my pathway, or if it did, it made no impression upon my steadfast soul.

My frame was calm, my faith serene, my mental vision fixed upon the unswerving path. If a patient died, as many did — sometimes unaccountably to me — the responsibility was thrown upon an inscrutable providence. If he lived under my ministrations, Quinine, Calomel, and their accessories were the gods which had brought him safely through.

Once in a great while a qualm was felt at the sudden demise of some mature man who bade fair to live out his allotted time, but I had treated him regularly, scientifically, according to the approved method, what more could be expected of mortal man?

After a sleepless night or two, and the oft-recurring wish that I had done something more, or less, or something else, I would become reconciled, charge the death to providence, the bill to the administrator, and with faith as firm as ever start out next morning seeking whom I might find to devour my prescriptions.

Occasionally it was entirely apparent that *too much* was done; that the patient got *too much* regular medicine; providence would *not* share the responsibility, and conscience would *not* down at my bidding.

One of these instances I now recall. The patient, a young man of twenty-four years, was a perfect Apollo in form and figure, a Hercules in physical strength, with a mental endowment of no ordinary kind, improved by close application to study in one of the finest institutions of learning in the land.

At the close of the college year he came home, not sick, yet not quite well; had had, a few weeks before, a slight attack of articular rheumatism; had still some wandering pains about the joints, of no great severity; went where and when he pleased and did what he pleased. Soon, however, he began to have some trouble referable to the cardiac region, attended with a sinking sensation, which distressed and alarmed him. These attacks at first came at intervals of fourteen or twenty-one days, later they become more frequent; intervals were shortened to five or seven days. They were accompanied by great weakness in the chest, so that he was scarcely able to talk. His heart would beat violently, though not very rapidly, especially when lying down. Rising or even turning in bed would accelerate it. The pulse at the wrist was small, slow when lying quiet, extremely slow at times, and often irregular, missing sometimes for hours every third beat, at other times every fifth or seventh beat. He often complained of heaviness of his arms and of numbness or tingling of the fingers. His attacks (at least the severe symptoms) were of short durations, so they were always well nigh over upon my arrival, as my office was two miles distant from his residence.

So the case ran on through the spring, through the summer, into the autumn. I had numerous consultations, but they neither brought light to me nor relief to him. Finally, at a meeting of our county medical association, composed of twenty-eight physicians (not a *militia* man among them) all *regulars,* it was determined to invoke the aid of a celebrated physician of a distant city, whose specialty was disease of the chest and its contents, notably the heart, and whose reputation as a skillful diagnostician and prognostician was deservedly great. Accordingly, with the acquiescence of my patient, who was present, the celebrated physician was summoned and arrived the next day but one. Immediately upon looking at the patient, and before further examination, he told me aside that we should find organic heart disease. After making a careful examination he diagnosed pericarditis, thereby agreeing with a majority of former examiners. The prognosis was doubtful, and the treatment Mercury, until the constitutional effects became manifest, with Digitalis tr, ten drop doses, thrice daily.

Previously, through the instrumentality of our youngest member (a follower of Dr. Ringer), he had taken this remedy in drop doses at six-hour intervals, but grew so manifestly worse during its administration that we had abandoned it. Through our remonstrance the dose was changed to eight drops, which was administered at once.

Then we took our leave, our counselor departed on the train for his distant home, the rest of us went our several ways.

Scarcely had I reached my office when a messenger came in hot haste, saying my patient was dying. I rushed to his bedside and found him almost dead. I antidoted *Digitalis* in every possible way. I worked with him many hours, plied him with stimulants and applied external heat. A sudden flush of heat would be followed by coldness, prostration, pinched features, blanched lips, lustreless eyes and deathlike expression. At times, one side was cold, the other burning hot. After midnight the paroxysms ceased and he slept quietly.

For several days he was better than for weeks before. Of course the drug was discontinued. I wrote the consultant, carefully detailing the symptoms, and telling him that to my mind it was clearly a case of *Digitalis* poisoning. He replied: "It was a coincidence; repeat the dose; continue the remedy." I gave the reply to the patient and to his father, who was himself an intelligent man, assuring them that I would not take the responsibility of a repetition of the "dose," advising them to continue the remedy only upon the condition that they release me from any responsibility in the case — that I would not, *could* not, share it. For days they hesitated and debated; finally they determined in favor of Digitalis. Luckless conclusion! That dose was his last. In precisely the same time as before, the same untoward symptoms began. When the messenger reached my office I was away. Before I could be found and reach my patient he was too far gone for help or hope.

With bitter reflections and a sad heart (for I loved him), I saw him die. Just before his death, between gasps, he said, "Tell Dr. — never to give Digitalis to another case like mine."

Years passed by before the mystery of this taking off was understood. It is all clear now; but the book which would have revealed it — aye, and prevented it, too — was a sealed book then, and my stubborn prejudice was the seal which locked it from me. Many problems then are now solved, many mysteries revealed, many dark places flooded with light.

I recall another case which occurred in the same community. A farmer boy, twenty years old, stalwart and strong, with an inherited constitution which betokened defiance to disease, awoke one morning with slight throbbing headache and vertigo. He was feverish, but ate a light breakfast and as usual went to the field to work. Towards noon the headache had so increased that he went home. After bathing his head in cool water and sitting quietly in the shade, he felt better. During the afternoon he remained at the house, and early in the evening retired, but could not sleep. He made no complaint, however, until morning, when a physician was called, who prescribed Bromide of potash. He grew worse through the day and at nightfall the physician was again summoned. He continued to grow worse, and at midnight I was called in consultation. I found him suffering with excruciating pain in the head, the carotid and temporal arteries were throbbing violently; his face was red, head hot, eyes injected, and pupils dilated. His temperature was 104°; he was very restless, slightly delirious, often sat up in bed, and sometimes attempted to get out. While sitting he would fall asleep and awaken with a sudden start. When lying down he could not sleep.

Bromide of potash had been abandoned in favor of some other remedy; we resumed it in larger doses, reinforced by Valerian.

A homœopathic *student,* with a vial of Belladonna, would have saved this boy, but how were we to know that? *We were regular physicians!* So we bathed him, bled him, gave him Hydrate of chloral, Bromides in larger doses, and Morphine hypodermically. Not all of these at once, but as one combination failed we tried another. Certainly! What else *could* we do? Seeing nothing more to be done, and no good from what *had* been done, I left him to his fate and the other doctor.

As I rode home under the fading stars, I congratulated myself that it was not my case; albeit, I could not banish the sense of personal responsibility. My prognosis was unfavorable.

A few days before I had witnessed the death of a young man under very similar circumstances. Good counsel, too, of the kind I had; but in spite of all that we could do he had gone straight down to death. Slowly I rode and pondered. How could such powerful and applicable remedies fail to cool that fevered brain. My conclusion was that they were not so applicable as they seemed, and that somewhere there was a right remedy, if we could only find it, or a right combination if we could only make it.

The next afternoon I was again called. The symptoms had all deepened; restlessness had given place to wild tossing, the mild delirium to furious rage. He was fighting, biting, striking, bounding continuously from side to side of the bed, and making such frantic efforts to rise that his strength seemed almost superhuman. Four strong men were scarcely able to control him. His temperature was the highest I had ever known. Drug after drug, opiate after opiate had been given to no purpose, except that it seemed to add fuel to the flame. Through the long hopeless night we did what we could and all we could, but the struggle was an unequal one. Our weapons opposed no barrier to the sharp scythe of death, and in the grey light of dawn he claimed for his victim one who had made a gallant fight for his life. Such magnificent manhood deserved a better fate than to grapple with the monster unaided. Would heaven that we, whose business it was, should have known how to furnish the aid. Alas, the stricken youth was the idol of his mother's heart, her staff and stay, and she a widow. She still lives, but the blush of shame for my ignorance then, would mantle my cheek even now, should I confess to her how easily her son might have been saved, could we only have known how.

The intervening years, with more and better light, have shown me why Digitalis slew the one, and how Belladonna would have saved the other; but all the years can scarcely dull the keen remorse I feel when contemplating the ignorance which, substituted for knowledge, permitted such needless calamities.

The same light was then shining and the same gospel being preached as now, but we neither saw the one nor heard the other.

May the Great Judge hold him guiltless whose prejudice obstructs truth and forgive all ignorance not absolutely wilful.

Occasionally I blundered upon a remedy which cured with such amazing celerity as left my diagnosis doubtful and my prognosis a delusion.

A case of inflammatory rheumatism for which my partner in practice prescribed six weeks in bed, as the only remedy, was cured within two days by small doses of Aconite alone. The patient was so anxious and restless that she could not keep still, although every movement was painful, and so apprehensive of death that she terrorized her friends by repeated predictions of its occurrence at a certain hour.

I remember a case of stranguary which had resisted every remedy ever found efficacious in such cases, to which, in sheer desperation (one day guided by Heaven knows what impulse), I gave a few drops of Tr. cantharides, in four ounces of water, teaspoonful every two hours. The patient returned the following day saying: "For God's sake, doctor, don't forget the remedy you gave me yesterday, it is the only thing that ever did me any good." I had no occasion to remember it for him, for he was cured and remained so. But it set me thinking. Unfortunately, thought could not pursue straight lines beyond a cable tow's length until it met a barrier hoary with age and firm as the everlasting hills, composed of custom, habit, tradition, superstition, ignorance, and prejudice, which turned it back into the old circle, the end of which is the beginning of the same.

One day in 1880, at a dinner, I met a homœopathic physician. The party was a small one, he and I were the only physicians present. After dinner, very naturally, we two engaged in conversation. Equally natural, we talked medicine. Hitherto I had considered homœopathic physicians wilful humbugs; their supersititious patrons I had thought were unwittingly humbugged. I had prepared some stunning questions to propound to the first homœopathic doctor to whom etiquette, common politeness or circumstance should compel me to talk.

I found in my new acquaintance a dignified, intellectual, scholarly man. At the beginning of the war he was brigade surgeon in the United States Army; at the close of the war, he was chief surgeon of one of the country's largest hospitals. All this, of course, as an allopath. Shortly after the war he had been converted to Homœopathy. I had often heard of him as an illustrious representative of that school. I found him a foe-man worthy of my steel. I propounded my questions. I expected to up-set his theories, demolish his sophistries; in short, as Mr. Macawber says, "floor him," and march triumphantly over his prostrate form. I had un-dersized my opponent, undervalued his theory. He answered my inter-rogatories! Shall I say satisfactorily? He walked away with them like Samson with the gates. He gathered them together and dumped them at my feet; he took them up and dissected them; plucked them to pieces and scattered them like chaff to the winds. He knew all that I knew of my own school, and apparently all that I did *not* know of his. He led me into a new field; he explained the theory of potency, the law of cure, the division of the superfices of drugs, and the dynamic power of rem-edies. My critical, carping inquisitiveness was satisfied. In his presence I sat abashed, confused, confounded. By and by I began asking questions for *information;* he answered clearly, concisely, logically. He talked to me two hours, and at the conclusion of the conversation invited me to his house. Possibly he fancied that mixed up with ignorance, egotism and prejudice, there might be something of me worth saving. That thought occurred to me at the time. I have always hoped that it was so. I accepted his invitation, I went to his home. He invited me to see a patient with him, saying that it would illustrate a subject of which we had talked. Again I accepted his invitation. We found — what shall I call it? To this day I do not know what his diagnosis was, but I do know there was a leaking heart, and one of the symptoms was the worst general dropsy that, up to that time, I had ever seen benefited.

The patient, a prominent citizen, had been sick several weeks. Three representative allopathic physicians, one of them a man of renown, had regularly attended him. Their prognosis was death, inevitable death, and soon.

When this announcement was made, some mutual friends of the patient and Homœopathy advised that the homœopathist be called, which was accordingly done. The visit in which I accompanied him was the third, and upon the third consecutive day. The patient's measurement around the abdomen was four inches less than three days before, and the water was leaving the limbs so rapidly that the integument was shriveled like a washerwoman's hands. From a sitting posture, which for days before he had been compelled to assume, he was reclining comfortably in bed, and the erstwhile drowning heart was doing its work agreeably to itself and satisfactorily to its possessor.

As we drove away from the house I said: "Doctor, what did you give that man?" He replied: "I gave him Hyoscyamus."

"Well," said I, "I have heard Hyoscyamus lectured upon, read it in text books, often administered it, but certainly should not have thought of it in this case." His reply was that perhaps the next dozen similar cases would not demand it; but in this case it was *the* remedy, no other or any combination of others would suffice or substitute for it. He then explained to me that the remedies formerly administered — diaphoretics, diuretics, and hydragogue cathartics — were useless and worse than useless; that even tapping, which had already been several times resorted to, could be of only temporary benefit, since none of these did more than remove the already accumulated fluid, while many of them were positively injurious, since they weakened and exhausted the patient; whereas this remedy, being the appropriate one, through its influence upon the vasomotor system of nerves, controlled seepage of fluid, and the cure at once began. And it was so. The man recovered without once turning aside, and the doctor afterward assured me that he never had occasion to change the remedy.

That day I went home somewhat wiser and, strange to say, a much sadder man. In my first tilt with a homœopathist I, a regular, had been vanquished, routed, utterly routed, horse, foot and dragoons; I was not chagrined; I was sad. How could I reconcile it to myself to investigate a theory of medicine wholly antagonistic to all my previous training? Was it possible that the great authors and teachers of our school were mistaken?

I tried to believe that the cure I had just witnessed would have ocurred anyhow. But how about the answers to my questions? And what of the arguments which supported the answers? I determined to revisit the doctor. I did so. I stayed a week; saw him treat other cases, witnessed other cures; saw him cure an ague which had resisted large doses of

Quinine, with Ipecac 30x. I remembered, as if it were but yesterday, how the examination brought out the characteristics; chill without thirst, worse in warm room, vomiting in all stages, thirst and cough during fever, etc. I examined the medicine for some hint of the drug, but there was no hint of Ipecac in taste or odor, and yet there were no more chills.

On the very next day another case of the same disease, of fourteen months standing, presented for treatment. Again a few questions elicited the following condition: Thirst only during chill; chill usually only on left side; constant sense as if stomach and abdomen were full of gas. This case got Carbo veg. 200x, two powders; one while in the office, the other to take in the event of another chill. He reported one more light chill, and that was the last one.

These two cases of genuine, old-fashioned ague, cured with what I considered "the little end of nothing," were unexplainable by any law of logic at my command. The first year of my practice had been devoted almost exclusively to ague cases. No matter how many diseases the patient had, ague was one of them. It was indigenous to the soil. It originated there, stayed there the year round, feasted and fattened upon the lean, lank, lantern-jawed, sallow-complected, stoop-shouldered inhabitants of that God-forsaken land. I knew what ague meant. I had met it at all hours of the day and night, in ambush and in the open field, on the skirmish line and in the death struggle. Sometimes the death struggle was very brief, for when ague assumed the character of congestive chill, got on its war paint and hoisted the black flag, it was as likely to overthrow its victim in the first as in the third attack. Many a bilious woodcutter of the swamps gave up the ghost before reinforcements could arrive, the doctor coming too late to help him in his last prayer. When it didn't mean sudden death, I knew what it did mean. It meant Quinine, and lots of it, before breakfast, dinner, supper, at bed-time and between meals. Quinine was the remedy — the one only true remedy that a first-class regular physician would think of using in a bad case. Cinchona or Cinchonida might answer if the chill only lasted four to six hours, and the fever following only reached 105° or 106°; but if it was a *bad* case, nothing ever invented, or that might, could, would or should be invented, would ever, ever substitute for Quinine. And Quinine would often break the paroxysm and sometimes prevent its return for seven or even fourteen days. But the cases which worried me most were those which Quinine could not break and which ran on and on. "Men might stay, or men might go," but they

went on forever. To such cases I gave Fowler's solution of Arsenic. This
they took until they were puffed up like poisoned rats. " 'Twas all that I
could do." And now to see these two cases cured — one with colorless
charcoal, the other with tasteless and odorless Ipecac — suggested a line
of investigation foreign to my former habits of mind.

This was enough to cogitate upon for awhile, so I went home and was
shortly afterwards called to attend a youth of twelve years, who had been
treated heroically during a long-continued low fever, and who, at the
time of my call, was in his fourth month of illness. He was in a pitiable
condition; for although the fever had succumbed, the patient was in a fair
way to succumb also. From crown of head to sole of foot he was dropsical.
The skin over the abdomen looked like a full-blown bladder, ready to
burst at a touch, or to collapse from the prick of a needle.

Not only water but wind had accumulated, and with these were pain
and tenderness. The stomach was so irritable that but little food was
retained. There was almost complete suppression of urine — the little
voided being muddy and offensive. The expression of face was that of
anxiety and alarm, sometimes of terror, and he could scarcely be induced to
attempt to speak, so intent was he on supervising the process of breathing.
He seemed to feel that unless constant and undivided attention was given
to respiration, it would cease. The temperature was subnormal, the pulse
small, weak and rapid. The heart's action was scarcely perceptible and
its sounds nearly inaudible. The complexion was ashy pale, the lips
purple, the fingernails lead-colored. The long-continued fever had consumed every ounce of adipose tissue, and protracted decubitus had worn
the bones through the skin. Such an emaciated, bloodless, cadaverous,
hopeless-looking object I have rarely seen. Three or four physicians had
treated him before I was called, and had been dismissed, or had dismissed
themselves. My immediate predecessor had made but a single visit, prescribed a coffin and left, saying that he could not raise the dead. I was not
in the resurrection business myself — had not been since I left college.

I did not prescribe; but I wrote a history of the case, made a careful list
of the symptoms and sent them by mail to my homœopathic doctor friend,
with the request that he would send medicine and directions. Next day
the medicine came, and I gave it as directed. I did not know what it was,
nor did I care. It was easier to give than mine, so I gave it. I knew mine
would not stay on his stomach, and would do no good if it did. I knew
his would do no harm, so I gave it and reported the case every day, re-

cording the appearance of every new symptom, and the subsidence of any old one. I told the parents that I was in close conference with a great doctor or a great humbug, I was not sure which; but if his medicine would accomplish anything it would do more than mine. So I simply played the part of an automaton. What an agreeable, indolent, enjoyable position to fill! No responsibility, no consumption of midnight oil, no cudgeling of brain, no halting between two opinions as to the efficacy of Acetate of Potash, Buchu and Elaterium as a diuretic; Nitrate of Potash, Opium and Ipecac, as a diaphoretic; Iron as a blood-builder, or Digitalis as a heart-strengthener. Nothing to do but give little sugar pellets, watch and report the result.

The patient was 'as pleased as a pack of bones could be at the change from obnoxious drugs to dainty doses, and about the first sentence he found breathing time to utter was: "I like that stuff, gimme more." The parents were well-nigh hopeless, though not indifferent. The doctrine was new, the doctoring new, but whether both were from heaven or hell, they were at a loss to say. I did not publish to the interested community my position in this case. I was willing that it should be a family affair; yet it was known, discussed and dissected by layman and doctor, neighbor and stranger, and if the results had been different, perhaps I should have been dissected also. As long as the patient lingered between life and death, the opinion of his friends was divided as to whether I was more knave or fool; but when improvement began, they had all known and predicted all along that I would "bring him through." I cannot make a long story short, but I can prevent it becoming longer. I need not follow this patient through a tedious convalescence. Suffice it to say that he recovered, that Homœopathy got the glory and God the praise, while I got more of both than I deserved.

Two years ago, among the hills of Kentucky, I met this whilom skeleton. He is a man of family now, "broad of chest and brawny of arm," six feet two in his stockings, a match for most men of his inches, and, when medical aid is needed, sends to Shelbyville, twenty miles away, for Dr. Bryan, because there is no homœopath closer; although the woods are full of allopaths, he will not employ them. After this patient's recovery, I turned my attention to Hahnemann's *Organon*. Later I procured other homœopathic literature — Hughes's *Pharmacodynamics*, Dunham's *Materia Medica*, and others. These books alone should convince the most skeptical, but such is the force of habit, such the power of prejudice, that although my reason must have been convinced, the old fetters still bound me, and while my faith in my beloved school was terribly shaken, I could not "ring out the old or ring in the new." Although the old was hopelessly declining, the tendrils of the new were too fragile to take tenacious hold of anything. I could not go from "big pills" to "little pills" at a single bound. If I reached infinitesimals I must do it by easy stages. If I had made a mistake in the first place, I must not make a greater one in the second. If allopathy was one extreme, Homœopathy must be the other. If both are extremes, the truth must be in the middle.

After much casting about and many anxious inquiries in search of it, I thought it might be found in the eclectic school. Accordingly the next September found me in Cincinnati, and a matriculant of the Eclectic Medical School of that city. Permit me to say, to the credit of that institution, that some of its teachers and many of its alumni "are not far from the Kingdom." The modern eclectic, who keeps close up with Prof. John M. Scudder and abreast of his teachings, is next best to a crude homœopath.

While in this college I visited all the others in the city. I had matriculated chiefly for the lectures on practice; these I was careful to attend; at other times, when I chose, I went visiting. Some of my visits were to the Homœopathic College; perhaps a good many of them. Possibly I visited there more frequently than strict rules of etiquette demanded. But, oh! I went with a song of rejoicing in my heart, and left with a sigh and a wish that I might remain.

The college session ended; I returned to my home and my practice. My Hughes and my Dunham were doubly dear. I studied them, pondered them, committed much of them to memory, brooded over them through the day and dreamed of them at night.

My plan was to thoroughly study one remedy at a time, put it into my case, and when I found it indicated, use it. In this way my medicine cases gradually changed complexion. Sulphate of Quinine was supplanted by China, Santonine by Cina, Nux vomica took the place of Strychnia, and Belladonna that of Atropine. Morphine was in much less demand than formerly — albeit, I still carried my hypodermic syringe, lest some day I might need it; like a pistol in Texas.

To be sure, my remedies were very crude; I was very crude myself. I never rose above the first dilution, rarely above the mother tincture. But I prescribed as best I could, according to homœopathic indications, when I could see any, and sometimes met with success, which astonished me

more than it did the patient. He expected me to cure him; had called
me for that purpose; but sometimes I cured him much sooner than had
been my wont, or than under the good old way, I had any reasonable
right to expect.

I shall never forget one of my first experiences. I had been called in
consultation with one of my former colleagues. The case was one of
vesicular erysipelas. The patient (a married lady) was very restless,
constantly moving a limb or changing position. The inflammation had
begun on the chin, spread over the entire face, and was rapidly invading
the scalp. Her eyes had entirely closed by swelling; her temperature was
105°, she was somewhat delirious, and in every way growing rapidly
worse.

Through some misunderstanding as to time, the other doctor had not
arrived. I was several miles from home and a heavy road between us.
The night was coming on and promised to be stormy.

The picture of Rhus tox. was so perfect that, tyro as I was, I felt sure
of it. I put one drop of the *mother tincture* into twelve teaspoonfuls of
water, ordered one teaspoonful every hour till she slept (which she had
not done for forty-eight hours), wrote an apology to the doctor for the
ethical breach, explained to him what I had given, and ventured the
opinion that by morning the inflammation would be fading out. At midnight, after seven doses of medicine, she fell asleep, slept sweetly until ten
o'clock next morning, awoke refreshed, opened her eyes to the sunlight
with neither photophobia nor acrid discharge. The inflammation had
subsided, the fever had abated, and neither returned. To this day I have
never done better work, or witnessed better results.

Years after this my friend, the doctor, asked another of my doctor
friends if he knew what I gave for erysipelas. He had not yet learned
that we have more than one remedy for one disease.

* * *

I had been practicing Homœopathy about three years, with success
proportionate to my ability for selecting appropriate remedies, when one
day a young lady, who had suffered for fourteen years with an intermittent
neuralgia, applied to me for relief. She was then twenty-eight years old,
though she looked much older. Suffering, not age, had furrowed her
brow, and the expression of her face was sad and anxious — almost

despairing. She assured me that half her life had been spent in pain of the most excruciating character. Her ill health began when she was fourteen years of age, and every week since then had brought three or four days and nights of torture. She said the attacks came in the early morning, increased during the forenoon, reached their acme at noon, decreased with the declining sun, ceased at nightfall, returned about ten o'clock in the evening and lasted until three or four next morning. She described the pain as jerking, shooting and burning, usually in the left eyeball, sometimes spreading in all directions on left side of face and head, but rarely crossing to the right side. The height of the paroxysm was attended by a profuse flow of tears from the affected eye, and she declared the pain to be almost unendurable. In addition to this, during damp weather she had asthma accompanied by rheumatic pains all over the body, especially severe in the intercostal muscles, with sudden shocks of pain in the left chest, and violent palpitation of the heart.

In the earlier years of her ailment she had consulted many celebrated physicians. Later, she had been gulled and bled by advertisers. Then, losing faith in men, though not in medicine, she procured and took each new patent anti-neuralgic as soon as she could hear of and obtain it, until finally, hearing of the novelty called Homœopathy, she determined to try that. I gave her Spigelia 30x, night and morning. An appropriate sequel to this story would seem to demand that after many months' persistent use of the remedy she was greatly benefitted. But the fact is that she was permanently cured within one week. During the two following years I saw her frequently, though never professionally.

Four years later, while traveling through the State, I stopped at a village some thirty miles from this young lady's home. During the day I was called professionally to see a girl of thirteen years, whom I found suffering with prosopalgia.[1] The mystery of the call was explained when I found as a visitor in this family my former patient, who, hearing of my arrival, had persuaded the parents to send for me. I learned from her then, that neuralgia, rheumatism or apprehension of their return had ceased to trouble her. I thought and still think of this as one of the most convincing proofs of the beauty, truth and simplicity of Homœopathy, and the irresistible force of a properly chosen remedy. Here was a chronic disease which had resisted regular physician and quack, officinal preparation and

[1] Headache.

proprietary medicine, during all these years — cured, absolutely cured, and entirely eradicated, by a few doses of a simple plebeian plant, which has never aspired to a high position, or been ranked as a polychrest in our school of medicine. It is but an additional proof to the many already adduced that there is no such thing as substitution. That as with men, so with inanimate things, each has its sphere of action in which it must work, or its niche which no other can fill.

How passing strange that our brethren of the antiquated school should lose sight of and destroy the individuality of remedies by mixing into heterogeneous masses the homogeneous affinities which nature has been at infinite pains to prepare and unite. In nature's laboratory no mistakes are made. The law of elective affinity makes no faulty combinations. Each plant is a family in and of itself, in which the most perfect homogeneity and harmony prevails. Growing side by side in the same soil, under the same sunlight, pink root and plantain, poke root and poppy, select and arrange in definite proportion the molecules of soda and lime, potash and iron which each individual plant needs and must have to preserve its identity and individuality. Man cannot separate these families without doing them injustice and impairing their usefulness. Nor are any two families sufficiently congenial to be associated together without discord. This being true, it follows that no two remedies should be administered at the same time to any patient under any conditions.

Neither should medicines be alternated, for although conditions of disease may change quickly and demand a change of remedy, they do not turn to and fro, hour by hour. Whoever saw a rheumatism flying like a weaver's shuttle, back and forth, from Rhus tox. to Bryonia? Who would give one remedy each, for the different stages of intermittent fever, or to a cholera case "the big four" at a gulp? Camphor, Cuprum, Arsenicum and Veratrum are the great cholera remedies; but it is not wise to combine or alternate them. A master prescriber will not select Aconite for the chill, Gelsemium for the fever, and Belladonna for the sweat of an intermittent, but he will select that remedy which *covers the totality*. Study your remedies, dear young doctor, and study your patient. Study until the features of disease and its remedy are alike luminous and transparent. Learn to diagnose diseases, but fail not to know how to apply remedies. Study disease until your head aches — remedies until your heart aches. Earth furnishes the matter, study will make it yours.

Man is made of earth. The elements of earth compose his body. From the earth comes his nutriment and his medicament. Food sustains the entire body and keeps it in a normal condition. Medicine corrects errors in limited areas.

Health is the normal action of every part of the body. Disease is the abnormal action of some particular part. A pound of meat may be necessary to furnish nutriment to every bone and muscle, while the hundredth part of a grain of medicine may be sufficient to correct disease originating and localized in a group of microscopical cells, or in a nerve center no larger than a mustard seed. While in the chrysalis state, during the period of transformation into a full-fledged homœopath, my faith was severely tested by the haunting spectre of small doses. It was a comfort to learn that the law of similars had nothing to do with doses. Selection of the remedy is one thing, determination of dose another and entirely different thing. My study of microscopical anatomy so far had been to very poor purpose, for I had been able to make of it but little use. I had learned that all life is cell life, but this knowledge had not taught me that all disease is cell disease. I renewed my researches, and found that in the human body there are myriads of cells smaller than the thirtieth decimal attenuation. To reach these cells the remedy must be equally fine. To affect them it must enter them, to enter them it must be smaller than they.

Food, to be appropriated by the body, must go to the stomach, and be digested, pass from the stomach and be assimilated. Medicine, to be effectual, should not travel this route. Digestion would destroy it. It should be so minutely divided that the open-mouth absorbents swallow it as soon as it comes in contact with the mucous membrane of the mouth. Thus unchanged it enters the circulation. No need then of further concern or anxiety. If the doctor has selected well, the drug will reach its destination.

A group of cells in a remote corner of the anatomy are hurt and crying out for help. Help is on the road. Over the trunk lines, past the way stations, out on the local road, recognized by every road official, *en route* and hurried unerringly to its destination.

The trouble may be a lack of lime or silica or salt. It may be a disturbance of the molecular motion or a lost balance in any way. It may be that Schuessler's theory is true, and yet it does not follow that Magnesia phos., administered as such, will cure all cramps, or Ferrum phos. subdue all inflammation. It may be that these remedies must be arranged as plants arrange them to be efficacious.

Awhile ago I had a case of abdominal cramping, for which I prescribed Mag. phos., which was given several hours without beneficial result. Being called again, I gave Colocynthis, which gave prompt relief. Colocynth grows only upon magnesia soil. Possibly Magnesia was the remedy, but to be effective it had to be prepared in the Colocynth pharmacy.

Who shall locate the initial lesion of disease, or who determine the dose for its relief? My theory may have been very faulty and very wide of the mark, but it furnished a solution to the vexed question of dose; and what it did for me possibly it may do for some other. I was easier in my mind after figuring it out, and I soon passed the place where faith staggers at infinitesimals. As to dose and potency, I have nothing to recommend save the smallest and highest capable of accomplishing the desired result. As to the selection of remedy, only this: "Let similars be treated with similars." If there be a "higher life" in Homœopathy I am ready for it. In back of bone and brawn and blood and brain there exists the real man, I am ready to treat him, if he is sick and I can find him.

We may not be able to locate the origin of or always diagnose disease to our entire satisfaction, but this need not, *does* not, prevent intelligent and successful treatment of the sick. Every disease or condition of disease will photograph its appropriate remedy, and every remedy true to the picture will accomplish the object designed. In the midst of uncertainty and doubt regarding exact pathological conditions, we can at least be sure that disease is not an entity. That it cannot be expelled by emetics, cathartics, diuretics or diaphoretics. That it is wrong life, perverted life; inharmonious, discordant life; and that while it may be coaxed back into tune and harmony, it will not, can not be coerced.

A recent writer has said that the osseous structure alone, with every bone in proper position, makes a fairly good picture of man. The same is true of the muscular, vascular and nervous systems. Each, if separated from all the others and kept *in situ,* would form eyes, nose, ears, mouth, size, weight and form of a man. But that which ties them all together, blends them all into one, directs, governs and controls, makes the eye to sparkle, the cheek to blush, the tuneful tongue to sing; that invisible power whose departure is the signal for decay, and whose absence means what we call death — this is the man, the real man, the monarch whom all the rest obey. Is this king immortal? Is he part of the Infinite and Almighty? If so, is he subject to disease? Does he suffer pain? Shall remedies be addressed to him for his use, or will he, through brain and nerve, those loyal subjects nearest the throne, distribute to servant and vassal throughout his kingdom as each has need? Whether, as has been prophesied, we shall all at some time agree that all disease must be treated through the nervous system, or whether his majesty, the keeper of the house, the watcher at the windows, the ethereal essence, the vital force, shall demand our attention and receive our aid, is a question which I cheerfully leave to the prophets among us. Prophecies may fail, and speculation avail nothing, but this one thing, thank God! we know: while humanity inhabits the earth, while conditions which now surround it continue to exist, while "pestilence walketh in darkness, or destruction wasteth at noonday," *the law of cure,* THE ONE ONLY LAW OF CURE, shall endure unchanged and unchangeable, and shall take deeper root within, and firmer hold upon, the hearts of nations yet unborn. Disaster cannot overtake, catastrophe overwhelm, or oblivion engulf it. Even now, in its infancy, it gives promise of power. If its friends are faithful they will find it true. If its representatives are conscientious and careful, it will not disappoint them.

Be disease acute or chronic, simple or complicated, it must yield if met by the right remedy. This statement is made after due deliberation. If, after careful investigation, the doubter is still incredulous, I envy him not his incredulity. Let not him who fails attribute his failure to the law, but to his own inefficient application of it. Permit me, patient reader, in support of my proposition, to examine one or two other witnesses. There be those who need no "further witness," they have proven the truth and are satisfied. But I would fain reach those of other faith. If any such should read this testimony, I pray you accept it not as final — nor my word, nor the word of any man for that which you yourself may prove. Fairly and perseveringly investigate until the truth or falsity of the proposition be settled.

I was once called to see a patient whose disease was diagnosed by the attending physicians to be typhoid pneumonia. Two of these physicians, both reputable and "regular," had treated the case from its incipiency, and during its progress had summoned other advisers, both "regular" and reputable, but in spite of these, the patient had slipped deathward, until all agreed that certain death was nigh. After commending the sick man's soul to God, who gave it, and bidding the weeping family farewell, the counselors departed upon other missions of mercy and condolence. The two regular attendants remained to see, as they said, "what a homœopath would attempt to do for a man in the hour of death." Upon arrival I found appearances indicating the prognosis to be correct. The drawn and shrunken features, livid complexion, fixed and expressionless eyes, cold perspiration, and stertorous breathing gave unmistakable evidence of approaching dissolution. Without waiting for other symptoms than those perceptible at a glance, having already gleaned some others from the messenger on the way, I at once gave a dose of Veratrum album. Then, apart from the assembled friends, the doctors gave me a brief history of the case; told me what remedies they had administered, and inquired what I had given. Upon being informed they replied: "Why, he has had exhausting alvine discharges for the past forty-eight hours, which, during the last eight or ten hours, have been involuntary."

That, I replied, is a bad symptom, but it indicates Veratrum. "But," said they, "Veratrum is one of the most prostrating of remedies, and this patient is already prostrated beyond the power of voluntary motion."

"Very true," I answered, "and for that very reason Veratrum is all the more suitable."

Again they replied: "But doctor, the dew of death is upon his brow; he is sinking every moment; within two hours he will die unless something be given which shall induce reaction, for which purpose we have given the strongest stimulants, with no results."

I said, "Your position is well taken, gentlemen, and if this remedy fails to arouse the sinking vitality, it cannot be done, and we must lose our patient." I admitted that my hope, even in this remedy, was as slight as the patient's chance of life; but that as long as he could take it I should continue to give it.

As soon as this brief colloquy was ended, I gave the second dose, and continued to repeat it at intervals of fifteen minutes for two hours, at the end of which time the unexpected reaction was perceptible. The interval of dose was then extended to one hour, and we watched by his bedside until six doses were taken, at the end of which time the improvement was apparent even to non-professional eyes. The livid hue was giving place to a hopeful glow, and the death-damp to warm moisture. The lusterless eyes began to hint of returning expression, and some incoherent muttering announced that the sluggish stream of life was receiving a fresh supply from the fountain, and with this came the capacity to feel and the return-ing consciousness of suffering. The friends took courage and rejoiced. The homœopath was elated, but undemonstrative, and the allopaths, amazed beyond expression, muttered and grunted, but never swore an oath, and even forgot, for the time being, to take the credit of the change, though they did say, afterward, that "the patient was just ready to turn" (which indeed he was, in the wrong direction), "when the homœopath was called." After turning in the right direction, the patient slowly but steadily improved until convalescence was established through which he passed into ordinary health, in which condition he still remains.

One witness more, but one, shall be called. Indeed, the forthcoming evidence need not appear except for the attempt to invalidate the testimony just given by the assertion that the recovery was due to ammonia and whiskey previously administered, rather than to Veratrum, which every homœopathic physician would at once recognize as the true and only remedy in such condition as the one described.

At the time to which I now refer, I was the only homœopathic physician in my town. The local physicians opposed me because they considered me an impostor; the druggists opposed me because their craft was in danger, and many of the dear people, taking their cue from physician and pharmacist, supposed that Homœopathy was a myth and its representatives the shallowest of pretenders. Thanks to the influence of a true system of medicine, as compared with a false, these same people who had at first been fond of deriding me became in time my personal friends and the earnest advocates of Homœopathy.

I had been so often called just at the turning point — in fact, I can say truthfully, and I hope modestly, that I had so often been instrumental in turning the very sick from glory back to grace, that such turnings had ceased to be considered coincidences, and had begun to be believed the legitimate results of properly applied remedial measures. About this time there was sent to me for treatment, the shadow of a man — for he was scarcely more — so wan and wasted was he by the consuming fire of consumption. This had been the diagnosis of his physicians any time, and all the time, for the past twelve months, and they had now limited his span of life to six weeks. This was also the diagnosis of other physicians who saw him upon his arrival and afterward. He was brought from a neighboring town in bed, from which he was unable to rise without assistance, and lodged at his sister's, who, dear soul, had faith like a saint, and believed that Homœopathy could save her brother. It was through her instrumentality that he was brought and I was called.

He had hectic fever, night sweats, hollow cough and difficult expectoration of heavy, purulent, offensive matter. When propped up in a sitting posture the cough was less severe, but this position could be maintained but a short time on account of extreme weakness, which was greatest in the evening. The whole chest, especially the right, was sore and painful. The odor of the sputa was atrocious and was recognized and complained of by the patient himself. The extremities were usually cold, the finger nails blue, and the feet often bathed in cold perspiration. No search was made for bacilli tuberculosis, the physical signs being amply sufficient for a positive diagnosis. Such was the condition of this patient on November the first, when homœopathic treatment was begun. The treatment consisted of Sanguinaria six days in each week, with a single dose of Calcarea on the seventh. In seven weeks from the administration of the first dose, he walked alone down stairs and ate his Christmas dinner with the family. The first day of the following May he went fishing with the boys, and when last I saw him he assured me that he had neither cough nor pain, and that he had gained seventy pounds since his illness two years before.

Living witnesses, peers of the realm, would willingly attest to the truth of the statements herein made, and cheerfully certify that the pictures are not overdrawn. Scores of cases might be presented in proof of the superiority of Homœopathy over other methods of medical practice. The law itself is perfect; but, alas! he upon whom its application depends is fallible. Could hands unerring apply a law unfailing, age, not disease, should cause death. Mortal injury alone should loose the "silver cord," or break the "golden bowl," until the "grinders cease because they are few, and those that look out of the windows be darkened." High noon should fulfill the promise of life's bright morning, and the lengthening shadows of declining day should warn the traveler of approaching night, ere he prepares to seek repose. Made in his Maker's image, man travels heavenward, but his journey thither should cover threescore miles and ten on life's highway, nor end until weariness compels him to lie down and rest.

FROM TRADITIONAL MEDICINE TO HOMOEOPATHY
Eugene Underhill, Jr., M.D.

From my earliest recollection it seemed a foregone conclusion that I was going to be a physician. There simply was no doubt about it. If family predisposition means anything, I had the professional background of two generations as both my father and grandfather were physicians.

After graduating from college the question of what medical school to attend was next in order. Although Father was a graduate of Hahnemann Medical College, his advice was to investigate all the medical schools in Philadelphia.

Accordingly I assembled the catalogs, visited the colleges and interviewed the deans of the respective institutions. My decision was in favor of the University of Pennsylvania.

I well recall the look of disappointment on Father's face when I told him of my preference, for I was, in fact, turning my back on the system of medicine which Hahnemann of Philadelphia still represented in those days. However, Father's vision was not confined to the walls of any institution, nor even to any so-called system of medicine. He said, "I think you have made a wise choice," but added, "Some day you will be practicing Homœopathy." Those words were forgotten until years later their prophecy was translated into fact.

So I went to the medical department of the University of Pennsylvania and graduated and to this day have never regretted it. If I had it to do over again I would go back to Old Penn and battle it through. After completing my internship and passing the State Board examinations I was at last a "regular" doctor ready to begin the practice of medicine.

Just how a prejudice against Homœopathy was acquired during my medical course and internship, it is even now impossible to tell. Prejudice is infectious and contagious and few are they who are immune to it. For over three years I practiced regular medicine "untainted" by any Homœopathy whatsoever.

Father and I applied together for membership to a fraternal organization. On the evening of our initiation we met Dr. George H. Thatcher, a leading Homœopathic physician of Philadelphia. From that first meeting a friendship was formed which grew and deepened with the years until the doctor's death in the spring of 1930.

One day when in his office I asked Dr. Thatcher in what he was specializing. He answered, "You won't have any more time for me when I tell you. I am one of those high-falutin', high-potency Homœopaths."

Some months later I was in the doctor's office, and he asked, "Have you any interesting cases on hand?" Previous to this we had talked about almost everything except medicine. It just happened that I did have an interesting case on hand. In fact, it was getting too interesting, and I had begun to have visions of being dismissed almost any day.

The patient was sorely afflicted with acute arthritis which had begun in his feet and was now involving the knees as well as the feet. The limbs were swollen and the skin mottled. His one relief was to sit with the feet and legs in a tub of ice water, and he insisted on having plenty of ice floating in the water. In all my experience I have never seen this case duplicated. Motion greatly added to his suffering. He was much worse at night and could not endure any covering on the feet, legs, or knees. I soaked him with salicylates, gave him colchicum, purged him, gave him diuretics and applied evaporating lotions to the inflamed joints with only slight temporary relief. I called at the house every day and each time found him more discouraged, more grumpy, and his feet and legs still parked in the ice water.

So, when Dr. Thatcher asked about any interesting cases, naturally I told him about this man. I had no sooner recited the main feature of the case when he said, "Why, that man needs Ledum". (Ledum palustre, or wild rosemary, marsh tea or labrador tea. The plant grows in cold, swampy regions, particularly in Canada. *Ledum,* from the Greek ledon, a resinous juice and *palustre,* a swamp.)

The doctor appeared to have such certain assurance that it was truly amazing. He asked, "Do you mind if I fix up a few powders of Ledum for him?" It is said that necessity knows no law, and I was ready to give the man anything from soothing syrup to dynamite, and so welcomed the offer and agreed to discontinue all other medication both external and internal, in order to give the powders a chance, as Dr. Thatcher put it.

I saw the patient the same afternoon, and he was about ready to call it quits. However, on seeing a radical change of treatment and thinking that I had been studying up his case, he finally consented to give the powders a chance. His wife was not very enthusiastic and I thought, well, they will soon call another doctor. The next day he was just about the same, but they did say that he was no worse, but added, "I guess no better either." However, my "get away" that time was not quite as unsatisfactory as before. The following day told a different story. The wife greeted me with a pleasant good morning and promptly announced that our patient was better. For the first time I found him without his tub of ice water, and he said, "Doctor, why didn't you give me those powders before? They have done me more good than all your other dope put together. Don't let me be without them." I told him that was a medicine I rarely used and would have to go back to the office to get it. Dr. Thatcher was much interested and pleased with the report and doled out more powders. The patient was able to return to work in two weeks, and remained well for over a year, then the family moved away and I have never heard from them since.

On looking back on that case, I realized that Dr. Thatcher and the white powder soon faded out of the picture. It was about time for the patient to get well anyway.

Months later when in the doctor's office, came the same question. "Any interesting cases on hand?" For months I had been treating an eighteen year old girl for severe dysmenorrhea. She suffered most severe cramping pains and had to spend the first day of the periods in bed. The only relief I had succeeded in giving her was by prescribing Viburnum prunifolium compound and whiskey. Each time she seemed to require larger doses. As to preventing recurrence of the trouble, I had already considered and suggested dilatation and curetage and the family had about decided in favor of the operation. I told Dr. Thatcher about this case, but he was not so sure this time. He said, "I think we can help her, if you wouldn't mind getting the answers to some questions so we can tell just what remedy she needs." I agreed to do this without any particular interest or enthusiasm, more as a favor to the doctor than for the sake of the patient.

He wanted to know: Whether the pain preceded the flow or only came on after the flow was established. What kind of pain it was, whether bearing down, cutting, cramping, burning, etc. Was the pain continuous or intermittent? What gave the most relief? What was the effect of heat, cold, motion, pressure, etc., on the pain? What position in bed did she assume during the pain? What did she think caused the trouble in the first place? When was the first menstruation and did she suffer in this way from the very first time? Just where was the pain most intense, back, front, or on which side? Did she want more or less covering than at other times?

I sent for the patient to come to the office and got answers to as many of the questions as I could. Found out that the pain almost always preceded the flow, that the flow was slow and sluggish in starting and relief only came — usually on the second day — with the establishment of a free flow. The pains would shoot all over the abdomen, but were always worse over the right ovary. Pains came in spasms and were cramp-like and almost drove her frantic. The only relief was by bending almost double and holding a hot water bottle tightly to the lower abdomen. Several times she had burned herself with the hot water bottle. The pains were worse from any uncovering and she wanted the room warm. Trouble began after a long exposure to cold during menstruation.

After reading over this data, Dr. Thatcher said with all the assurance in the world, "That girl needs Magnesia phos. Do you mind if I fix up a few powders for her?" Of course, I didn't mind. As I left his office, he said, "You might stop all other treatment so as to give the powders a chance. Let her start them at the first onset of the pain, and tell her to be sure to take the special powder marked X first." So I carried out his suggestions and gave the patient the medicine. It was some time before I heard from her. One day she came to the office and said, "Doctor, I want more of those powders. They were wonderful. I have had the easiest time I have had for years. Don't ever let me be without that medicine."

Naturally I had none of the medicine on hand and had to invent an alibi. Told her that it was very special medicine and I would have to send away for it. Again, nothing to do but go to Dr. Thatcher, report and ask for more powders. Somehow there was a feeling of annoyance associated with the idea. Again the pleased expression on the doctor's face and more powders, but very little was said about the case. If I recall correctly, I was in more of a hurry than usual that day. However, I appreciated his kindness, in words if not in fact, and sent the medicine to the patient. After three months she was completely cured, and never really suffered during menstruation afterwards.

Even after these outstanding demonstrations I gave Homœopathy no serious thought and did not mention these experiences to anyone. The next time Dr. Thatcher asked about interesting cases I had none, and soon turned the conversation to the first World War which was still raging in Europe. In fact it was some time before I felt inclined to discuss professional matters with him, although he always showed a genuine and sincere interest in my progress.

However, one day he asked the same old question again, and I was having real trouble with a case, a man of middle age suffering from gastrointestinal disorder, and I was beginning to fear cancer of the pylorus with possible metastasis to the liver. He was very sallow, could eat only the least food. He would feel hungry, but a few mouthfuls would fill him up and he could eat no more. There were almost continuous eructations of empty gas. He had a sticking feeling in the gall-bladder region and was very sensitive in the lower right quadrant of the abdomen. This man was about to give up his work. He said, "Doctor, if quitting time only came at three I would be all right, but by four o'clock I am all in and don't pick up until nearly time to go to bed." I had given him Nux Vomica and Tinct. Gentian, also iron and arsenic; likewise a little Hg. and K. I. on suspicion although his Wassermann was negative. The x-rays were also negative and there was no palpable mass in the abdomen. Still he simply did not respond and continued to lose ground. I outlined the case to Dr. Thatcher about as I have described it here. He asked, "What else does he complain of?" Then I recalled that the man suffered from severe right-sided headaches and would either wake up with this headache or else it would come on late in the afternoon. Dr. Thatcher said, "You have a very interesting case here. Let's see, his complaints are mostly right-sided — head, liver and lower quadrant of abdomen. He has easy satiety or sudden repletion, when eating a few mouthfuls fills him. He suffers from a great amount of gas. His time of aggravation is from 4:00 p.m. until some time in the evening. You say he is very sallow in appearance. Why, that man needs Lycopodium."

The doctor could not have named a more helpless or hopeless remedy according to my way of thinking. Then he took a book and showed me the symptoms listed under Lycopodium. Then he said, "Doesn't that look like your man?" I read over the symptoms and sure enough, not only were the ones there that I had told him about, but to my amazement a number of others almost in the very words the patient had used in describing them. "Fits him like a glove," said Dr. Thatcher. "Do you mind if I let you have some of the remedy to give him?" This was really interesting and I said, "Sure, I will give it to him."

Never have I seen more prompt, clear-cut results or a more appreciative patient. When the time came to ask for more powders I was in a vastly different frame of mind. The other two cases now stood out with this one in sharp contrast to the indifferent results I was usually getting. I said, "Doctor, you have cured three cases for me sight unseen and they have been such striking cures I cannot ignore them. I thought it was time for the first man to get well, medicine or no medicine. The second I thought was a fortunate coincidence, but three is one too many for me. I would like to study Homœopathy."

My good friend, the doctor, wasted no time in handing me two books and said, "Read these over. I'll start you so you won't get mental indigestion." Those books were *Leaders on Homœopathic Therapeutics* by E. B. Nash, and *Homœopathy in Medicine and Surgery* by Edmond Carleton. I studied these books and talked Homœopathy early and often. Soon I had a pocket case containing thirty remedies and started in earnest to try my hand at Hahnemann's proposition that "Like cures like," and found as he did, and as every other man finds who will give Homœopathy an intelligent and honest trial over a reasonable period of time, that the Law of Similars is indeed one of the fundamental laws of Nature, and one of the most easily demonstrated of those laws. But to understand and comprehend this law requires an earnest and sincere effort of mind. It requires the laying aside of personal prejudice and conceit, a truly Herculean task.

Thus did the writer finally become like his preceptor, "a high-potency Homœopath."

CHAPTER 6

The Nature of Disease

The present generation has been imbued with many strange and fallacious ideas about sickness. First of all, you must thoroughly discard the
idea that all diseases are caused by germs. Remember that germs are a
concomitant of disease. They are present in a sick person *because* of the
disease, the disturbed function. Having been taught from earliest childhood that germs were the cause of disease, this will be pretty hard for you
to believe, but it is true. What are germs, anyway? They are not vicious
little animals; they are small vegetative growths and will grow only on or
in suitable soil and under suitable conditions.

I am not expostulating a new theory when I say this. At this point I
would like to quote from a book entitled *Béchamp or Pasteur* by E.
Douglas Hume (The C. W. Daniel Company, Limited, Ashingdon,
Rochford, Essex, Great Britain):

In spite of the hold of Pasteurian dogma over the Medical Faculty, scientific
minds here and there confirm fragments of Béchamp's teaching, without
knowledge of it, from their independent studies. In this connection may be
quoted the evidence before the Royal Commission on Vivisection of Dr. Gran-
ville Bantock, whose great reputation needs no comment.

"Bacteriologists," he said, "have discovered that in order to convert filth
or dead organic matter of any kind into harmless constituents, Nature employs
micro-organisms (or microbes) as her indispensable agents . . . In the modern
septic tank it is the action of the micro-organisms, whether aerobic or anaerobic,
that dissolves the sewage, and it is the continuous action of these microbes
that converts all manurial matter into the saline constituents that are essential
for the nutrition of plant life." After several examples Dr. Bantock continued:
"The microbe in its relation to disease can only be regarded as a resultant or
concomitant"; and after quoting many instances of error of diagnosis through

reliance on bacterial appearances he quoted: "Is it not therefore reasonable to conclude that these micro-organisms . . . are certainly *not* causative of disease?" He also said: "I am bound to accept as a matter of fact the statements made as to the association of the Lœffler bacillus with diphtheria; but to say that their presence is the *result* of the disease appears to me to be the more sound reasoning."

Then, again, we may quote the practical observations of the great pioneer of nursing, Florence Nightingale.

"Is it not living in a continual mistake," she said, "to look upon diseases, as we do now, as separate entities, which *must* exist, like cats and dogs, instead of looking upon them as conditions, like a dirty and clean condition, and just as much under our own control; or rather the reactions of kindly Nature against the conditions in which we have placed ourselves? I was brought up by scientific men and ignorant women distinctly to believe that smallpox was a thing of which there was once a specimen in the world, which went on propagating itself in a perpetual chain of descent, just as much as that there was a first dog (or pair of dogs), and that smallpox would not begin itself any more than a new dog would begin without there having been a parent dog. Since then I have seen with my eyes and smelt with my nose smallpox growing up in first specimens, either in close rooms or in overcrowded wards, where it could not by any possibility have been 'caught,' but must have begun. Nay, more, I have seen diseases begin, grow up and pass into one another. Now dogs do not pass into cats. I have seen, for instance, with a little overcrowding, continued fever grow up, and with a little more, typhoid fever, and with a little more, typhus, and all in the same ward or hut. For diseases, as all experience shows, are adjectives, not noun substantives."

It was she who said also: "The specific disease doctrine is the grand refuge of weak, uncultured, unstable minds, such as now rule in the medical profession. There are no specific diseases: there are specific disease-conditions."

Such was her teaching based upon far-reaching personal experience, upon opinions that are understandable in the light of Béchamp's microzymian doctrine, which thus gains confirmation from Nature's everyday lessons. It seems that causative disease-entities must give place to disease-conditions following upon bad heredity, bad air, bad food, vicious living and so forth, and, *provided our ancestry be good, our surroundings sanitary and our habits hygienic, our physical status lies chiefly in our own keeping, for good or evil, as our wills may determine.* Instead of being at the mercy of extraneous enemies, it rests principally with ourselves whether our anatomical elements, the microzymas, shall continue on the even tenor of their way, when our conditions will be those of health, or, from a change of environment in their immediate surroundings, develop morbidly, producing bad fermentative effects and other bodily calamities. Thus, while our own shortcomings are first reflected on them, so their ensuing corruption afterwards revenges itself upon us.

It has been argued in answer to Miss Nightingale's sound reasoning that she was only a nurse and therefore not qualified to express medical opinions. This objection comes oddly from the devout adherents of men, such as Jenner, who bought his medical degree for 15 pounds, and Pasteur, who managed to obtain by a majority of just one vote a place among the Free Associates of the Academy of Medicine!

In Dr. Farr's Annual Report to the Registrar-General in 1872 (p. 224) he says: "The zymotic diseases replace each other; and when one is rooted out it is apt to be replaced by others which ravage the human race indifferently whenever the conditions of healthy life are wanting. They have this property in common with weeds and other forms of life: as one recedes another advances." This substitution theory is adopted by Dr. Charles Creighton, who in his *History of Epidemics in Britain* suggests that plague was replaced by typhus fever and smallpox; and later on, measles, insignificant before the middle of the seventeenth century, began to replace the latter disease.

It is interesting that the replacement of disease-conditions noted by Florence Nighingale in unhealthy huts or wards, according to their changing degree of unhealthiness, exactly bears out what Dr. Charles Creighton shows to be the testimony of historic records. And this evolution or retrogression, as the case may be, of disease-conditions is surely explained by Béchamp's microzymian doctrine, which teaches that upon the anatomical elements, whether called microsomes or microzymas, the actual builders of the body-cells, depends our state of well-being or otherwise, and that a morbid change of function in these may lead to disease conditions in us, the latter altering as the former varies, and the former influenced by surrounding conditions, whether insanitary or unhygienic.

If the microzymian teaching thus sheds light upon zymotic mysteries, how much more upon hereditary tendencies, too much overlooked by modern medical orthodoxy. Since the microzymas perpetuate life from parent to child, so they carry with them parental characteristics for good or evil which may lie dormant throughout generations or be made manifest, according to the microzymas that carry the preponderating influence, thus explaining the Laws of Mendel. Yet again, disease-conditions due to abnormal growth, of which cancer is an obvious example, seem to bear out Béchamp's doctrine that upon the status of the microzymas depends the status of the whole or any part of the corporate organism.

In place of the modern system of treating that phantom shape, a disease-entity, and trying to quell it by every form of injection, scientific procedure on Béchamp's lines will be to *treat the patient* . . .

Dr. Royal E. S. Hayes, writing about *Béchamp and Pasteur* in *The Homœopathic Recorder*, August, 1952, says:

Béchamp proved that bacteria in the air, earth or water are not preexistent, but are the living remains of organisms which have been destroyed or have disappeared. Normal air never contains morbid microzymes or so-called germs or microbes. Disease cannot be taken from the air but may or may not be from a patient at some certain moment of contact. Pasteur's ridiculous theory of invasion of living tissues and causing disease there was the beginning of the modern dark ages of therapeutics. Proliferation is not possible by inoculation.

During the years when Béchamp was getting all this straightened out, Pasteur was watching with great interest the progress of his own fame and plagiarizing Béchamp's work.

. . . something happened that took all the wind out of my sails. I chanced to get a book from the C. W. Nelson Co., England, written by E. Douglas Hume, 259 pages, fifteen shillings. After reading this fascinating book through twice, let me emphasize that it is a morally compulsory item to have for several reasons. The information that it contains is indispensable truth that has been covered up by Pasteur's villainy, tied in with contemptible social circumstances and popular gullibility. The book tells practically the whole story of Béchamp's marvellous work, recorded in many years' proceedings of the scientific societies of France. It tells also of the so-called scientific labors of Pasteur, his intrigues, plagiarisms, false practices and representations: of his crude experiments, beastly cruelty, inoculations, falsifications with thoroughly documented exposures of his so-called preventative medicine. I repeat, the information, the truth of principles and facts exposed in this book are an indispensable source of awareness for every physician. One reviewer says it is the most sensational work of biology for several generations, if not for all time. Another says it is an amazing, overwhelming exposure of Pasteur with documented facts. Another, "Probably one of the most important books on medicine or science published during recent years." Another, "This book has erected a monument to truth." I will add that the facts in this book have been shown to biologists with the result that they have no reply to them. Through the incontrovertible facts which will spread from it and from *The Blood*,[1] it will become the nemesis of the present below-the-belt therapy which contributes to deficiencies of the young, insufficiencies of elders and hastens and originates the degenerative diseases.

The central truth which Béchamp has taught is that disease originates within the organism, including heredity, and is individual even as are the chromosomes. Then, as vitality is disturbed by insufficient reaction to influences of the

[1] By Professor Pierre Antoine Béchamp.

environment, individual disease appears. The time is coming when commercial and bureaucratic medicine will be forced by economic and revolutionary forces to adjust its ministrations to humane considerations in general and to individual considerations in particular. Then the whole loathsome, putrid mass of animal and human experimentation and practice will be sloughed off. The great soul of Béchamp and its influence on human welfare during a dark period will be recognized as one of the great benefactors of the races in an age of well-nigh therapeutic helplessness and insanity. The story must be told frequently.

Endless streams of so-called germ killers continue to come from the chemical makers. The doctors are likely to depend on the representations of the chemical houses. It would take a very large book to contain the names of the immense numbers of chemical substances that have been concocted and sold as germ killers even during the years that I have practiced medicine. So far, in my opinion, nothing in either prevention or cure of any kind of illness has resulted but on the contrary, as I have said before, an immense amount of *harm* has resulted — harm in prolonging the original sickness and harm from the drug poisonings which result in many other ailments.

So think it over. Divest your mind of the fear of germs and give your attention to the development of good natural living habits. You will be amply repaid by good health.

I have done very successfully a lot of surgery for a long time, and during all that time I had to deal constantly with certain aspects of germ danger. It would take too much time to argue all aspects of the germ subject, so I will just say that the danger from germs comes generally when they are forcibly introduced into the body or bloodstream and especially into some delicate structure.

Surgery opens up such avenues of invasion, and suitable precautions, of course, must be taken. Forcible introduction by accidents is unavoidable and unfortunate. Even in such cases the cure is not effected by the direct killing of the germ by germicides, but by the proper internal remedy which *helps the vital force* to *prevent* the *growth* of the *germ* and production of its poison.

Hundreds of thousands of people receive cuts, bruises, skinned knuckles every day, which are subjected to contact with all the various germs which inhabit the skin and are encountered on whatever agent caused the injury. Yet, how many of those people develop serious infection? How many get a real case of blood poisoning? A very small percentage. Why?

Why don't you all get the same kind and degrees of infection? It is because each person is different and a law unto himself. Those who suffer severely, or die, lack that imponderable "something" that was present in others and which was their protection. The remedy for all infected cases is not germicide but the Homœopathic constitutional remedy for the patient.

Infection by the tetanus ("lockjaw") germs sometimes happens. It is deadly and does not show its presence until it is almost too late. This deadly germ has to be *forcibly introduced* into the body deep in the tissue away from the air.

Whether or not every case that is infected by this germ results in "lockjaw" and death, or whether it occurs only in those whose blood lacks the power of defense against this particular germ will probably never be known. I have seen some cases recover under the Homœopathic treatment, and I have seen others die, but I have never seen any other method, including the use of tetanus antitoxin, succeed. It is fortunate indeed that this infection is comparatively rare.

I was called to a nearby sanatorium one day, a couple of years ago, to see a patient who was suffering from a very large carbuncle which had started on the back of the neck, and which finally involved the entire nape and had continued to the face and shoulders. This patient, a woman, was my first patient of years gone by. That was probably the reason I was allowed in that non-Homœopathic institution. I examined the patient and found her to be a very sick woman, with high temperature and severe pain. Well, everything was ready for me to do a bit of surgery — instruments nicely laid out, plenty of sulfa drugs, etc., and nurses ready and waiting. Of course, under Orthodoxy, surgery was the only thing. I smiled and very politely explained that none of that would be necessary, as it was, according to my philosophy, purely a medical case.

Well, you should have seen the polite and surreptitious eyebrows raising. I was in an extra good mood that day and I took time to explain my reasons, choice of a remedy, etc. I had quite a problem to differentiate four remedies which might have been indicated, but finally chose what I deemed to be the one for her, and subsequent events proved my choice to be the correct one. I handed the little white pills to the nurse and gave directions as to how they were to be given, and I took my departure, requesting them to call me in a day or two to report on the patient's progress. As I was leaving, I thought I could see pity (or was it contempt?) in the expression on the nurse's face for my awful ignorance.

Next day, over the telephone, it was a different story. I knew immediately that there was a great improvement in the patient by the unmistakable note of respect in the nurse's voice. She said they had never seen such a remarkable improvement, couldn't understand it, etc. Naturally, I was pleased. I thanked her and asked that she call me again in the morning to report the patient's condition. With great surprise in her voice, she asked, "Why, Doctor, aren't you coming to see her today?"

I said, "No, it isn't necessary, I'll be over in a day or two."

To make a long story short, the patient made a most beautiful, quick and complete recovery without even a scar. She was nearly seventy years of age. I might add, too, that in all my years of practice as a surgeon, I have never operated upon a carbuncle, and I never had a patient die from one, and I have seen many patients with carbuncles.

A doctor friend of mine, for whom I did surgical cases for many years, came into the hospital with a carbuncle of pretty good size on the back of his neck. He asked me to cut it out. I refused to do it, but instead I suggested that he take some of my good Homœopathic pills. He was a confirmed and stubborn allopath and replied, "No, I do not want your d——d pills! Either you operate or I'll get someone else."

I said, "I'm sorry, but if that's the way you feel about it, you'll have to get someone else."

He got a so-called "big shot" from Boston, who proceeded to carve him up good and proper. He seemed quite proud of his technique at carbuncle operations. Well, too bad, but "Digger O'Dell," the friendly undertaker, came in a few days later and took him away. I'm sure that is what would have happened to my little old lady had she been subjected to surgery.

You see, the *system which allows a carbuncle to develop* lacks something. It isn't so much that the operation itself kills the patient, but the *failure to receive the proper remedy* is the real tragedy. If the system can allow a carbuncle to develop, it can also reverse the process with the help of the proper remedy and the carbuncle will just disappear. I have seen it happen many times. It is the cause which should be removed — not just the result of a cause.

In the Medicine section of *Time,* May 8, 1950,[2] an article entitled "The Dangerous Doctors" stated:

[2]Courtesy *TIME,* The Weekly Newsmagazine, copyright Time, Inc., 1950.

Doctors seldom mention the fact that an illness can be iatrogenic, i.e., caused by the doctor.[3] Yet many forms of sickness are created or made worse by the doctor's own emotional shortcomings. So says Psychiatrist Franklin Gessford Ebaugh of Denver in the *Journal of the Michigan State Medical Society.*

"Usually," says Dr. Ebaugh, expanding earlier reports by a colleague, Dr. Frank R. Drake (*Time*, March 1, 1948), "such illnesses result from the doctor's failure to recognize or treat the *emotional* factors in the case. The doctor may be too busy looking for possible physical and mechanical causes: Not infrequently some innocent anomaly . . . is falsely honored and burned at the diagnostic stake. Lo, the tipped uterus, the flat foot, the infected tooth, the evil adhesion!"

"One-third of all the people who go to doctors suffer primarily from emotional disorders," says Dr. Ebaugh. Often a doctor can find *nothing organically wrong* with the patient, but is afraid that another physician may. So he hedges his report to the patient, leaving him confused and worried. Dr. Ebaugh calls this the "mug-wumping technique of trying to be right in any event."

Dr. Ebaugh warns physicians against using psychiatric jargon or other technical lingo on patients: "Hiding your own ignorance behind the mask of scientific verbiage is more frequently depressive rather than impressive to the patient . . ." The patient should have his illness straightforwardly explained.

The article finishes with some of Psychiatrist Ebaugh's pet peeves. Among those he is particularly scornful of is the doctor who "has so much self-love that he must preserve the illusion of omnipotence . . . the doctor who plays God." His patients, if they do not get better or do exactly what he says, "must bear the brunt of a revengeful Jehovah and assume full guilt for their failure to recover."

There seems to be a growing tendency to debunk the claims made by present Orthodox medicine. This manifests itself in the various articles and books that have been written, such as "Why Are There So Few Good Doctors?," "How To Pick A Doctor," "What's Wrong With Doctors," "Unnecessary Surgery," etc., which to me is a good sign, because it shows that a few individuals here and there are beginning to do some thinking, as the above *Time* article would attest.

Health is usually described as a condition of the organism in which there is freedom from all those changes in the structure of the body that endanger life or impede the easy and effective exercise of the vital functions, and freedom from pain and uneasy sensations.

[3] From the Greek: *iatros* (physician) and *gen* (producing).

Departures from this happy state present themselves to us, both in form and degree, in infinite variety. As a matter of fact, *health in perfection* is perhaps never seen. All the infinite variations from the healthy state are made manifest by symptoms which the patient can feel in uneasiness and pain. The symptoms may occur in many people with a sufficient similarity to enable physicians to classify and put a name to each grouping. Thus arose medical diagnosis. While diagnosis should be used for purposes of nomenclature only, unfortunately each name has, in the mind of orthodoxy, become a *disease entity at which they throw their strong drugs*. Even autopsies show that 50 per cent of diagnoses were wrong. What chance then, under this regime, does a sick person have when treatment depends on such kind of diagnosis?

All diseased conditions begin as a simple derangement of function and as such, may be quickly cured by the proper Homœopathic remedy. If sickness were inevitable and unavoidable and curable only by Orthodox medicine, then the human race would have long since vanished from the earth. That the race did survive is conclusive proof that Nature can overcome and cure most natural sicknesses.

Before the Law of Cure was discovered, Orthodox doctors had no recourse but to pursue their deadly measures. They had to do whatever orthodoxy bid them to do and mostly for their own protection. But during the last 150 years there has become available the wonderful method of Nature which pointed the way to prescribe curative medicine for all sickness, and in my opinion it was and is stupidity, bigotry, and laziness to continue to prescribe deadly drugs.

A wise doctor once said that if a man or woman, having reached the age of forty, is not by that time his own doctor, he or she is a fool. What did he mean by that? This is what I think he meant.

If a man hasn't learned in all that time what constitutes adequate clothing and what kinds of food disagree with him, that he is likely to get indigestion if he loses his temper, especially while eating; if he hasn't discovered the harm in staying up late night after night, steeping himself in nicotine, poisoning himself with alcohol; if he remains unaware of the harm of worrying about things that cannot be helped; is consumed with jealousy, hatred or anything that upsets the emotions, and many other things too numerous to mention, then to use a common expression, he is just plain stupid.

CHAPTER 7

How Are Drugs Sold?

Snap on your radio or television set at any hour, any day in the week. What do you hear? Well, about eighty per cent of the time you can hear or see what may be classified as entertainment, but the rest of the time you are on the receiving end of what is known as "the pitch." Along with soap, cigarettes, and cosmetics, what gets pitched at you with the greatest frequency? Drugs. Drugs which, I have concluded, will at best do nothing, and, at worst, may make you a chronic invalid.

Each week every doctor's wastebasket is filled by an immense amount of literature extolling the virtues of an endless stream of drugs. Much of this literature is accompanied by samples of the drugs. I have been unable to find a single one of these products that has any curative action whatever, yet fourteen billion or more dollars are spent yearly for their purchase.

The drug industry has one of the highest markups for its products of any industry in the nation. Its advertising budget is a sizeable percentage of the consumer price. Why spend so much for advertising? Because a market has to be created. You have to be made to believe that you must take such and such a pill at the first sign of a headache and such and such a pill at the first sign of stomach distress.

Perhaps you will remember the first anti-histamine which proved so deadly that the Government stepped in and stopped the kind of advertising which sold so much of the stuff.

Well, now, the drug houses are advertising and selling in great quantities a new anti-histamine (under another name) which is more deadly than the first one, only this time it is advertised as giving *symptomatic relief* — but no cure — of influenza and "virus" colds, thus avoiding Government interference. This is the way they say the relief is accomplished:

1. Good symptomatic results from anti-histaminic action, particularly in cases where there is an allergic factor (thenylpyramine hydrochloride).

2. Effective relief of associated headache and body aches (acetophenetidin, salicylamide).

3. Nasal dripping checked (atropine sulfate).

4. Depression overcome by stimulation of the central nervous system and circulation (caffeine, camphor).

5. Diarrhea and intestinal cramps, often complicating virus infections, rapidly controlled by the small amount of opium.

Now all this mess of deadly drugs (yes, every one is deadly) is advertised, recommended and sold to the people of the world right now, and no one seems to care how many people it will kill or make into chronic invalids, or who will develop the morphine habit from the opium, nor how many hearts will be affected and damaged by the caffeine this foolhardy prescription contains.

A common cold will not kill anybody if Nature is allowed to carry on, as she will always do, to a cure. A dripping nose is a sign that cure is already on the way. Those who recommend drugs of any kind to stop such discharge are doing a wicked and dangerous thing. Lo, the poor patient! He seems to believe everything he hears about it via televized dramatizations. His family doctor will prescribe such drugs even though he knows nothing about what such a combination of drugs will do to his patient. Each drug is supposed to offset or counteract the bad effects of the others. Each drug has a suppressive effect depending on its own poisonous action. Surely Nature knows what she is doing. The prompt elimination of the natural body poison is essential if health is to be preserved.

Should anyone be allowed to suppress a discharge of poison through the bowels by giving opium? Who knows how many get their start as narcotic victims by the use of such prescriptions? It is a known fact that a large percent of drug addicts get their start from physicians' prescriptions containing opium, heroin and allied drugs.

Now let us look carefully at the ingredients of this "wonder" prescription:

1. Thenylpyramine hydrochloride has as one effect the power to shrink the nasal mucous membrane, thus allowing easier breathing, even though this is temporary. It also causes headaches of varying severity by stopping the discharge.

2. Acetophenetidin and salicylamide (the latter being a drug formerly used in acute rheumatic fever and which caused heart complications) knock out the headaches (sometimes) but do not remove the cause.

3. Atropine sulfate, which is an alkaloid of belladonna and is a deadly poison, has the power of drying up the nasal dripping. This interferes with Nature in her efforts to relieve the patient of a deadly body poison, which never should be done.

4. Now something further must be added to overcome the depression which ensues, so Ingredient No. 4 comes along in the form of caffeine and camphor, both of which are poisonous "heart stimulants," so-called (a better wording would be heart irritants).

5. By this time, Nature having been frustrated in the attempt to eliminate through the mucous membranes of nose, and throat, as her second choice, has had to resort to the bowels as the next best way — third choice. The result then is the usual combination of cramps and diarrhea. So opium is the fifth ingredient, as it has the poisonous action of relieving the pain temporarily and suppressing the elimination of poisons via the bowels.

That makes a total of nine different (ipecac is also listed in the formula) and harmful drugs in this new anti-histamine, which is referred to in the advertising as a "doctor's prescription."

Think it over, my friends. Who could even imagine that in the present day of so-called medical research, which entails the spending of millions of dollars of the people's money, such deadly prescriptions should be allowed to be advertised and sold to sick humanity.

This, mind you, is only one of many that are equally bad. This is the kind of stuff for which $14,000,000,000 of the people's money goes every year.

An article in *Time*,[1] May 20, 1957, indicates that at last some thinking "researchers," as they are described, know that something is decidedly

[1]Courtesy *TIME; The Weekly Newsmagazine*, copyright Time, Inc., 1957.

wrong with present-day Orthodox medicine and condemn most emphatically much of the current procedure.

The *Time* article is entitled "Combination Dangers" and states:

Every week U. S. physicians are being bombarded with samples and ads of prefabricated antibiotic combinations — penicillin with novobiocin, neomycin with bacitracin, oleandomycin with tetracycline, and dozens more. In addition, antibiotics are offered in combination with the sulfas or with unrelated items — anti-histamines, hormones, vitamins. Just how good are these package drugs?

Very good indeed, holds one school, led by Henry Welch, a microbiologist with the Food and Drug Administration. Dr. Welch and some physicians insist that treatment with combinations is no "old-fashioned 'shotgun' approach, but a calculated, rational method of attacking the problem of resistant organisms."

Research physicians, by and large, take the opposite view. In a series of scathing editorials in recent medical journals, several groups have attacked the combination drugs. In the A.M.A.'s *Archives of Internal Medicine,* nine doctors list and refute the claims made for the combinations. With the most widely agreed answers, these are:

Claim: mixed infections caused by two kinds of bacteria may need mixed antibotics. *Answer:* such infections are rare, except in wounds, and can best be treated then by proper choice of drugs in the right amounts — not by trusting to luck that a manufacturer's choice of items and dosage will turn out to be right.

Claim: when a patient's life is in danger, and there has not been time to identify the disease-causing bacteria, two or more drugs provide insurance. *Answer:* this is only true if both are used in full doses — the danger is that in a fulminating infection a patient will get a packaged combination containing only half doses of each antibiotic.

Claim: two antibiotics may be synergistic; i.e., have a combined effect greater than the sum of their separate effects. *Answer:* no proof of this in patients (except those with heart inflammation caused by the enterococcus and a few other microbes).

Claim: a second antibiotic may delay the emergence of bacteria which are resistant to the first antibiotic. *Answer:* this may be true in test tubes, but generally there is no proof that it works in human patients.

Experts agree that three combinations are justified: 1) streptomycin with other drugs (such as isoniazid) to discourage the appearance of resistant tubercle bacilli; 2) penicillin with streptomycin for inflammation of the heart lining (endocarditis); 3) tetracycline (or related antibiotics) with nystatin, not routinely but in some cases, to guard against secondary infection with the fungus monilia. Granting exceptions such as these, the *Archives* editorialists conclude: "It is our firm conviction that the promotion and sale of such combinations should be discouraged."

A curative remedy is one by which definite, careful and painstaking experimentation on healthy people has been proven to be curative when correctly applied. It may be years before a patient comes along who requires a certain particular remedy, but it is the only one that will cure this particular case. With several thousand remedies on hand, the Homœopathic doctor can take care of almost any kind of curable disease, but how would it be possible to advertise any one of these remedies as a cure for any disease without going into a long description of the symptoms, plus the type of patient who presents such symptoms? It can thus readily be seen that to advertise a drug as a cure for any sickness with no more identity than an arbitrary diagnosis is absolutely ridiculous and dangerous. Unfortunately, that is the way Orthodox medicine is practiced today.

CHAPTER 8

"Miracle" Drugs

Let us go back just a few years to the time when the "miracle" drug, *Sulfa,* was getting well under way. I shall present four cases which were reported in a publication of a large national medical association by a prominent doctor. These case reports contain a very carefully prepared microscopic detail of the diseased tissues, autopsy findings, etc., too long to record here; therefore, I shall give only the case history and summary of autopsy findings.

CASE NO. 1

HISTORY: R. N., white girl, aged 15 years, was admitted to hospital May 14, 1941. She had had acne and irregular menses for the past 18 months. Since February, 1940, she had been treated with hypodermic injections of an estrogenic substance in the first half of her menstrual cycle, and gonadotropic substance in the second half. For the acne, she was given desiccated thyroid, ferrous sulfate and heliotherapy until April 12, 1941, without relief. On that date, she was given 25 tablets of sulfathiazole, each containing 7.5 grains, to be taken once a day. The ferrous sulfate was discontinued. Up to May 9, she had taken 22 tablets, at which time another series of 25 was begun. Three days later, shortly after taking a tablet, she began to complain of "grippy" generalized aches and pains, chilliness, headache and burning sensation in her eyes. The next morning her temperature was 104 F. Her physician ordered continuance of the sulfathiazole, increasing the dose to 15 grains every 4 hours! She took six doses on May 13 and in addition to her other symptoms became delirious. The next morning she vomited after three attempts to take the tablets. It was noticed that she had not voided since 4:30 p.m. the previous day despite forcing of fruit juices and fluids. On the way to the hospital in the ambulance she had generalized convulsions. She died on May 15 with a diagnosis of uremia due to sulfathiazole.

SUMMARY: A young girl after three weeks' treatment for acne with sulfathiazole had chills, fever and pyrexia. Despite the absence of positive physical manifestations to corroborate an infection cause of the symptoms, she was given increased doses of the drug. This was followed by anuria and coma. High concentration of sulfathiazone was found in the blood and crystals of the drug in the urine. In spite of discontinuance of the drug, administration of fluids intravenously and ureteran catheterization, the patient died fifty hours after onset of the anuria.

The anatomic diagnosis was acne vulgaris, sulfathiazole urolithiasis, petechia and hemorrhage in the pelvis and ureter, edema in the bladder, focal necroses in the liver, spleen, lungs, kidney and bone marrow, nephrosis, and splenomegaly. The final impression was acne vulgaris with sulfathiazole intoxication showing visceral focal necroses and nephrosis.

CASE NO. 2

HISTORY: H. K., a white man, aged 60, was first admitted to hospital three weeks before the present illness for the repair of a hernia. His course was satisfactory until the tenth post-operative day, at which time his temperature rose to 102 F., and a few rales were heard at the base of the left lung. He was given sulfathiazole and two days later his temperature was 99 F. He was discharged in good condition except for a few residual rales at the base of the left lung. A sulfathiazole determination on his blood before discharge showed a total concentration of 8.6 mg. per hundred cubic centimeters. At home the drug was continued. On August 8 he had a chill and a temperature of 105 F. and a generalized maculopapular erythematous rash developed. The sulfathiazole was continued because it was thought that the rise in temperature indicated an infection. His temperature remained high, and he gradually lapsed into coma, becoming incontinent of urine and feces, and was readmitted to the hospital the following day. Up to this time he had taken 660 grains of sulfathiazole. He died several days later.

SUMMARY: An elderly man who had been operated on for the repair of a hernia had a slight temperature and vague pulmonary signs on the tenth post-operative day, for which he was treated with sulfathiazole; the drug being continued after his discharge. Eight days later he had a chill, his temperature rose to 105 F., and a maculopapular rash had appeared. He lapsed into coma and became rapidly anuric. Catheterization and renal decapsulation with pelvic drainage were resorted to in attempts to stimulate and re-establish kidney function, without avail. On discharge from the hospital his blood showed a total sulfathiazole level of 8.6 mg. per hundred cubic centimeters. Two days before death it was 8. mg. per hundred cubic centimeters in the free state.

The anatomic diagnosis was nephrosis;[1] focal necroses in the liver, kidneys, adrenal glands and bone marrow; deposits in kidney tubules (sulfathiazole?), splenomegaly; interstitial hepatitis, dermatitis, acute conjunctivitis. The final impression was sulfathiazole intoxication with visceral focal necroses and nephrosis.

CASE NO. 3

HISTORY: A white man aged 71 had had hypertension for ten years, albuminuria and pyuria intermittently for the past two years, and some frequency and nocturia. Two weeks prior to admission he had an attack of chills and fever with pyuria, and was given sulfathiazole. Nine days later his temperature was normal and examination of the urine showed a few clumps of leukocytes and a faint trace of albumin. His prostate gland was moderately enlarged. Intravenous pyelography revealed a picture suggestive of polycystic disease of the kidneys. Cystoscopy showed cystitis and trigonitis. Both ureteral orifices appeared normal. The middle lobe of the prostate gland was definitely enlarged and both lateral lobes were moderately enlarged.

On the day before admission he complained only of slight frequency of urination, but during the night chills and fever developed. On admission he appeared acutely ill. His temperature was 104.2 F., the pulse rate 96, and the respiratory rate 20 a minute. There were a few rales at the left base, but no dullness or bronchial breathing. The clinical impression was polycystic disease of the kidneys with pyelonephritis. Sulfathiazole 15 grains (1 gm) every four hours was continued and 2,000 cc. of 5% dextrose in saline solution was given parenterally. The next day his temperature was 104 F., and he appeared lethargic. Catheterization yielded 4 ounces (120 cc.) of residual urine with a faint trace of albumin and a few leukocytes

[1] Destruction of kidney.

and erythrocytes. Escherichia coli was cultured from the urine. Culture of the blood was sterile. The blood urea nitrogen was 11.5 mg. per hundred cubic centimeters. Portable roentgenograms of the chest suggested broncho-pneumonia infiltration throughout both lungs. On the second day he was comatose, but lumbar puncture the next day yielded no additional information. Sodium sulfathiazole was administered by venoclysis.

Neurologic examination indicated definite cerebral involvements which was interpreted as being due to the continued pyrexia. On the fourth hospital day the total blood sulfathiazole was 6.7 mg. per hundred cubic centimeters. He died approximately 50 hours after admission. During hospitalization he received a total of 250 gm. of sulfathiazole.

SUMMARY: An elderly man who had intermittent symptoms referable to the prostate gland for about two years, two weeks before admission had an attack of chills, fever and pyuria and was treated with sulfathiazole. He apparently responded favorably to the treatment. Five days before admission the abnormal urinary findings were slight. His temperature was normal. However, the drug was continued and on the night before admission chills and fever occurred. In the hospital, the urinary changes were slight with the exception that escherichia coli was cultured from the catheterized specimen. Roentgen examination suggested broncho-pneumonia, and because of this diagnosis, together with a possible suppurative nephritis, full doses of sulfathiazole were given. The patient continued feverish and rapidly lapsed into coma and died.

The anatomic diagnosis was focal necroses in the liver, kidneys, spleen, adrenal glands, lymph nodes, urinary bladder, trachea, coronary artery and bone marrow; sulfathiazole urolithiasis, edema in the bladder, abscesses and overgrowth of the prostate gland and kidneys; nephrosclerosis; polycystic kidneys, nephrolithiasis (left side); splenomegaly; necrotic tracheobronchitis; and terminal pneumonia with sulfathiazole intoxicaion.

CASE NO. 4

HISTORY: A white woman, aged 32, was admitted to the hospital, Jan. 27, 1942. In April, 1940, she was treated for sinusitis with sulfanilamide. In September, 1941, she complained of fatigue and vague symptoms which occurred intermittently. At this time her urine contained faint trace of albumin and occasional red and white blood cells. Chemical examination of

the blood revealed nonprotein nitrogen 50.7 mg. per hundred cubic centimeters and urea 23.5 mg. Six days prior to admission the patient noted a
dry non-productive cough and three days later malaise and pain low in the
back. The night before admission she had a chill and the next morning her
temperature was 102 F. Her physician prescribed 15 grains (1 gm.) of
sulfathiazole every three hours. By that evening she had taken 52.5 grains
(3.4 gm) of the drug and her temperature had risen to 106 F. She now
complained of severe headache and pain in the back and was referred to
the hospital.

SUMMARY: A woman who had received sulfanilamide about a year prior
to her present illness apparently had some renal disease, as evidenced by
albuminaria, the presence of red and white blood cells in the urine and
some nitrogen retention in the blood, six months prior to hospitalization.
Her present illness began with signs suggestive of bronchopneumonia, for
which she was treated with sulfathiazole. After having taken 52.5 grains
(3.4 gm.) of the drug, her temperature rose from 102 to 106 F. She was
then hospitalized.

Sulfathiazole was continued and she took an additional 45 grains (3 gm.)
of the drug before it was noted that she had a generalized cutaneous rash.
Because she had not voided since admission, catheterization was performed,
yielding 60 cc. of turbid urine containing albumin, casts and white blood
cells. She died about nine hours later. Before death, a blood sulfathiazole
determination showed a total concentration of 13.9 mg. per hundred
cubic centimeters.

The anatomic diagnosis was nephrosis; focal necrosis in the kidneys,
liver, spleen and adrenal gland; acute, focal myocarditis with necrosis, toxic
dermatitis with focal necrosis; chronic pyelonephritis, and chronic bronchitis. The final impression was bronchitis and chronic pyelonephritis and
death during sulfathiazole therapy.

*   *   *

These four people were admittedly killed by the "miracle" drug. The
autopsy findings in these four cases, reported in the greatest detail at a
meeting of a powerful Orthodox medical society, showed that *nearly every
vital organ in the body was diseased* — yes, practically destroyed — by the
"miracle" drug, a drug being prescribed at the time in large doses for every
conceivable sickness by Orthodox doctors all over the United States.

The AMA has since repudiated its previous acceptance of this drug. But did this report put an end to further use of the drug? Not at all. The report was received merely as an item of interest showing in what organs of the body the drug produced its deadly effects.

Doctors "fell" for these "miracle drugs" because the first dose has the deadly effect of knocking down a fever — literally knocking it down. Most doctors still labor under the misapprehension that a fever is harmful. On the contrary, a fever is the sign that Nature is on her job and a cure is on the way. No one ever saw a fever in a corpse. After fever has done its part in curing, it subsides. *Any measure that kills Nature's power to produce a fever* only too often *kills* the sick person.

Even Hippocrates said: "Give me fever and I can cure any disease."

In the following cases both patients were dying when I was asked to see them. One look at their charts told me the reason. There was nothing I or anyone else could do. Here is a list of the drugs administered:

CASE NO. 1

Alophen	Codeine ½
R tab 1	Terpin Hydrate
R tab 1-9-3-	Sulfathiazole tab. 2
R tab 1	Sulfathiazole tab. 2-9-1-
Seconal 1	Luminal 1½ grs.
MS ¼ sq.	Sulfathiazole tab. 2
Luminal ¼ - 10-2-6-	Nembutal 1
Luminal ¼ - 10-2-6-	Sulfathiazole tab. 2-9-1-
Luminal gr. 3-9	Allonal 1
Luminal gr. ¼ - 10-2-6-	Allonal 1
Luminal gr. 3	Allonal 1
Boric Acid Irrigation 10-6-	Sulfathiazole 2 tab.
Luminal gr. ¼	Luminal 1½ grs.
Sulfathiazole tab. 3-9-2-	Soda Bicarb.
Luminal tab. 2-8-5-	Sulfathiazole 15 grs. 8-12-4-
Sulfathiazole gr. 3	Sulfathiazole 15 grs. 8-12-4-
Soda Bicarb. 9-3-	R 1 teasp.
Luminal gr. 3	Sulfathiazole tab. 2-8-12-
MS ¼ sq.	Acceserone
Intravenous 1000 5% G	Sulfathiazole tab. 2-8-12-
MS ¼	Nembutal 1
Seconal 1	DSD 12½

R teasp. 1
Sulfathiazole 2 tabs.
ACR 2 teasp.
Digitalis grs. 1½ - 10-
Sulfathiazole tabs. 3
Nembutal
Sulfathiazole tabs. 3
Digitalis
Nembutal 1½ gr.
R 1 teasp.
R 1 teasp. 11-4-
Nembutal 1
Nembutal 1
R 1 teasp.
ACR 11-4-
Digitalis 1½ grs. 10-4-
MS 1/6
Nembutal
ACR teasp. 11-4-

Digitalis 1½ grs. 10-4-
Nembutal 1/1
R 1 teasp.
Sulfathiazole tab. 2
Bicarb grs. 10, 10-1-4-
Sulfathiazole tab. 6.
Nembutal 1
R 1 teasp.
R 1 teasp. 11-4-
Digitalis 1½ grs. 1-4-
Nembutal grs. ½
Aspirin 10 grs.
Digitalis ½ gr. 10-4-
ACR ½ teasp. 11-4-
Nembutal 1
R 1 teasp.
R 1 teasp.
Digitalis ½ gr.
Caffeine Sodio-bensoate ampules 1

CASE NO. 2

Codeine ½ gr. PRN.
Digitalis 1½ grs. tbs.
  9:30 a.m. 4 tablets
  1:30 p.m. 4   "
  5:30 p.m. 3   "
  9:30 a.m. 2   "
  1:30 a.m. 2   "
  5:30 a.m. 2   "
Digitalis ½ gr. 4 ID
Nembutal 1½ grs. at bedtime
  — repeat if necessary
Digitalis 1½ grs. bd. IL
500 cc. 5% Saline
500 cc. 5% Saline
MS ¼ sc.
500 ¼ cc.
500 ¼ cc.
MS ¼ sc.
500 cc.

Whiskey 1½ teasp.
MS ¼ sc.
Digitalis 1¼
Whiskey 1 teasp.
Citrate of Mag.
Citrate of Mag.
MS ¼
Whiskey
Citrate of Mag.
Whiskey
Digitalis 1½ grs.
Whiskey
Whiskey
MS ¼
Digitalis 1½ grs.
Mag. solution
MS ¼
Whiskey
MS ¼

Sulfathiazole tab. 2	Sulfathiazole
Whiskey	Sulfathiazole
MS ¼	Sulfathiazole
Sulfathiazole	Whiskey
Whiskey	Sulfathiazole
Sulfathiazole	Digitalis
MS ¼	Whiskey
Milk of Mag.	

Both patients died. In the first case there had been performed a prostatectomy (removal of the prostate gland). The operation itself was successful. The patient in the second case had had a fracture of the tibia (shin bone). Both patients, in accordance with current Orthodox medical practice, had received the "miracle" drug. They died, but no complaints were made by their relatives. Had not everything been done? Had not large doses of the famous drug been administered? Then, the families concluded, it must have been the "Will of God."

But there was nothing godly in this all too common tragedy. In my opinion it was nothing but ordinary mortal stupidity that put these victims in bed and made them absorb a lethal volume of drugs and chemicals until their constitutions could take no more. Even a perfectly healthy body would have been overwhelmed, let alone one weakened by illness.

The physicians who were treating these two patients confessed they could not understand why the patients appeared so sick, that they could discover no reason for these deaths. They never suspected that this *criminal drugging* they had resorted to was the *actual cause of death*.

A bit of grim humor is attached to one of these cases. When the prostate case died I called the surgeon into my office, and before three witnesses, I asked him if it was his habit to approve the kind of drugging his patients received from the family doctor following an operation.

His answer was, "Of course I do."

I then said, "Here is a case that died. I want your opinion of the drugging this case got after an operation."

I brought out the chart (of course, the name was concealed).

"Well", the surgeon said, "the doctor who gave that amount of junk should lose his license to practice; that stuff would kill anyone."

When I broke the news to him that it was his own case, his reaction was awful. His face became florid as he ranted and raved and lambasted the family doctor.

It may be difficult for the layman to appreciate fully the significance of such cases as these. The man in the street is only too apt not to want to appreciate it and face the situation. He does not want to recognize the sinister implications in the fact that despite repeated reports to various medical societies concerning the deadly effects of the "miracle" drugs by the very physicians who prescribe them, nothing has been done by any medical society to stop their use.

Now let us compare three more cases. The first case is an example of empiric prescribing, using the drugs in style at the moment, in maximum doses, often repeated. This is Orthodox, allopathic medicine. The other two were prescribed for according to the Law of Cure (Homoeopathy), using small doses of a remedy chosen because its pathogenesis corresponds to the symptoms.

First Case:

A young married woman came to our hospital to have her baby. She was the patient of a well-known Boston doctor, who decided she needed a Caesarean operation. We shall assume the indications were correct. She had the operation June 9 along with the following drugs which totaled one hundred and ninety-five doses.

CASE 34871 — LIST OF DRUGS ADMINISTERED, COPIED FROM HER CHART

6/10/45:

4:30 A.M.   Morph. Sul., 1/6
8:00 A.M.   I.V., 1.000 5% Glu.
            Ergotrate, 1cc. at 6-8-12
            Morph. Sul., 1/6 s.c.
            Ergotrate
            Pantopon S., Gr. 1/3 s.c.
10:30 A.M. Sulfadiazine Tab. IV at 10:30, 2:30, 6:30

6/11/45:

3:30 A.M.   Pantopon, Grs. 1/3 sc.
            Sulfadiazine Tab. II at 10:30 A.M.
9:00 A.M.   I.V. 1,000 5% Glucose
10:15 A.M. Pantopon S., Gr. 1/3 sc. at 9:30 A.M.
10:30 A.M. Ergotrate Tab. I at 10:30
12:00 Noon Penicillin 20,000 Units I.M. at 11:30 A.M., 2:30 P.M.
            Sulfadiazine Tabs. IV at 2:30

4:00 P.M.   Ergotrate I
5:30 P.M.   Caff. Sod. Benz.
6:00 P.M.   1,000 cc 5% Glucose. 10 min. Adrenalin
8:30 P.M.   Caff. Sod. Benz.
             Penicillin, 20,000 Units
10:00 P.M.   Ergotrate Tab. I at 4-8

6/12/45:
2:00 A.M.   Penicillin 20,000 Units at 11:30 P.M., 2:30 A.M.
             I.V. 1.500 cc 5% Glucose
             Penicillin, 20,000 Units, last at 5:30 A.M.
8:30 A.M.   Penicillin, 20,000 I.M. at 8:30 A.M.
9:30 A.M.   I.V. 1,000 5% Glucose.
             Penicillin, 20,000 Units I.M. at 11:30 and 2:30
5:30 P.M.   Penicillin, 20,000 Units.
             1,000 cc. of 5% Glucose I.V.
8:30 P.M.   Penicillin, 20,000 Units.
9:10 P.M.   Pantopon, Grs. 1/3 sc.
11:30 P.M.   Penicillin, 20,000 Units.
11:45 P.M.   I.V. 1,000 cc. 5% Glucose

6/13/45:
2:30 A.M.   Penicillin, 20,000 Units.
5:30 A.M.   Penicillin, 20,000 Units.
2:00 P.M.   Pantopon S., Grs. 1/3 sc.
5:30 A.M.   Penicillin, 20,000 Units.
8:30 P.M.   Penicillin, 20,000 Units.
9:30 P.M.   Pantopon, Grs. 1/3 sc.
11:30 P.M.   Penicillin, 20,000 Units.
             Penicillin, Units 20,000 I.M. at 8:30, 11:30, 2:30

6/14/45:
7:30 A.M.   Penicillin, 20,000 I.M. at 8:30, 11:30, 2:30
5:30 P.M.   Penicillin, 20,000 Units.
8:30 P.M.   Penicillin, 20,000 Units.
9:15 P.M.   Pantopon, Grs. 1/3 sc.
11:30 P.M.   Penicillin, 20,000 Units.

6/15/45:
2:30 A.M.   Penicillin, 20,000 Units.
5:30 A.M.   Penicillin, 20,000 Units.
             Penicillin, 20,000 Units I.M. at 8:30, 11:30, 2:30

5:30 P.M.	Penicillin, 20,000 Units.
6:30 P.M.	Paragoric
8:30 P.M.	Penicillin, 20,000 Units.
9:15 P.M.	Pantopon, Grs. 1/3 sc.
11:30 P.M.	Penicillin, 20,000 Units.

6/16/45:

2:30 A.M.	Penicillin, 20,000 Units.
8:00 A.M.	Penicillin, 20,000 Units I.M. at 8:30, 11:30, 2:30
10:30 A.M.	Pantopon S., Gr. 1/3 sc.
3:30 P.M.	1,000 cc. of 5% Glucose.
8:00 P.M.	Penicillin, 20,000 Units.
9:00 P.M.	Prostigmine.
11:00 P.M.	Plasma, 150 cc.
	Prostigmine.
	Penicillin, 20,000 Units.

6/17/45:

1:00 A.M.	Prostigmine
2:00 A.M.	Penicillin, 20,000 Units.
2:30 A.M.	Pantopon, 1/3 sc.
5:00 A.M.	Penicillin, 20,000 Units.
	Prostigmine.
8:15 A.M.	Penicillin, Units 20,000 I.M. at 8-11-2.
5:00 P.M.	Penicillin, 20,000 Units.
8:00 P.M.	Penicillin, 20,000 Units.
8:45 P.M.	Pantopon, 1/3 sc.
11:00 P.M.	Penicillin, 20,000 Units.

6/18/45:

2:00 A.M.	Penicillin, 20,000 Units.
5:00 A.M.	Penicillin, 20,000 Units.
8:00 A.M.	Penicillin, Units 20,000 I.M. at 8-11-2.
8:30 P.M.	Penicillin, 20,000 Units.
9:10 P.M.	Dilauded, grs. 1/32.
11:15 P.M.	Penicillin, 20,000 Units.

6/19/45:

2:15 A.M.	Penicillin, 20,000 Units.
5:15 A.M.	Penicillin, 20,000 Units.
	Penicillin, 20,000 Units at 8.
5:00 P.M.	Dilauded, Grs. 1/32 sc.

6/20/45:
12:15 A.M.   Dilauded, Grs. 1/32 sc.
8:30 P.M.   Dilauded, Grs. 1/32 sc.

6/21/45:
11:00 A.M.   Prostigmine, 1-4,000 c11.1-3
3:00 P.M.   Caff. Sod. Benz.
8:30 P.M.   Sulfadiazine Tab. III.
9:30 P.M.   Plasma, 200 cc.
10:00 P.M.   Dilauded, Grs. 1/32

6/22/45:
12:30 A.M.   Sulfadiazine III.
4:30 A.M.   Sulfadiazine III.
9:00 A.M.   Sulfadiazine Tabs. II at 9-1
9:30 A.M.   Tinc. Opii.
12:15 P.M.   Penicillin, 25,000 Units I.M. at 11:45, 3.
4:45 P.M.   575 cc. of Blood.
5:45 P.M.   Adrenalin, 10 M.
6:00 P.M.   Caff. Sod. Benz.
6:30 P.M.   Adrenalin, 10 M.
6:45 P.M.   Coramine, 1 Amp.
7:00 P.M.   Morp., Grs. 1/6 sc.
8:00 P.M.   Penicillin, 25,000 Units at 7-10.

6/23/45:
1:00 A.M.   Penicillin, 25,000 Units I.M. at 1 A.M.
             4 A.M. — Dilauded (1:15).
8:00 A.M.   Penicillin, Units 25,000 I.M. at 7:15, 10:15, 1:30
             Sulfadiazine Tabs. II, same at 9-1.
5:00 P.M.   Sulfadiazine Tabs. II at 5-9.
6:00 P.M.   Penicillin, 25,000 Units at 4-7-10.
9:00 P.M.   Dilauded, Grs. 1/32 sc.

6/24/45:
1:00 A.M.   Sulfadiazine Tabs. II.
5:00 A.M.   Sulfadiazine Tabs. II.
9:00 A.M.   Kaomagma IV at 8:30
             Sulfadiazine Tabs. II at 9-1.
11:30 A.M.   Multicebrin.
5:00 P.M.   Sulfadiazine Tab. II.
8:00 P.M.   Kaomagma.

9:00 P.M.　Sulfadiazine Tab. II.
9:45 P.M.　Dilauded, Grs. 1/32 sc.

6/25/45:
9:00 A.M.　Multicebrin at 10.
5:00 P.M.　Kaomagma.

6/26/45:
6:00 A.M.　Kaomagma.
8:00 A.M.　Kaomagma.
11:30 A.M.　Kaomagma.
2:00 P.M.　Sulfadiazine Tabs. II at 2.
6:00 P.M.　Sulfadiazine Tabs. II, 6-10.

6/27/45:
2:00 A.M.　Sulfadiazine Tab. II.
6:00 A.M.　Sulfadiazine Tab. II.
　　　　　　Sulfadiazine Tabs. II at 10-2.
10:30 A.M.　Kaomagma.
6:00 P.M.　Sulfadiazine Tab. II.
10:00 P.M.　Sulfadiazine Tab. II.

6/28/45:
12:40 A.M.　Cod., Grs. ½
2:00 A.M.　Sulfadiazine Tab. II at 2 A.M., 6 A.M.
9:00 A.M.　Sulfadiazine Tabs. II at 10.
11:00 A.M.　Cod., Gr. ½ at 10:40
1:35 P.M.　Dilauded, Gr. 1/32 sc. at 12:45 P.M.
3:30 P.M.　Caff. Sod. Benz.
6:30 P.M.　Sulfadiazine Tab. II.
9:00 P.M.　Caff. Sod. Benz.
9:15 P.M.　Dilauded, Grs. 1/32
12:00 M.　　Caff. Sod. Benz.

6/29/45:
2:20 A.M.　Plasma, 250 cc.
3:30 A.M.　I.V. 1,000 cc.
5:30 A.M.　Caff. Sod. Benz.
6:30 A.M.　Digifolino.
8:30 A.M.　Caff. Sod. Benz.
1:30 P.M.　Dilauded.
1:45 P.M.　Sulfadiazine Tab. II.

3:00 P.M.	Caff. Sod. Benz.
	R. T. Bsp.
6:00 P.M.	Caff. Sod. Benz.
6:00 P.M.	Coramine.
	Dilauded.
7:00 P.M.	Caff. Sod. Benz.
	Digifolino.
8:00 P.M.	1,500 cc. of 5% Glucose.

6/30/45:

2:00 A.M.	Coramine.
10:00 A.M.	1,500 cc. 5% Glucose.
9:00 P.M.	Dilauded, Grs. 1/32 sc.

7/1/45:

12:15 A.M.	Dilauded, Grs. 1/32 sc.
8:30 A.M.	1,500 5% Glucose.
10:00 A.M.	Coramine, Amp. I at 8:45 A.M.
10:30 A.M.	Dilauded, 1/32 sc. at 10:30 A.M.
6:30 P.M.	Dilauded, Grs. 1/32.

7/2/45:

7:00 P.M.	30,000 Units Penicillin I.V.
	1,500 cc. of Plasma
11:20 P.M.	Penicillin I.V. 30,000 Units, Plasma

7/3/45:

2:20 A.M.	Penicillin, 30,000 Units.
3:45 A.M.	Coramine, I Amp.
5:00 A.M.	Digifolino.
5:20 A.M.	Penicillin, 30,000 Units.
8:00 A.M.	Penicillin, Units 30,000 IM at 8:30, 11:30; 2:30.
10:30 A.M.	1,500 cc. of 5% Glucose.

Died July 3, 1945

All prescriptions were ordered either by the family doctor or the so-called specialists who were used as consultants.

Of course, this young woman died! Not even a strong, robust person could survive such drugging, surely impossible for a sick one.

There is no question in my mind that under Homœopathic treatment this patient would have lived. I am convinced that she died from drugs.

At the very least, the results under Homœopathy could not have been worse, for, whatever the medication, it would have been orderly and according to rule. The patient would have been spared at least the torment and suffering incident to the one hundred and ninety-five administrations of drugs, mostly by mechanical means. At various times during the progress of the case, a number of consultants made these varying diagnoses: bronchial pneumonia, rupture of uterus, pyelitis, septic endometritis, metritis, parametritis, adynamic ileus, previous pneumonia, wound sepsis and arthralgia, all of which were wrong. Yet, none of the attending physicians or consultants had any orderly medical procedure to offer except to sedate and to push whatever drug happened to be in fashion at the moment. She received a total of 1,070,000 Units of Penicillin along with all the other drugs. Not one of them ever suspected that she was suffering from drug poisoning, but kept right on giving more and more until her system could stand it no longer.

One is reminded of the words of Marcel Proust: "Medicine being a compendium of the successive and contrary mistakes of medical practitioners, when we summon the wisest of them to our aid, the chances are that we may be relying on a 'scientific truth,' the error of which will be recognized in a few years."

In this case the consultants who were called in had absolutely nothing to offer in the way of curative medicine, nothing that had been tried and found true, even from a seven-thousand-year experience. Some of them advised continuing the sulfa, others advised penicillin, then a combination of both. Why? Where is there a trace of science in their system? What chance has a patient then who needs a real curative medicine? None whatever, unless he is fortunate enough to get a doctor who knows curative medicine. Who is *your* doctor and why?

Second Case:

Many years ago I was called to Cambridge, Massachusetts, to see a patient. When I arrived I was met by quite a number of anxious relatives who were concerned over the condition of the young patient.

I was shown upstairs where I saw lying unconscious on the bed a young woman waterlogged to such an extent that eyes, ears, nose and mouth were hardly discernible. Her arms were larger than thighs and her legs were almost as large as the body. I found that she was pregnant and that her kidneys had practically ceased functioning. Something had to be done quickly. I had to convince the relatives that she should go to the hospital at once. They finally, reluctantly, consented. The ambulance carried her to my hospital where I quickly made an incision through the abdominal wall and into the uterus and extracted two little premature baby girls. They weighed less than two pounds apiece. I quickly handed them to the nurse to put into the incubator and then directed my full attention to the patient. I chose the indicated homœopathic remedy, which was Ars. Alb. 200x.

Within a few hours her kidneys resumed their function and in about ten days there emerged from the almost unrecognizable human being that first met my gaze the most beautiful blonde girl one would wish to see.

Well, time marched on and I soon more or less forgot the whole incident. Many years later I was window-shopping in Hollywood, California, when I felt a tap on my shoulder. I looked around and who do you think it was? Yes, the little blonde, the mother of those little "preemies." Naturally I was delighted to see her. She was well and looked it. I asked about the little girls and found that they were well and healthy, both married and each the mother of five children. Every Christmas now I receive a card showing the children as they develop.

That case was and is probably the most satisfactory piece of surgical and medical work I ever did. I feel that if I never had done anything else, it alone has justified my being a doctor and surgeon. Just the slightest deviation in what was done, I am sure, would have resulted disastrously.

This young woman was not well and healthy when brought into the hospital as was the woman in the other case. She was unconscious and in a dying condition, but compare the outcome of these two cases.

Third Case:

The third case was a woman who came in for strangulated umbilical hernia (rupture), following a Caesarean operation performed in Germany many years before. After much persuasion she reluctantly consented to the operation, which proved quite difficult as there were many adhesions. The intestines were blue, a portion of omentum was beginning to turn gangrenous, and the mesentery was studded with dark, small infarcts (clots). After the operation her temperature began to climb. On the fourth day it reached 103°, with a remission on the fifth. The

pulse meanwhile climbed to 180 and became fibrillating; it became intermittent, almost impossible to count. On the sixth, seventh and eighth
days, the temperature rose and fell. The patient was nervous and apprehensive. Pyrogen, a homœopathic remedy, was prescribed in three
doses of 6x, and then one dose of 50M. Pulse, temperature and respiration rates came down immediately to normal and stayed normal. The
patient was transformed; she was smiling and cheerful, with a wholly
different outlook on life.

This patient was brought to me by a physician of the old school who
insisted violently that sulfa be given for the temperature and digitalis
for the heart, but which, of course, I refused to give. His observation of
our handling of this case changed his whole attitude and established his
interest in Homœopathy.

The cost of the drugs given to the patient who died was several hundred dollars. The medicine given the patients who lived cost them absolutely nothing at a cost to me of but a penny or two, and no consultants'
bills to pay either.

From the point of view of the scientific Homœopath, there is but one
course to pursue and one medicine only which suits the particular case.
That is the kind of medical treatment to which the whole world is entitled even if it threatens to eliminate a $14 billion per year drug cartel.

Some years ago a patient in Honolulu wrote me a pitiful letter in which
she said she was "at the end of her rope." She was told that she had
incurable cancer. One breast had been removed and her doctors wanted
to remove the other. She wanted my advice. I wrote I could give very
little satisfactory advice without seeing her, so she and her husband flew
to Boston to see me.

This is what my examination disclosed: a healthy woman of forty-
five, with no organic trouble whatever, who had been employed as a
librarian in Honolulu. One day the steel bow of her spectacles broke,
leaving a sharp end; this end accidentally caught in her dress and went
through and scratched her right breast. Here is where "a little knowledge"
proved a dangerous thing. She feared blood poisoning and immediately
went to the clinic where she was congratulated for her intelligence in
coming there as they had a "sure fire" drug which would prevent blood
poisoning. The drug was called the "wonder" drug, Penicillin. Given
a "shot" every day for five days, she did *not* get blood poisoning but
something worse. In a week's time her breast began to swell and many

hard lumps began to appear on the neck and under the arm. This so frightened her that she went back to the clinic. Again she was praised for coming because *now* she had a "galloping" cancer (whatever that is) and they were just the ones who could cure her. First the breast must come off immediately, they told her, and then, because the condition had advanced so far so rapidly, it would be impossible to remove all the lumps, so she must have deep X-ray therapy. At the end of a month her arm had swollen until it had almost doubled in size and was so painful they resorted to injection of novocain. It was then she was told that the source of the cancer must be in the other breast and so they wanted to take it off too.

I found no cancer nor any suspicion of it. I did find, however, the unmistakable results of *penicillin poisoning*. I gave her some medicine and advised her to go to her old home in New Hampshire and to see me once in a while, that I could quite guarantee in five or six months she would be all right. She was much pleased. In two weeks she came to visit me again, very happy about her progress. I told her recoveries from this drug were slow but advised that all was going according to schedule, but I noticed an uneasiness in her husband. He wanted to get back to Honolulu and I could see that he wasn't satisfied with the present treatment. He took his wife to someone else in one of our prominent hospitals. There they were told an immediate operation was necessary, which was done. The patient died three days later.

No one at the hospital recognized the condition as penicillin poisoning. It has happened only too often. I cannot understand why it was overlooked. This patient *did not have cancer;* furthermore, she was on the way to recovery.

At this same time I was called to see a patient whom I had known intimately for many years. The first words he uttered were, "Oh, doctor, don't let me die of this cancer." He presented a large, hard, red, shiny and somewhat painful tumor the size of a football, beginning at the lobe of the left ear and occupying the entire side of the neck, down to and including part of the shoulder. He was very frightened and afraid he was going to die. I didn't say, "You have a galloping cancer and I am the only doctor who can cure you and it will cost you a thousand dollars."

I did say, "Well, what can you expect? You made a fool of yourself again."

He said, "What do you mean?"

I said, "I mean that you got a cold, developed tonsilitis and then you went to your pal doctor who shot you full of penicillin, didn't you?"

He said, "Yes."

Then I said, "That is what I meant when I accused you of making a fool of yourself — I have warned you many times against the drug, yet you paid no attention to my warning."

It was difficult to convince him that he did not have cancer. I told him to go back to work, get plenty of sleep, take some medicine which I gave him, and promised that in six months the tumor would absolutely disappear. Well, in just five months he was perfectly normal again and has remained well since, and that was ten years ago.

These tumors which are produced by penicillin all have about the same consistency although they may vary in size. In the early days of penicillin, such side effects were unsuspected. No warning had been given; in fact, even today many cases of such growths are removed by operation, the surgeon never suspecting that they were artificially produced by the drug. Now, do you want to risk penicillin?

This Week Magazine,[2] March 31, 1957, contains a graphic description of the dangers of antibiotics in the article entitled, "Antibiotics: Handle With Care." This is No. 78, they tell us, in *This Week's* "Good Health Series," authorized by the American Medical Association. The article is written by Perrin H. Long, M.D., Chairman of Department of Medicine, State University of New York Downstate Medical Center. Selections from the article follow:

QUESTION: Arnold Troy, of Barrington, R.I., writes: "I have just been through more than six weeks of the most miserable torture of my life from penicillin poisoning. I wonder whether you could print an article about this problem and also mention all the other commonly used antibiotics in relation to their bad side effects."

The American Medical Association suggested that we take Mr. Troy's question to Dr. Long. Here is his reply:

ANSWER: Many things that are useful to men may, under certain circumstances, be very dangerous. This is true in medicine, because drugs which help many people may turn out to be poisonous to others. . . . Competent authorities estimate that between *200 and 300 people will die* in the United States *this year* from what are called anaphylactoid reactions to the penicillins.

[2] Reprinted from *This Week* Magazine. Copyright 1957 by the United Newspapers Magazine Corporation.

These reactions occur in people who have become sensitized to penicillin, and occur within a few minutes after the injection or swallowing of penicillin.

Other antibiotics also have their perils. Streptomycin has produced uncontrollable dizziness, permanent deafness, fever and skin rashes, in a number of people. The tetracycline groups of antibiotics, while rarely producing reactions of sensitivity, do produce nausea, vomiting and diarrhea in certain patients. Also, by killing off the bacteria which are normally present in the bowel, they may permit the overgrowth of other disease-producing microorganisms, thus unfortunately producing another disease in the patient.

Chloramphenicol is charged with causing disturbances of the blood in a few patients. Bacitracin has caused kidney damage in certain individuals. Erythromycin has been responsible for skin rashes; and currently about 10 per cent of the patients receiving novobiocin, one of the newest antibiotics, are having fever and rashes. It should be clear to all that antibiotics are not harmless, and, like most drugs, some people react badly to them. . . .

It is well known that penicillin has *no curative effects* in the common cold, influenza and "virus" infections, other than those produced by the viruses of psittacosis (parrot fever) and trachoma. Regardless of this knowledge, patients insist on having penicillin, and doctors give it, when the patient has a "cold" or "flu" or a "virus." Doctors say if they don't give it, their patients will go to a doctor who does, and, of course, doctors don't like to lose their patients.

Every doctor should know that penicillin must be used with the greatest care in patients who are already allergic, such as individuals who have hay fever, asthma, or certain types of eczema. These individuals easily become sensitized to penicillin, and serious reactions may occur when this antibiotic is given.

People who don't know they are allergic may get a minor reaction to their first dose of penicillin. This is a *red danger signal,* and they should remember to inform any doctor treating them in the future of their sensitivity.

Recently a physician told me a sad story which illustrates the problem: He was called to see a patient who suffered from asthma and who had just developed a common cold. She demanded that he give her an injection of penicillin, stating that that was the way her colds were always treated, and she would get another doctor if he didn't. He refused, and was immediately dismissed.

Another physician was called, who administered the penicillin. The patient died of an anaphylactoid reaction within three minutes after the drug was injected.

Who was to blame? Both the patient and the second doctor were at fault. She for demanding treatment with the threat of getting another doctor; he for permitting the patient to direct a type of treatment which he should have known was *valueless* and might even be dangerous.

What can be done about the increasing number of reactions to antibiotics?

First, the patient and his physician must realize that antibiotics are not completely harmless agents.

Second, physicians must administer antibiotics only when the indications for their curative effects are clear.

Third, the public must rid itself of the notion that antibiotics are cure-alls.

Why then must sick people have to submit to the dangerous methods of Orthodox medicine today? The article which I have just quoted was instigated by the complaint of a man who was made ill by penicillin. The situation is such that even the AMA cannot ignore it, but the explanation which they give falls far short of any legitimate excuse for their continuing to give such stuff to sick people.

All through this book I have criticized the present Orthodox medical setup. I have also said that all down through the ages thinking men have criticized the then existing medical measures, but up until the time the Law of Similars was discovered, there was nothing in the way of *constructive* criticism.

Now the world knows, or should know, that there is a Law of Nature to direct the choice of *curative* remedies for all kinds of illness, remedies which have no action but to cure. There are no dangerous and fatal side-effects, and, as I have said before, this knowledge is free to the world.

CHAPTER 9

Some Current Medical Practices

A prominent woman was brought to my hospital one day unconscious. She had suffered a brain concussion as a result of an automobile accident. She had no open wound, had lost no blood. She remained unconscious for several days, a not uncommon occurrence in such cases. The husband was, of course, fearfully worried. He called in a specialist from a hospital of which he, the husband, was a trustee. He wanted the doctor to do something and to do it at once. The poor doctor was "on the spot." He consulted me. He suggested transfusions. That would satisfy the husband and show him that something was being done.

I said, "No, a blood transfusion is dangerous."

The husband insisted. A transfusion was performed by the doctor. The reaction was marked. It was unfavorable.

In a few days the patient had managed to eliminate the foreign blood and went back to her former condition, which was good and satisfactory and consistent with a severe concussion. Her temperature had returned to normal. All was well except that she still remained unconscious. Again her husband became impatient, and again the doctor was "on the spot."

He again consulted me, and my answer was still the same: "Let her absolutely alone. She will come out of it in a few days." (I once had had a patient who had remained unconscious for twenty-one days and then recovered beautifully.)

The pressure from the husband was too great, however, and another transfusion was performed. Death occurred immediately. It is impossible to prove or disprove that the transfusion killed her. My conclusion, based upon many years of experience and observation, is that it did.

In the December 8, 1947, issue of the *New Republic,* Leonard Engle, Science Editor of *Readers Scope,* and a regular contributor on scientific subjects to *Science Illustrated,* the *Toronto Star Weekly,* and *Science Correspondent to the Nation,* pointed out that certain states have the good fortune to have plenty of whole blood for tranfusions and medical purposes, free of any expense except the doctor's fee. In other states and cities a snag was struck which prevented the fulfillment of this "great humanitarian project." He also called tragic anything that thwarts the Red Cross' attempts to succeed in its endeavors to secure blood. He said that at the present time three million Americans will be treated with some form of blood this year and that its use will grow within five years to ten million annually. He made the flat statement that tomorrow's blood therapy will help eight to ten million Americans per year back to health, but only if blood is available.

He warned against a dwindling supply and gave a formidable list of endorsements from the Army, Navy, Health Boards, American Medical Association, etc.

He criticized the practice of some who buy blood for five dollars per pint and sell it for fifteen dollars. He characterized as scandalous the alleged practice of bleeding over and over again whiskey-soaked bowery bums, poorly fed derelicts, etc., and stressed that damage is being done to those poor, unfortunate donors who manage to exist somehow with the help of the five-dollar fee which they receive as often as they can build up another pint of blood, wherein lies the scandal. He expects you to take for granted that all of this blood is necessary for the health of the nation.

Nothing is less true. The author misses the most glaring flaw in the whole argument and that is: *the blood itself that comes from the veins of drunken derelicts, blood in which alcohol, tobacco and perhaps other narcotics are not the only deleterious substances.* The blood in any person is in reality the person himself. It contains all the peculiarities of the individual from whence it comes. This includes hereditary taints, disease susceptibilities, poisons due to personal living, eating and drinking habits.

Every individual has his own type of blood and since *no two are exactly alike,* you cannot with impunity put another person's blood into your veins no matter how well typed. Your system has to get rid of it and begins to do so *immediately* and continues to do so until it has all been eliminated.

If a person is doomed to ultimate insanity, the cause of it will be found in his blood. If one is headed for diabetes, cancer, tuberculosis, etc., the *poisons which eventually produce such diseases are in the blood first and remain there.*

The poisons that produce the impulse to commit suicide, murder, or steal are in the blood. Hepatitis, boils, abscesses, carbuncles, anemia, any systemic disease, the venereal diseases, malaria — the causative poisons of all of these are in the blood even before the symptoms appear. There is no way of determining beforehand whether such poisons are present. Even the test for syphilis is untrustworthy.

A lot of propaganda is circulated about purifying the blood and only using the clean residue. It cannot be done. The bloodletting of yore has been superseded by blood transfusion. Of all the ridiculous medical practices of the past and present times, this present blood craze is the worst. It is not only useless where fractional blood is used, but often deadly where whole blood is used. Blood once removed from the living body becomes a dead, abhorrent, loathsome substance no matter how fractionized or preserved. It can serve no purpose whatever in sickness of any kind. In place of blood transfusions, one should use normal saline, which is the natural basis of all blood — the saline of the ocean where man first started.

In performing upwards of twenty thousand surgical operations, I never gave a blood transfusion and never had a patient die from lack of it.

I have given many "transfusions" of normal *Salt Solution*. It is better and safer. I have used it in cases of all degrees of exsanguination and none died. Some were white as chalk and cold as stone, but they lived.

*   *   *

A young woman came to me not so long ago for an operation. She was actually beaming as she related her experience at one of Boston's well-known clinics. She said, "I have just been thoroughly examined at the wonderful X clinic. It is such a beautiful place. I was there seven days, and it cost $190, but it was really worth it."

She handed me a stack of laboratory reports and final diagnosis, and now she was ready for the operation. I listened patiently and then said, "My, my, what an experience; and whom did you meet at the marvelous place? Not God by any chance?"

She gasped, "Why, what do you mean?"

"Of course, it is a nice place," I said, "but beautiful furniture and high prices won't tell you what is the matter with you. Neither will a machine-made diagnosis help much. The question is who made the diagnosis. Is it reliable? Can it be depended upon? Not by me, at least. I never operate on another man's diagnosis, especially if the diagnosis is made by laboratory and instruments alone. I learned to make diagnoses long before all these so-called instruments of precision were invented."

"Now," I said, "if you will go with my nurse, she will get you ready, and in five minutes, not seven days, I will tell you just what is really wrong, if anything."

The examination was made and a condition was found entirely different from that claimed by the X clinic. An operation was necessary, which I performed, and the patient went home entirely cured at the end of ten days. She also had a chronic eye trouble for which she had been treated by numerous doctors without benefit. She was reconciled to it and considered it incurable. She received the proper Homœopathic remedy while convalescing from her operation, and it too was cured. You never saw such a happy patient.

Why did the clinic overlook the eye trouble and why did it fail to make the correct surgical diagnosis? I'll tell you. It was because apparently not a single doctor connected with this well-known clinic is capable of making a diagnosis through his own personal skill, which is only acquired by careful observation and experience. Neither have they any knowledge of curative internal medicine. They rely entirely on instruments of precision and laboratory findings, and that is not good enough. The patient's symptoms, about which he complains, are Nature's cry for help and are usually ignored by the doctors. Without careful consideration of these symptoms, correct treatment is often impossible to give.

I know the value of the laboratory as well as any man. I also know its limitations probably better than most doctors. The general public has accepted it as the great streamlined advancement in scientific medicine, as was expected of them, along with transfusions, miracle drugs, etc., and are perfectly willing to pay the price for such service and abide by it. If subsequently the case dies, who is to blame? Wasn't everything known to medical science invoked? You can't gainsay the Laboratory! No indeed!

For medical purposes instrument-made diagnoses are of very little value, if any. Remedies seldom can be chosen for sick people through laboratory findings. Remedies are chosen through the patient's symptoms. True, the laboratory helps diagnose diabetes, for instance. Insulin is therefore prescribed, but insulin is not a *cure* for diabetes; it does not stimulate the body to secrete its own insulin.

The number of cases of this disease is greater today than at any time in medical history. Diabetes does not obtain until after a previous disturbance of function somewhere in the body which the laboratory cannot detect until too late. (The same may be said of tuberculosis.) A good Homœopath may be able to prevent diabetes by prescribing the constitutionally-indicated remedy when the disturbance of function first occurs, symptoms of which are present long before the laboratory can shed any light on the case.

At the moment the people are being lured by hundreds of thousands to submit to X-rays of the chest, allegedly for the purpose of determining whether or not they have tuberculosis, and at what stage. The claim being made is that X-ray will determine in time to make a cure in cases just beginning. It sounds very reasonable, and the public is responding gladly and willingly, and someone — the taxpayer — is paying indirectly for millions of dollars worth of film. It is extremely doubtful that any good will come of this measure, and very likely a lot of harm will be done.

X-ray will *not* show the beginning of a sickness, which at first is only a disturbance of function, but which may in some cases eventuate as tuberculosis. Many people have had some trouble with their lungs at one time or another in their lives of which they were not aware, and which healed spontaneously, leaving a scar or spot which will cast a shadow on the X-ray plate. This may erroneously be diagnosed as being trouble that something should be done about, even if the patient is perfectly well. It is difficult for even a so-called expert to determine whether it is an old scar or an active one. If it is determined to be active, what is the doctor going to do about it? Although he knows little or nothing about its treatment, you may be assured he will do something, and that something is usually wrong. Today's doctors still try to treat disease, instead of treating the patient who is sick.

A young man who took the test was told that the X-ray revealed a spot, and something must be done for it. It came as a great surprise to the young man, because he had been feeling perfectly well. He had just gone for a check-up as the public was advised to do. The last I heard from him he was in a hospital, helpless and completely deaf, all as a direct result of the "something" that was done for him.

If the advocates of this actually very foolish and dangerous procedure are earnestly concerned about the tuberculosis "situation" — the safeguarding of the people — they would do a much better job if they would use their influence to insist on the teaching of real curative medicine by the medical schools, along with the correct philosophy of disease, all of which would produce real physicians who could recognize at once any signs that any ailing individual may be heading for ultimate tuberculosis, and would know what to do about it. Homœopathic doctors could recognize impending tuberculosis and knew how to prevent it long before the X-ray was discovered.

X-rays are not only often inconclusive, they are also dangerous as is shown in the following item by Frances Burns in the *Boston Globe,* May 16, 1957 (reprinted by permission):

There's a tendency in modern medicine to make more X-rays than are necessary, particularly for people who always think there's something the matter with them, Dr. Dameshek and Dr. Frederick W. Gunz say in a guest editorial in the *Journal of the American Medical Association.* Dr. Gunz, from Bart's, London, formerly a fellow at the New England Center Hospital, now is at Christ Church, New Zealand.

Studies in connection with atomic radiation have demonstrated that radiation accumulates for a lifetime in the body, *even when there are small doses of it.*

Doctors are trying to find out why Leukemia has "shown a striking increase in the past 20 years," Dr. Dameshek points out.

"This increase," he said, "was apparent well before the recent increasing use of radioactive isotopes, atomic bomb tests, etc.

"Is it possible that one of the reasons for the increase is the great expansion of the use of diagnostic and therapeutic X-ray procedures during the last few decades?"

There is one thing physicians and researchers are sure of, say the physicians. Leukemia comes as a result of ionizing radiation. This is shown because:

(1) Radiologists or doctors who take X-ray themselves have leukemia eight to 10 times as frequently as other doctors,

(2) Leukemia occurred 12 times as often in those who survived the atomic blasts near the center in Hiroshima and Nagasaki, as in those on the edge of the area.

(3) There is a relatively high incidence of leukemia in persons in Britain and Holland treated with X-ray for spondylitis, a disease of the spine.

(4) Leukemia develops often in persons treated by X-ray for enlarged thymus, a chest gland.

(5) Possible leukemic effect has been noted on babies of mothers who have had X-rays to determine the size of the baby and its position in the womb.

One patient, Dr. Dameshek explained, had been given X-ray treatment for one kind or another of skin disease four times in 10 years. Such treatment might deliver as much as 1000 to 1200 roentgen rays; for rheumatic spondylitis, several thousand rays.

It is by no means proved, comment the doctors, that diagnostic and treatment X-rays are clearly related to leukemia in human beings. But it is time to take precautions, nevertheless.

They propose that there be a "strict evaluation and eventual limitation" of the use of X-rays in treating non-cancerous skin disease, bursitis, rheumatoid spondylitis and enlarged thymus in infancy. This involves the setting up of committees by medical society and specialty groups.

Unnecessary and frequently repeated diagnostic X-ray procedures should be limited. "Many of these procedures are routine and at times seem to be carried out solely for the purpose of completeness of the examination. Many neurotic persons or diagnostic 'problem' cases go from clinic to clinic and each clinic almost invariably feels impelled to take its own X-rays," the doctors said.

Finally, each diagnostic and therapeutic X-ray procedure should be recorded in a suitable booklet to be kept by everyone as a permanent record of his dosage.

This booklet would tell the doctor at a glance whether the patient was beginning to exceed his lifetime quota of permissible X-ray dosage. It would have the psychological effect, say the doctors, of tending to curtail the use of unnecessary X-rays.

The Massachusetts Division of the American Cancer Society has called attention to the importance of this record by the two physicians.

It is very gratifying to me to see that there are now some thinkers who have devoted considerable study to the matter of the dangers of X-rays and who are at last revealing the dangers to the public.

Yet at the present moment many obstetricians insist that a series of X-rays be taken during pregnancy to show the relative size of the baby's head, the outlet of the pelvis and position of child, etc.[1] If such procedures were necessary, one might well ask what did the people do before the advent of the X-ray? Who is your doctor and why?

[1] See chapter on Having A Baby.

CHAPTER 10

Vaccination

If the general public were presented honestly with the abundant medical data available proving the most harmful effects of vaccine, they could understand why cancer, tuberculosis, heart disease, etc., can and quite often do result from these poisonous substances introduced directly into the blood by pointed needles. The inoculations lay the foundation for such diseases as syphilis, tetanus, cerebrospinal meningitis, glandular abscess, erysipelas, cancer, tuberculosis, polio, encephalitis, and many other manifestations of pathology.

England had compulsory vaccination for many years and during such time had many cases of smallpox causing death among the vaccinated. The law was repealed some years ago, and there ensued almost a freedom from the disease. The death rate dropped to nearly zero.

It might be enlightening to read the opinion of some prominent Englishmen, lay as well as professional, which eventually resulted in the abolishment of the compulsory vaccination law in England:

John Walter Carr, M. D., C.B.E., in his Presidential Address to the Medical Society of London, on the 8th of October, 1928, said: "Our views about vaccination are changing: they would probably change even more quickly had it not become part of the official creed, established by law and therefore as dogmatic and as difficult to alter as the Athanasian Creed [1] itself."

Major Greenwood, D.Sc., F.R.C.P., F.R.S., Medical Officer (Medical Statistics) at the Ministry of Health, stated: "A dreadful amount of nonsense was perpetually talked about vaccination, and that was the

---

[1] The symbol of doctrine called after Athanasius, 298?-373 (one of the fathers of the Church and patriarch of Alexandria), and formerly ascribed to his authorship, but now assigned to a later date: sometimes called the "Quicunque vult" (Whosoever will) from the first words of the Latin text.

difficulty. In Jenner's classical paper no mistake was omitted that could possibly have been made and there was a good deal of evidence that Jenner had been a rogue." (*Lancet*, February 2, 1929, P. 233)

Charles Creighton, M.D. was described by Professor William Bulloch, F.R.S., in an obituary notice published in *The Lancet* on July 30, 1927, as "the most learned man I ever knew," and his *History of Epidemics in Britain*, as "the greatest work of medical learning published during the nineteenth century by an Englishman." Dr. Creighton told the Royal Commission that he never questioned his early teaching on smallpox and vaccination until preparatory to writing the article on Vaccination for the 9th edition of the *Encyclopaedia Britannica*. Ultimately, he described vaccination as a "grotesque superstition."

The following extract from the obituary in *The Lancet* gives food for thought on this question:

The issue between Creighton and general professional opinion on vaccination was not thrashed out there and then as it ought to have been. It was deemed more expedient to drop Creighton into oblivion, and if he was ever referred to at all it was as "Creighton the Anti-Vaccinator." All his other work was forgotten in the debacle, and he was a doomed man. . . . In the opinion of many he was harshly treated by the world for holding views that did not conform to standard. Perhaps this very world has become more tolerant than it was in Creighton's time, because even in his own subject there are epidemiologists who express with impunity today views as heterodox as those for which Creighton was pillorized and ostracised forty years ago.

Edgar M. Crookshank, M.D., Professor of Pathology and Bacteriology at King's College, London, said that when Sir James Paget directed his attention to one of Dr. Creighton's works, "at that time I accepted and taught the doctrines current in the profession and to be found in the textbooks of medicine." After two years of intense laboratory work and investigations, here and on the Continent, he issued imposing volumes on *The History and Pathology of Vaccination,* in which he fully supported Dr. Creighton's contentions, saying that the abandonment of vaccination altogether would show the great advance made in Pathology and Sanitary Science.

Sir Benjamin Ward Richardson, M.D., FRS., when reviewing Professor Crookshank's "History and Pathology of Vaccination," in *The Asclepiad,* 1890 said: "The life and letters of Jenner comprise an analysis mortal to the scientific reputation, and even to the morality, of that much be-lauded man. We have set up the idol and the world has lent itself to the idolatry, because we, whom the world trusted, have set the example. But the world nowadays discovers idolatries on its own account; and if we continue the idolatry it will simply take its own course, and, leaving us on our knees, will march on whilst we petrify."

Sir W. D. Collins, M.D., M.S., ex-chairman of the London County Council, for seven years a member of the Royal Commission on Vac-cination, stated: "There are members of my own profession, whose reputa-tion and standing cannot be disputed, who are profound sceptics in re-gard to Vaccination." (House of Commons, February 15, 1907)

C. C. Okell, M.A., M.C., D.Sc., F.R.C.P., late Bacteriologist to Uni-versity College Hospital said: "Compulsory Vaccination once had the suffrage of the Nation, but now it has hardly a serious supporter." *(Lancet, January 1, 1938.)*

Expert criticism of vaccination is generally stifled by reason of the fact that non-acceptance of the Orthodox views may prevent medical men from obtaining official positions and honors in the profession. A few examples are now given.

W. Scott Tebb, M.A., M.D., DPH, was appointed Medical Officer of Health for Penge, but was not allowed to accept the post when the Local Government Board found that he was the author of a scholarly work entitled, "A Century of Vaccination and What it Teaches."

Charles Ruata, M.D., Professor of Materia Medica at the University of Perugia, wrote a long letter on "Vaccination in the Italian Army," in which he gave the statistics of the terrible ravages of smallpox among the Italian troops, in spite of their most thorough vaccination. The letter was published in the *British Medical Journal,* May 27, 1899, and resulted in Dr. Ruata's being prosecuted for medical heresy!

Walter R. Hadwen, M.D., J.P., of Gloucester, for twenty-two years President of the British Union for the Abolition of Vivisection, wrote, lectured and debated against the practice of Vaccination. He was black-balled out of the British Medical Association after having spoken against vaccination at a public meeting. As a result of his opposition to treat-ments derived from vivisection he had to endure boycott and misrepre-sentation which ended in his being tried on a charge of manslaughter, of which he was duly acquitted.

The 14 *Medical Vice Presidents* of the National Anti-Vaccination

League. These, and some other fifty or sixty fully-qualified medical men, have all been trained in the faith. They, of course, realized that, when openly declaring themselves against vaccination, they were abandoning all hope of attaining any professorships or other official positions.

Alfred Russel Wallace, LL.D., F.R.S., who, at the same time as Darwin, evolved the theory of natural selection, was strongly opposed to the practice of vaccination, and said that he regarded his books on vaccination as the most important of his scientific works. *(My Life, page 333)*

Catherine Booth, wife of the founder of the Salvation Army, observed the bad effects of vaccination during her extensive experience in visiting the poor. She wrote to a friend:

I send by this post a pamphlet on vaccination. Do read it, if only for the exhibition it gives of the prejudice of the "profession." It seems as though all advance in the right treatment of the disease had to be, in the first instance, largely in spite of the doctors, instead of their leading the way. I should sooner pawn my watch to pay the fines, and my bed, too, for the matter of that, than have any more children vaccinated. The monstrous system is as surely doomed as bloodletting was. Who knows how much some of us have suffered through life owing to the "immortal Jenner"? . . . There is nothing worse in this pamphlet than several cases I have come across personally. But these were the direct results. It is the indirect that I fear most. The latent seeds of all manner of diseases are doubtless sown in thousands of healthy children. *(Mrs. Booth of the Salvation Army*, by W. T. Stead, pages 204-205)

The doctors mentioned above were all allopaths.

Dr. A. D. Speransky, famous Russian scientist, conducted researches and experiments over a period of ten years and set forth his findings in 1934 in a book, *A Basis for the Theory of Medicine*. Speaking with complete candor on the question of immunization, Dr. Speransky says:

More than once, isolated voices of physicians have been raised in warning against the seduction of inoculations and of so-called diagnostic tests (the reactions of Pirquet, Schick, Dick, etc.), which are widely used in schools and children's clinics. Such voices have not been heeded as they should have been, since they only pointed out isolated facts and could not explain them. Indeed they met with numerous objections on the part of those who held the view that skin inoculation tests are harmless on the ground that in the vast majority of cases such operations are not followed by any immediate harm. . . .

Following the outbreak of encephalitis in the Netherlands, England and Wales in 1928, the Health Commission of the League of Nations sent a commission of inquiry into those countries. From the report of the Health Organization of the League issued on August 27, 1928, we collected the following illuminating report:

The post-vaccinal encephalitis with which we are dealing has become a problem in itself mainly in consequence of the events of the last few years in The Netherlands, England and Wales. In each of these countries the cases which have occurred have been sufficiently numerous and similar to require them to be considered collectively. Their occurrence has led to the realization that a new, or at least previously unsuspected or unrecognized risk attaches to the practice of vaccination.

In England and Wales in the 38 years ending December 1937, only 118 children died of smallpox, but 291 *died of vaccination,* according to a reply of the Minister of Health to a question in Parliament on July 13, 1938.

Investigations conducted in England and made public through *The Lancet,* and other publications, show that brain fever, spinal meningitis, lock-jaw and sleeping sickness result from vaccination. The germ supposed to be identified with smallpox has never been isolated and it is apparent that the viruses identified with the above diseases are non-filtrable and ultra-microscopic and find their way readily into laboratory vaccines. In infantile paralysis, for example, the common medical theory is that this disease is produced by an ultra-microscopic, nonfiltrable virus. This theory is set forth in the *Practice of Medicine,* edited by Dr. Frederick Tice, Julius Friedenwald, and L. F. Warren, and published by W. F. Prior Company. In it Dr. Tice says:

Microscopic examinations of the poliomyelitis tissues reveal no visible microorganism. Therefore the micro-organism must be beyond the range of the microscope. *The micro-organism of poliomyelitis is there characterized as a filter-passing ultra-microscopic virus.* Recent developments in the field of virus classification place it along with the smaller particle viruses such as the virus of foot and mouth disease.

It is now a matter of official Navy record that vaccination for smallpox can cause *syphilis.*

Reporting in the April, 1941 issue of the *Naval Medical Bulletin* on the results of tests on 20,000 recruits at the Naval Training Station, San Diego, California, between July, 1939, and January, 1941, Capt. G. E. Thomas of the Medical Corps of the United States Navy found that there was a relationship between cowpox vaccination and the "false" positive test. As an example, he cited a recruit who had a negative Kahn test on first arriving at the station. A first vaccination failed, but after a second vaccination he developed a marked vaccinia. Three weeks later the recruit was selected as a blood donor for a city hospital, and a Kline test performed there was found to be positive. A Wasserman and a Kahn test performed at the Naval Station were both positive. The recruit had not been on liberty since arriving at the station, and it was Capt. Thomas' opinion that the findings were the results of vaccination.

Having quoted almost exclusively from the brilliant men, past and present, of Orthodox medicine concerning their views on smallpox vaccination, I would like here to give you the viewpoint of one of the greatest Homœopathic doctors the world has ever seen — the late Dr. Stuart Close of Brooklyn, New York. The following is a selection from a paper read before the Homœopathic Medical Society of the County of Kings, February 19, 1901, entitled "Vaccination from a Homœopathic Standpoint."

It is time that vaccination should be studied from the standpoint of biology. Such a study will show that "pure virus" is an absolute impossibility in the very nature of the case.

Admitting that "vaccine has a natural tendency to degenerate," the question at once arises as to the point at which degeneration begins. Biology, reason and experience unite in declaring that the process of degeneration begins the moment the human element is introduced into the organism of a lower order of being — an animal. When we see a man fall from the top of a ten-story building we say he is lost. We say that before he has fallen a foot. The same principle that made him fall one foot will inevitably make him fall the rest of the way. He is a dead man from the very first.

When the human virus of smallpox is inoculated into an animal organism that organism is instantaneously affected. The disease which is set up is a mongrel thing, neither human or animal. It is the expression or manifestation of a union under which a reversal of the law of evolution takes place — a degeneration. It is a promiscuous mixing of diverse elements, and its tendency is rapidly downward from the beginning. Syphilis in its origin was possibly the result of a similar promiscuity between the sexes in different orders of being, causing a degenerative process that, once initiated, became rapidly more and more malignant until it assumed its typical form. Vaccinia therefore is degenerated variola.

The pathological analogy between vaccinia and syphilis is so close that many observers and students of the subject believe them identical; but into that subject time forbids me to enter, except to point out that, like syphilis and unlike smallpox, vaccinia or degenerated variola, is not acute, not definite and not self-limited. On the contrary, the condition set up by vaccination is chronic, is as protean in its manifestations as syphilis, which it closely resembles, and enters as a complicating and modifying factor into every state of the individual victim. It forms a dyscrasia, in other words, comparable only to that of syphilis, tuberculosis and cancer.

Of the two evils which is preferable? It would seem that an informed and unprejudiced mind, having to choose between the mere possibility of an acute, tractable, natural disease from which recovery is perfect, and the certainty of a chronic, degenerate, artificially produced disease, would have no difficulty in deciding which was the lesser evil.

The product of this mongrel disease, when reinoculated into the human organism, remains true to the principle of degeneration under which it has come into existence, and continues to act under that principle to the end. . . .

It was formerly thought that one attack of smallpox conferred immunity from subsequent attacks. Instead of that being true, it is now known that one attack predisposes to a second attack. The German investigator Vogt has shown that the liability to a second attack is sixty per cent greater than to the first, while at the same time the percentage of deaths from second attacks is much higher. This of itself is a powerful argument against ordinary vaccination and preventive inoculations, which are based on the supposition that one attack confers immunity from a second. If this is true, it explains why smallpox always appears first among the vaccinated, and why smallpox continues to infest the civilized world while its allied "filth diseases" of the middle ages have disappeared before the advance of civilization, through the good offices of hygiene, sanitation and isolation.

For the physician or layman familiar with the principles of Homœpathy, the problem is a simple one, and the solution is at hand. Once it is clearly perceived that the question is a medical one, and the substance used a drug, all is easy. Potentization and administration of the medicine by the ordinary natural channels follows logically and naturally. There is ample room here for individual differences of opinion as to the merits of low potencies and high potencies, as with all other drugs. The homœpathic low potency user who desired to prescribe arsenic or lachesis, would scarcely think of doing so by inoculating the crude substance directly into the circulating fluids by means of the lancet or scarifying needle. There are very few men who would dare give lachesis, or any of the nosodes, below the sixth potency, administered by the mouth, and even then they would be very careful to see that there was no crack or abrasion about the mouth, lips or tongue of the subject. Vaccine is a nosode, the degenerated animalized product of smallpox, a poison whose virulence is often quite as terrifying as that of the snake-poisons, and which should be treated with quite as much caution. Allopathic physicians and surgeons recognize this, and attempt, though very clumsily, to dilute and modify the various toxins used by passing them through several animal organisms before they dare use them. This is only a crude imitation of the simple, positive and truly scientific homœpathic potentization. This method is unscientific and uncertain because there is no way of measuring or controlling the modifying influence upon the poison of a living animal organism. Life is an indeterminate quantity, and no two living organisms are alike. It is dangerous because it introduces the principle of degeneration.

The theory that the animal organisms under the influence of a toxin of disease produces an antitoxin by which a degree of protection to life is obtained, and that they are able to separate this anti-toxic serum from the toxic fluids is mere assumption and wholly outside the real question.

The effect of such an assumption has been to befog the whole subject, to blind the eyes of all parties concerned to the essential truth and to prevent the slightest progress in acquiring better methods.

The living organism can in some measure protect itself against poisons introduced into it through the natural channels. Every secretion of the bodily organs acts upon and modifies to some extent the poison as it is brought successively in contact with them. The saliva, the gastric juice, the biliary and pancreatic secretions, the intestinal mucous and other mucous secretions all act upon it, diluting, modifying and changing it according to chemical and biological laws, while the reflex actions of vomiting, perspiration, diarrhea, fever and pain all play their part in aiding to expel the noxious matter and maintain the integrity of the organism. But when a poison is introduced by inoculation into the circulatory fluids of the body and through wounded terminal nerve fibres to the central nervous system, every *effort of nature is thwarted,* every safeguard is destroyed and the very centers of life are invaded. It has free course and full power to injure and destroy. The protective secretions themselves are poisoned, because their source — the blood — is poisoned.

Every argument in favor of the use of potentized medicines in the treatment of disease applies with equal force to vaccine virus, or any other nosode or "serum" — used either for prophylaxis or treatment. No exception can be made without violating and invalidating the fundamental principles of Homœpathy. If potentized medicines are effectual in any condition of disease they are in all. Potentization of medicines is logically and necessarily involved in accepting and applying the principle of Similars. The Homœopathic remedy must be similar to the disease in form or nature, as well as in effects or symptoms. As disease is a dynamic disturbance, immaterial, intangible, "spirit-like," as Hahnemann says, so must the remedy be also. The remedy may be used in high potency, low potency or any intermediate potency, but to be truly effective for healing it must be potentized — carried beyond the crude state where it is recognized by the physical qualities of color, taste and odor. It must be in such a state that it can only be recognized by the finer organic and psychic senses, as shown in the reaction towards health. Only thus do we get true healing action. The action of crude drugs is toxic, not healing. If healing ultimately follows, it is at the expense of an excessive and unnecessary initial pathogenetic disturbance, by which the vital powers are wasted and recovery retarded.

No man can be truly said to be susceptible to smallpox or any other contagious disease who is in a state of perfect health, because the healthy organism is always in a positive condition, and the balance of power is on the side of health and vigor. Such a state resists and repels the assaults of all external influences. In one sense he is susceptible, as he is to all influences, but it is a sensitive, vital, defensive reactibility, or irritability, by which all noxious influences are quickly sensed but as quickly repelled and resisted. That is normal susceptibility. An abnormal susceptibility — that state in which he is liable to contract a disease — is a negative state, a state of depression, of lowered vital resisting power, of passivity, as it were, in which he is open to assault and makes little or no defense. This is essentially a state of disease and requires treatment. The balance of power is on the wrong side. It will be manifested to the acute observer by some signs or symptoms, which will indicate the Homœpathic remedy. The organism in the language of these symptoms demands the corresponding remedy as hunger demands food. Some element necessary to the integrity of the organism is lacking — and that element is the similar medicine in such form as may be quickly and easily appropriated by the suffering organism — in other words, the potentiated (potentized) remedy. When that remedy is found and administered, health is restored, the balance of power is returned to the right side, morbid susceptibility is removed and the man is safely and naturally protected from all assaults.

It is only necessary to restore and maintain health, which is opposed to disease in the very nature of things. Nothing can be more opposite and antagonistic than health and disease. Therefore the best protective against disease is health.

To give you an idea of the nature of these vaccines — in a speech at The Caxton Hall, Westminster, on Thursday, October 2, 1952, relative to Inoculation Dangers to Travellers, M. Beddow Bayly, M.R.C.S., L.R.C.P., said:

. . . from the *Handbook of Infectious Diseases,* issued by the League of Nations in 1945. Briefly: blood from a human typhus case is inoculated into guinea-pigs; their brain-tissue or blood is injected *per anum* into lice; when these have been fed for 7-8 days on human beings, they are crushed up and squirted into the nostrils of white mice or into the wind-pipes of dogs. These animals die of pneumonia in a few days, when a mixture of the ground-up lungs (one part mouse, two parts dog) provides the final life-preserving concoction for immunizing human beings against typhus.

When we recall that vaccine lymph is derived, in the first place, either from the ulcerated udder of a cow, a smallpox corpse, or the running sores of a sick horse's heels, the choice depending upon the country of its origin and the firm which manufactures it, it is hardly to be wondered at that it has far-reaching ill-effects on the human constitution. Years ago, the *Lancet* declared that "no practitioner knows whether the lymph he employs is derived from smallpox, rabbit pox, ass-pox, or mule-pox." Our own Ministry of Health has long confessed to complete ignorance of the ultimate source of its own supply of lymph; but last year Dr. A. W. Downie stated in the *British Medical Journal* that "the strain of vaccinia virus used for the routine preparation of lymph in this country is believed to have been derived from a case of smallpox in Cologne during the last century." That, of course, disposes of the whole theory of cow-pox vaccination.

Whatever the source may be — and there is little to choose between them in filthiness — the virus is rubbed into cuts or scratches on the shaved abdomen of a calf or sheep; after several days the contents of the pustules which form are scraped out, mixed with glycerine, kept for two weeks at 4°C, and issued in glass capillary tubes as pure glycerinated lymph. Presumably it is called "pure" because, under the Therapeutic Substances Act (1943) it must not contain more than 20,000 extraneous micro-organisms per cubic centimetre. Some fussy people, of course, may think this too many and demur at the title. They will not be reassured when they learn, according to the *British Medical Journal* (November 4th, 1950) that "With the best of care, heavy bacterial contamination of vaccine lymph is inevitable during its preparation, and as many as 500 million organisms per ml. may be present, particularly in the tropics. They belong mostly to the cocci group, but may include also Bacillus subtilis, Bac. coli, Pseudomones pyocyanea, yeasts and fungi; anærobic organisms may also be occasional contaminants. None of the methods advocated to reduce the number of bacteria can be considered satisfactory."

It is rather alarming, too, to learn that it has not long been discovered that the blood of persons recently vaccinated against smallpox gives a positive Wassermann reaction. To many this will give rise to a mental flash-back to the time when arm-to-arm vaccination, compulsory for 45 years — from 1853-1898 — was abandoned on account of the large increase in the number of deaths from infantile syphilis to which the procedure gave rise.

No wonder medical textbooks gave a whole catalogue of diseases as possible sequelae of vaccination; among them: erysipelas, boils, eczema, gangrene, impetigo, pemphigus, and, last but not least, acute encephalitis, which was the subject of investigation by two British Committees some years ago. The evidence submitted established beyond a doubt the casual relationship between vaccination and acute inflammation of the brain. Who knows how much chronic and unidentified damage to the brain and nervous system is done in other cases?

It would require a book the size of Webster's Unabridged to present even a fraction of the evidence against vaccination. Enough has been said here, however, to warrant the contention that compulsory vaccination affords no protection against smallpox and indeed may possibly even invite it.

These are facts, soberly considered, and stated with a full sense of the seriousness of the question. Study them, discuss them, inform yourself as to their evidential value, and their effect upon *you* and *your children*. And then *act*.

I have purposely presented the subject of smallpox and vaccination at some length because vaccination against smallpox is the father of the general theory of immunization against other diseases. I want you to be able to draw your own conclusion as to whether the results of such procedures are good or bad.

This matter is serious business. Vaccination against smallpox is only a small part of the deviltry of the advocates of the theory of immunization. The greatest menace lies in the possibility of compulsory vaccination of our young children and babies for all sorts of conjured-up diseases. Enough harm is being done right now through voluntary consent of misinformed mothers to have their babies polluted by these poisons almost from the time of their birth.

Germs which live habitually in man are harmless when man is in good health. Sickness in the individual stimulates them, gives them food, and makes them grow and reproduce.

The following is quoted from "Challenge of Germ Theory of Disease," published by the Responsible Enterprise Association:

Edgar C. Dunning, Doctor of Medicine (Homœopathy) from the University of Michigan presented to a meeting of parents gathered together by the Responsible Enterprise Association, Organizers of the Order of Patrick Henry, November 27, 1946, at Detroit, Michigan, some interesting discoveries challenging the germ theory of disease.

He pointed out confirmation by the Mayo Foundation of the discovery that merely a change in the food (culture medium) of germs will completely change their form; as bees can produce drones, workers, or queens, by merely changing the food of the larva.

He explained how invisible viruses, too small for any filter to hold, or any microscope to show, can be changed into full-sized bacteria of different kinds, depending upon the balance of food and minerals in the culture medium (the human body), or upon the vibration frequency of the electro-magnetic medium pervading all things, making very clear that most folks instead of using those big words would merely say, "depending on the effect of light."

Warnings have been issued that those who are allergic to eggs are liable to get severe reactions to the Asian flu serum. Patients are exhibiting definite reactions in the form of diarrhea, inflamed lumps at site of infection, general malaise and all symptoms similar to bad colds. In fact many patients get the symptoms of flu in spite of vaccination. In these cases of course the diagnosis is "cold" not flu.

It reminds one of a serious epidemic of smallpox that occurred some years ago in Monmouthshire, England, at a time when people were uncertain about the value of vaccination. Among those who fell victim to the epidemic, those who were vaccinated were diagnosed as chicken pox and those who were not vaccinated were diagnosed as smallpox.

If you have noticed, you will be impressed by the fact that lately very little has been in the news about polio. Why? Have you thought about that?

During the past years we were told by press, radio, and television of the hundreds of thousands of polio cases. A state of near-hysteria was whipped up during 1954, 1955 and 1956. It had the desired result of causing people to submit to Salk vaccine to such an extent that all interested parties were satisfied. Now the only news released is that there are few cases. It would seem to me that if everything that was said about polio during the preceding three years is true and that the disease has been conquered, there should be a joyous celebration instead of silence. In my humble opinion, there is as much polio today as there has been at any time in the past, but some people have very good reasons for letting sleeping dogs lie. People are buying the vaccine in satisfactory amounts — so let them assume the vaccine is effective.

No one ever knows how many cases of any sickness exist except for what is published for definite reasons. Seasonal colds — most of them now being called Asian flu — would be accepted as they have been since time began and no one would be giving them a thought, had not publicity at the instigation of the vaccine makers changed it all.

CHAPTER II

The Common Cold

In the March 4, 1957, *Time*,[1] appears a picture of the President and Mrs. Eisenhower. *Time* says, "With proper punctilio, the President's physician, Major General Howard Snyder, diagnosed this ailment, 'not a cold at all, but a mild case of tracheitis', i.e. inflammation of the wind pipe, accompanied by persistent coughing. Ike picked up his trouble, said Snyder, while standing for hours in the brisk breezy weather of Inauguration Day last month. Not even Georgia's warm sunshine burned it off. As a precautionary measure, Ike slipped off to Walter Reed Army Hospital the day after his T.V. speech on Israel to get X-rays of his sinuses and lungs. The result: negative. 'The President,' said the attendant physician, 'is fine.'"

As a matter of fact, the President had a cold, nothing more, nothing less. He did not pick it up — he developed it because he got cold. Instead of manifesting it in the usual way — running nose, etc., it showed up in the form of irritation in larynx and trachea by an annoying cough. Homœopathy would have prescribed a dose or two of *Aconite* which would have relieved and cured the whole condition almost immediately. Has Orthodox medicine anything as effective to offer?

It was ordained by our Creator that in order to remain healthy our body temperature must be maintained at the proper degree. When? Every moment of our lives. Where? Everywhere on the face of the earth. How? By seeing to it that the body gets proper and adequate protection against cold whenever and wherever it is necessary. Man is a warm-blooded animal and *must* be kept warm. This isn't the easiest or

---

[1]Courtesy *TIME*, The Weekly Newsmagazine, copyright Time, Inc., 1957.

the most convenient task there is, but it is certainly easier than having to undergo the suffering and danger of ailments.

In health, man's body temperature is 98.6° F. This is made possible through the very sensitive and automatic vasomotor system which controls the flow of perspiration from the skin. The principle on which it works in controlling temperatures is the well-known phenomenon of evaporation. In the process of metabolism (living), wherein a slow combustion or oxidation is taking place, there is a tendency to an increase in body temperature; at the same time there is a production of poison, a waste product which must be eliminated promptly and continuously. Man's own metabolic poison is more deadly to man than is the poison of any other animal. A means is provided for the elimination of this poison, in the form of moisture, through the pores of the skin. In this way, not only is the poison eliminated, but the temperature is kept normal and everything goes along fine. But things can happen to this system so that occasions arise where its smooth and automatic dual function is upset, and then trouble arises.

Animals are not interested in style. Their natural instincts search for safety. Domestic animals in drafty barns are subject to rheumatism. Dogs forced to sleep in drafty places will also suffer the same way. These animals' natural "clothing" for protection against cold is not enough under such conditions. Probably a draft is the thing most animals fear — they always seek sheltered spots. Primitive man did the same. As I traveled about in Europe, I was much interested to see the sleeping nooks in many of the palaces and castles. They had large, drafty rooms and buildings, but the people retired to sleep in small alcoves or holes in the wall, completely protected from moving air.

As most people think a cold is caused by germs, it prevents them from knowing the real cause and so they go on and on, year after year, always "catching cold." You never "catch" a cold — you develop a cold because you got chilled too much. A cold is no more contagious than a toothache. Some people can stand more cold than others, some are not influenced much by drafts — or at least think they are not, but even the hardiest succumb if they ignore it too long.

Many people cannot stand air-conditioned working quarters. They develop a cold in one form or another. What deceives people is the fact that a cold is not necessarily a running nose. Lucky indeed is the one whose nose does run fluently, for he is the one who will not have complications, unless anti-histamines or other kinds of drugs are given to stop the discharge. They do not realize that the discharge contains the *poisons that should have left the body by the natural exits,* through the *skin.* This discharge is the *first step toward recovery.* It is really a life-saver.

Many years ago I was listening to the election returns at the Highland Club in West Roxbury. It was a cold, wet night in November. The room was hot and stuffy and full of tobacco smoke, so it was thought to be a good idea to air it out for a while. The doors and windows were opened wide. I was sitting with two friends and we were caught in the path of an awfully cold draft of air, but we endured it until the windows were closed.

What happened to us? I got a bad cold, one of my friends got pneumonia and the other one got Bright's disease and died. From the same "exciting" cause (getting chilled) there developed in three different individuals a sickness of sufficient variation in symptoms as to warrant, according to the habit of the medical profession, a different diagnosis in each case. *No germ was responsible for these illnesses.* Neither should any of us have suffered anything more severe than a cold. The difference was because of the manner in which each one lived his daily life. One, myself, a non-smoker, non-drinker, light eater with little if any meat, developed a cold — nothing more. The other two, smokers, drinkers, heavy meat eaters, producing stronger metabolic poisons, fared far worse when the chilly draft suddenly stopped the elimination of these poisons which were escaping via the sweat glands in the skin. In one, the burden of elimination was transferred to the lungs, and in the other to the kidneys.

That is the way of all diseases; first, the exciting cause, then a disturbance in the function of some organ, and eventual pathology. The kind and extent of sickness eventuating in any individual is determined entirely by the condition of the person at the time, plus personal, inherited or acquired weakness or susceptibilities of any organ or organs of the body, and it becomes his own private, personal illness of which no two are ever exactly alike. Germs have nothing to do with it.

Dr. J. Haskel Kritzer, in an article he wrote in the *Journal of the National Medical Society,* said:

However debilitating and annoying as the common cold is, it is nevertheless a beneficial effort of nature to relieve the body of accumulations of morbid waste. The cold is, therefore, a natural safety valve, a corrective measure to compensate for incomplete elimination. The time, effort and money spent in the investigation of the common cold; the attempts to identify the specific germs, have thus far been fruitless. The only accomplished results are the manufacture of an unlimited variety of cold nostrums, serums and vaccines that are not only worthless, but are infinitely more harmful than the cold which they are intending to cure. It leads into a blind alley where space is endless and the invisible ultra-microscopic lives therein are inexhaustible. What unlimited fields to search for new germs and antibiotic vaccines. For the trend in modern medicine is a vaccine for every germ disease, a most dangerous and fallacious practice.

In warmth there is life; in cold there is death. The whole body should be warm. An exception might be the face and sometimes for a short period, the hands. The feet should always be kept warm.

One may get facial neuralgia, however, even on a warm day, if one sits for very long with a fan blowing on the face. Also, cold hands and especially cold feet often cause a cold. Hands working for too long a time, or too often in cold water, may lead to neuritis or arthritis in the arms.

I used to treat many cases of bursitis of elbow and shoulder brought on by driving either in an open car or with the window of a closed car down and the left arm protruding from the window. This occurred even though a heavy fur coat was worn.

A friend came to my office one day to get some medicine for a cold. She had a mutual friend with her who had remained in the car. I asked why the friend had not come in. The reply was, "She isn't feeling very well today because she is going to the hospital for an operation tomorrow." Naturally, I was concerned because here was a friend going to *another* hospital, when I considered mine about the best — so I asked why. I was told that a renowned surgeon was there who was an expert in removing bursae from the elbow. Eleanor had been told she had bursitis and that an operation was the only way she could be cured. I said to my friend, "Go get her this minute; I want to talk to her." She came in and I asked if she wasn't afraid the operation would do more harm than good. She replied, "Yes, but what can I do?" The history of her case revealed that she drove her car with her left elbow always protruding from the window. She had a very painful elbow, true enough. After I talked to her, she cancelled her appointment and I gave her a Homœopathic remedy and told her to protect the elbow from cold. She recovered completely in three days. Four years later, I met her. She was perfectly well, had no return, and took from her handbag an envelope with a few remaining pills which she was keeping "just in case."

Office buildings are often built with long corridors with a row of offices on either side. Each office has one or more windows and usually one door opening on the corridor. This affords adequate ventilation, only too often more than is needed. In small offices the occupant sits at his desk which is located where he will receive light to best advantage, but there is always a current of air coming in the window on its way to the corridor, which serves as a very efficient chimney. It may not even be noticed by anyone sitting there, but the draft constantly carries away vital body heat, and to one who is sensitive, often causes pain in neck, arms, shoulders and back. An insurance-man friend of mine had such an office and he was continually complaining of such aches and pains. These stopped as soon as he removed himself from the draft.

Many people, believing that germs or virus are responsible for colds, feel that if they can toughen their resistance by vigorous living, they can escape the germs. They think that by wearing summer clothing in the winter they can produce a sort of immunity to the cold. If a man goes without long underwear in cold weather and he gets a sore throat, tonsilitis, arthritis, etc., and thinks his ailment is *caused* by a germ or virus which is "going around," then you may be sure that the original cause will be maintained, and with germicides and antibiotics, which he will use sooner or later, he will surely prepare the way for an ultimately serious sickness.

Those who force themselves to endure the cold pay for it. All animals have an automatic power to provide extra protection against seasonal weather changes. Man is supposed to have sufficient intelligence to do it by his own efforts. This provision is only too often neglected because the reasons for it are not recognized.

Proper body temperature is a *must* if we are to remain healthy. Disregard of this important environment causes a vast variety of symptoms as Nature manifests her distress. Some denote light and trivial disturbances of the vital force, some deep and dangerous, all accompanied by various diagnoses — as follows — and all first cousins to the common cold.

1. Coryza (the common cold)
2. Pharyngitis
3. Laryngitis
4. Bronchitis
5. Bronchopneumonia
6. Lobar Pneumonia
7. Tonsilitis
8. Mastoiditis
9. Sinusitis
10. Cerebrospinal meningitis
11. Poliomyelitis
12. Headache
13. Backache
14. Stiff neck
15. Bursitis
16. Myelitis
17. Rheumatism
18. Arthritis
19. Acute Nephritis
20. Chronic Nephritis
    (Bright's Disease)
21. Sciatica
22. Diarrhea
23. Facial Neuralgia
24. Otalgia (earache)
25. Cough
26. Diphtheria
27. Croup
28. Shingles
29. Coldsores, etc.

Some people seem to develop colds more readily than others. I think it is because the thermostat in their vasomotor system is highly sensitive. It shuts off the excretion of perspiration poisons at the slightest feeling of cold.

By personal experiments, I have found that undue oversensitiveness to cold and drafts may be helped by a gradual toughening of the sensitive skin by a gradual lowering of water temperature in one's bath, either tub or shower, so that often a person eventually enjoys a cold tub or shower — to be followed *always* by a brisk rubdown till dryness is complete and then one finds himself less susceptible to changes in weather and less prone to develop colds.

I found that a quick plunge each morning in a tub of cold water works wonders. I never had any kind of a cold while doing it. Try it. It may do you a lot of good. Do not use water *too* cold to begin with.

Children are sinned against sadly by their well-meaning but unthinking parents. Evidently style in clothing dictates that a child is more attractive when bare from its little bottom to its ankles. Submitting to it, the poor child suffers all kinds of ailments. It is conceded by doctors who know, that 76 per cent of all children's diseases are due to inadequate clothing. That includes such conditions as enlarged tonsils, mastoiditis, infantile paralysis (polio), rheumatism, etc.

I was called in to see three little boys one day. Their ages were 2, 4 and 6. The poor little fellows were the most woebegone creatures, all suffering from colds. They had received shots of antibiotic germ killers from their family doctor, which only made them worse. One had an earache, one had sore and swollen gums following the administration of these drugs.

The Homœopathic remedy was given and the earache was gone next morning and the gums of the other little boy cleared up during the day. The parents were discouraged because each year they "picked up the germs" and were sick nearly all winter. Each year the parents had large drug and doctor bills to pay and they could ill afford such expense. It was unfortunate too, because it was all so unnecessary.

I found that none of these children had ever worn long underwear in the winter. I had their mother feel their bare skin under their overalls; they were stone cold. The mother was really surprised. She had no idea that their poor little legs could get so cold with the long dungarees on. I explained that such clothing was inadequate. Overalls or pants are not sufficient. They act as chimneys which permit a stream of air to go up and down the bare legs, which is often harmful as it carries away that indispensable layer of warm air.

I personally went to a mill where long underwear was made and brought them home a supply. The boys were delighted and felt much better after putting them on.

Do your part for the sake of your children's health. A child's legs should be covered by snug-fitting stockings from his feet all the way up to and beyond the underwear. Remember that it is the thin layer of still air which lies next to the skin that keeps a body warm and healthy, and that the presence of this warm layer of air is made possible only by garments that fit snugly.

When children cough at night it is usually due to cold in some form or other. I know children who cough at night while sleeping as soon as their diapers are wet. That is the effect of cooling by evaporation and why dampness is dangerous. Many children cough when they kick off their blankets and stop when covered up again. That proves the very intimate connection between the outer skin and the mucous membrane and their quick response to each other.

What a wonderful thermostat the skin possesses and also what a valuable alarm system we possess. It sounds its first warning in the form of sneezing and/or coughing. If immediate attention to body protection by covering is given, then sickness will seldom ensue. If symptoms do occur, then real (homœopathic) medicine will cure it in a short time.

The desert in dry weather is devoid of vegetation. When the dry season ends and the rains come, plant life springs up almost overnight and grows luxuriously, only to die down when the dry season again approaches. So it is with the germs that lie dormant in men and only show their presence when conditions are suitable for their growth.

In answering the question as to how to cure sickness, the answer is "Tolle Causem" — remove the cause. I could recite literally hundreds of cases of backache, headache, sore throats, sinusitis, sniffles, coughs, etc., that were all cured by closing the windows and precluding drafts in the sleeping room.

One might comment on what was once in vogue when consumptives were kept in cold, airy sleeping rooms. This was just a fad and I don't know of any good that came of it. There is no more virtue in sleeping either out of doors or indoors with all the windows open in order to get fresh air, than in a man immersing himself in a pond because he wants a drink occasionally. A man needs only so much water to sustain life, and he needs only so much air for the same purpose. It isn't necessary to suffer the greater risks of cold, when warm fresh air is just as good. You may be sure many a consumptive died under the vigorous cold air treatment who would have lived had he been more gently treated. Tuberculosis can be cured more easily and comfortably in warm rooms than cold ones.

As a matter of fact there is very little difference in the oxygen content of air wherever it is found. This is a general statement and excludes for instance a deep closed mine full of poisonous gases, or other such unnatural situations.

Usually the people who suffer from the lack of oxygen do so because their physical condition fails to create a demand for it — they are lazy, inactive or lethargic — and therefore the individual just does not breathe any more than is necessary to supply the relatively small amount of oxygen that the system calls for.

When a man works hard and sweats, his system calls for water, and so it is with oxygen. In strenuous exercise the respiratory rate increases. You can sit all day in the purest of air and it will not do you any special good, for it is not getting into you because it is not needed.

Some years ago I was giving a lecture to a large audience, and during the discourse I made a statement that all the fresh air needed for breathing purposes could come in through a keyhole. Just that little statement caused the reporters to take notice and a lot of publicity ensued. I received many letters, some praising and agreeing with me, others calling me a "damn fool." Well, let's analyze my statement.

How do you get air into your lungs anyway? Through the nostrils, of course. There are two of them; each one the size of a keyhole. Half the time the air is going in and half the time the air is coming out, to say nothing of the pause between. So you can see for yourself that a keyhole is big enough to supply all the air you need. Especially is this true at night, because when you are asleep the need for air is reduced to the minimum. Some of you will say, "I just can't sleep in a warm room. I must have the windows open; I need a lot of air." That is all nonsense — you couldn't use it if you wanted to.

There were two maiden sisters who lived on a farm. Each had her own room. One kept the windows closed at night, the other wanted hers open. A death occurred in the family and they went to a city to attend the funeral. They stayed at a hotel, and to save expenses, occupied the same room. Difficulties soon arose over the window. When one fell asleep the other watched her chance to get up and open the window. The other awakened and closed it. This went on and on until finally getting tired of opening the window, the fresh-air lover threw her shoe through it in sheer desperation and immediately fell asleep happily and soundly. Next morning revealed that the shoe had gone through the mirror of the bureau and not the window as intended. So you see she only thought she needed the air.

You don't need a lot of air, but you may prefer to sleep in a cold room. It makes little difference how cold the room is, so long as the *air is not in motion* and you are sufficiently covered. No harm will come to you just because it is cold. In fact, it is often beneficial. If that is the way you want it, then shut off the heat, open the windows some few hours before retiring, and then you will have a cool room; but *close the windows when you retire.*

I have given much study to this subject and made many observations. It is amazing to discover how many disturbances are caused in a person's health from sleeping in a drafty room, even on the hottest nights in summer.

As the normal temperature of the body is 98.6° F., if the temperature of the room is 72°, some protection must be provided against this 26° difference. On a hot summer day with the outside temperature at say 90°, which is relatively high, there is still a difference of 8° plus for which some protection is needed. If the outside temperature is the same as normal body temperature, and a breeze is blowing, one needs protection even then, because moving air hastens evaporation and cools the body. All animals have their hair or feathers even in hot weather, because protection is always needed.

When one is asleep, his activity is reduced to its lowest ebb. One is practically "dead to the world." The bed covers are often kicked off to a greater or lesser degree, and if air is in motion, the vital body heat is carried off. The vasomotor system, which is jealously preserving the body temperature, feels the change and immediately stops the elimination of poison (sweat), and trouble begins (remember the usual constant perspiration is invisible and unnoticed).

Still-air is a non-conductor of heat, and no harm would come if one kicked all bed clothes off in his sleep, but air is never perfectly still. The process of convection, or the exchange of air in the room for outside air, where the temperatures are different, is always going on even in spite of closed windows, and one should do all that is possible to reduce air flow in the bedroom.

Air in motion is a very efficient conductor of heat. Just remember the fan in front of your car motor and why it is there. A draft doesn't necessarily have to be palpable — felt or seen. Just air in motion, however slow, is often sufficient to cause definite and often serious disturbances in the health of susceptible individuals. Strangely enough, this cause is rarely recognized; it is like a well-camouflaged enemy.

In the intricate and complicated process of living and growing, of repairing and replacing worn-out cells, etc. — which is all accomplished through the power which we have of converting all kinds of food into our own cells, our own blood, our own beings — there are of necessity lots of poisonous by-products to be eliminated.

The bulk of the food we use enters one end of the alimentary tract, and when its purpose has been served, it passes out at the other end. That does not constitute the whole story of elimination, however; the kidneys and lungs too excrete large quantities of these by-products. The deadliest poison of them all, however, leaves the body as sweat through the many thousands of highly organized sweat glands in the skin, secreted in a liquid form, and which usually evaporates as rapidly as it comes out, except where it is excessive. Nature seems to feel it is essential that the temperature of the body be kept right at all times, even at the risk of auto-intoxication.[2]

What we are concerned with right at this point is what effect moving air in the bedroom has on this marvelous vasomotor system and how moving air can cause disease. When in doubt, the skin ceases to excrete at the dictates of this system. The burden of eliminating the poison thus falls to some other organ, and often it is the internal skin, which is the mucous lining of the respiratory system — nose, throat, tonsils, etc. — or the poison just stops coming out temporarily and affects various locations.

In the former case, we wake up with a sore throat, a hoarse voice, a running or stuffed-up nose, and in the other case we may awaken with a pain in the neck, a lumbago, headache, rheumatic pains here and there, sinusitis, etc.

I was in an employment office once in search of a housekeeper. The lady who owned the place asked me if I could do anything for a peculiar headache that she had every morning on awakening. After due consideration, I advised her to close tightly all windows in her bedroom. Next morning she called me up to say I was a wonderful doctor, that she did as I suggested and she had no headache that morning. She has remained free of them ever since.

Years ago I went to see a little girl who suffered from a constant hacking cough from the moment she was put to bed until morning. She would cough in her sleep. It was one of my first cases, and I took it with fear and trembling as she had had all the local doctors, besides some "specialists" from the city. What was I going to do? It was obvious to me that there was some cause, and it must be in the immediate environment of the bedroom, as she did not cough during the day. In fact, she was well otherwise. Suddenly I saw it all. Her crib was in a direct draft. I moved the crib to a corner of the room and closed the windows, and said the child would not cough any more. And she didn't! Removing her from the draft allowed Nature to continue with the proper elimination of these poisons, which having been diverted to the mucous membrane of the nose and throat, caused irritation and cough.

Not long ago I was summoned to Los Angeles to see a woman who was dying of Bright's Disease. She was given up as incurable. She was about sixty-five years of age, and when I saw her I knew she could not be cured.

[2] Self-poisoning.

She was an intelligent person, but she had a set opinion on various subjects. In her early years she relied upon patent medicines to quite an extent. Later on she gave them up. She positively knew that she must have plenty of fresh air at night so she invariably slept beside an open window, in a constant current of air which carried away the body heat and stopped skin elimination of poisons. Besides many manifestations of cold, she developed a throat trouble that eventually affected the vocal chords so that she could talk only in a whisper. She became very thin. The kidneys, subject to the extra burden, eventually gave up and she had to die. The kidneys did not fail because of the extra work alone, but because the blood which keeps all organs and tissues alive and healthy contained poison which the skin could not eliminate. It was the combination that did it.

The poisons that are produced by any individual vary in strength and amount of toxicity from time to time, according to the way he lives, drinks, exercises, and it is this variation of poison which determines the kind and extent of ailments which will be produced when these adverse conditions obtain.

To summarize: man develops colds because he is subjected to cold. Man, a warm-blooded animal, tries to live in all kinds of climate. He has not yet learned how to clothe himself to meet various weather conditions and until he does, he will always pay in ill health. Cold is man's worst enemy. If he paid the same attention to keeping himself warm as he does to dodging germs (which do him no harm), then he would get somewhere and the common cold would be the exception instead of the rule. It is as simple as that.

CHAPTER 12

Polio[1]

Among the many public pronouncements that have been handed out regarding polio, the one that especially aroused my dander was the one which stated that the four billion dimes publicly contributed had now at long last provided a safe vaccine which would wipe out this disease. Then and there I predicted the greatest increase in the number of cases that Massachusetts has ever had. Subsequent events confirmed my prophecy. And why? For several reasons.

First, it lulled the people into a sense of security that was false and unwarranted. Without accounting for the fact that a big exciting cause of polio is exposure of the body to cold, it told the people that from now on they could drop any extra care of their children in the manner of clothing or food. A shot of vaccine would do the trick. One morning on the subway I overheard two women:

"Isn't it wonderful," said one to the other. "Now we can take our children to the beach!"

Secondly, though the vaccine is supposed to create immunity by introducing an artificial sickness, I know of no sickness that immunizes one from further attack. People may and do have repeated attacks of colds, bronchitits, pneumonia, cerebrospinal meningitis, venereal diseases, mastoiditis, malaria, smallpox and so on. Where does this leave the immunity theory? Why should polio be the exception? It too, so to speak, is a first cousin of the common cold. There are twenty or more forms of sickness, all with different names — diagnoses, that is — which are but peculiar individual variations of the so-called *common* cold.

Ordinary medicine has long looked upon the "common cold" as being caused by a germ. Lately the germ has been refined and become a

---

[1] Sections of this chapter are taken from an article of mine in *The Layman Speaks*, March, 1956, entitled "Polio."

"virus." In either case the cold was supposedly contagious. Researchers have tried to convey it from person to person and found that this would not work. They are less unanimous now but nevertheless they have searched long and diligently for a serum or vaccine which might prevent this common and prevalent ailment, but again to no avail. Just so long as ordinary medicine clings to the fallacy that sickness is "caused" by extrinsic agents such as germs or viruses, just so long will not only polio but all the ailments of mankind increase. Germs are secondary. They thrive on pathological secretions. It is the *cause* of these pathological secretions that medicine must reach whether the purpose is prevention or cure — not just the germs. Therefore I felt sure, in the third place, that reliance *solely* on a vaccine would result only in more cases of polio.

It was not so long ago that serum from the blood of patients who had recovered from polio was the sure preventive. Well, how did it turn out? Not only useless but very deadly. More recently the much vaunted gamma globulin was another dismal failure. Is it good reasoning to expect a different outcome from a vaccine built up on the very same theory? This is a fourth reason for my prediction.

Batholomew of Jefferson College in 1881 says in his *Practice of Medicine:*

Infantile Paralysis is a disease of early life — six months to fourth year. Older persons may develop it. Little is know as to its cause. The influence of summer heat seems established by Sinkler in the *American Journal of the Medical Sciences,* Vol. LXIX, P. 348. Diagnosis is established *only after* paralysis obtains.

It may be confounded with acute myelitis, hemorrhage into the cord, progressive muscular atrophy, paralysis from cerebral affections in childhood and paralysis from local nerve lesions. After diagnosis is determined, treatment consists of quinine, belladonna, strychnia.

Sir William Osler, in his *Modern Medicine,* calls it Polio Myelitis and says it occurs in the first six years of life, after which the liability diminishes progressively up to the third and fourth decade. He quotes a series of cases by Seeligmuth, Galbraith, Sinkler, Cowers and Starr. Taken together the figures show first year of life, 121 cases; 228 cases in second year; 158, third; 66, fourth; 46, fifth; 16 in the sixth year of life. The time of the year was during June, July, August, September, October, and all chief epidemics had been observed during the hot season. He says change of temperature and prolonged bathing or paddling may be predisposing causes.

He says it is generally agreed that the disease sometimes follows at varying intervals measles, scarlet fever, diphtheria and other fevers. All agree that diagnosis is *impossible* until *after* paralysis in its varying degrees ensues; also that it may be mistaken for several other conditions.

Osler refers to Pasteur's family epidemic:

Within ten days seven children were attacked by an acute febrile disorder, and three developed paralytic symptoms. Two of these were examples of acute polio and another became hemiplegic on the right side as a result of encephalitis. Transitory nervous phenomena were exhibited by the remaining members of the family.

Finally in many of the larger epidemics, cases of encephalitis have been found among the cases of polio, and paralysis of the cranial nerves has occurred either with or without spinal symptoms in the same inidividual.

He says, "No drug has any specific effect on the disease itself or on the regeneration of neuro-muscular tissue."

Osler presents fourteen full pages of all angles of this sickness, displaying an immense amount of study, accumulation of various forms of data, quotations and some statistics — but when it is all said, it has accomplished absolutely nothing worthwhile as far as the cause, prevention and cure are concerned. It is a formidable discourse and would frighten and discourage anyone who did not know better.

According to Osler, an allopath, the prognosis is not good. According to Halbert in his *Practice of Medicine,* under Homœopathy mortality is rare if ever. Halbert treats the sick patient. Osler treats, or would treat, if he knew what it was, a disease-entity.

If a patient shows symptoms which vary from those which arbitrarily determine the diagnosis of polio, then the *variation* is due to *another disease-entity* and not the patient — according to Orthodox concepts. Strange concept, indeed, when just a slight change in the patient's symptoms makes a *new disease* for the doctor to treat. No wonder then that there has been no better understanding or treatment of this illness under Orthodoxy since time began.

Scientific, curative medicine prescribes remedies that Nature needs from the moment the patient shows signs of sickness. In this way of prescribing, all ailments can be "nipped in the bud," so to speak. The Orthodox method of waiting for a diagnosis to be made allows an illness to go unhelped until it progresses to a point where it has reached its height, at which time, according to the ideas of the individual doctor, a name is given to it. It then becomes to him a definite "entity." Now the disastrous drugging begins. The sick patient has then the original sickness to overcome as well as the poisonous effects of the drugs.

Remember — *no* ailment presents itself to a doctor with a label on it. No one ever saw a sick child with the mystic words written on it somewhere, "This is Polio," or "This is Pneumonia." No, my friends, diagnosis — the name of any illness — depends on the imagination of the doctor himself. Often doctors will dispute with each other in favor of their own diagnoses.

It is a well known and accepted fact that at least 50 per cent of all diagnoses on death certificates are wrong. Where does that leave you?

It must also be remembered that when the polio season is on, especially when there are signs of an epidemic, the family doctor is prone to suspect every case of fever, colds, headaches, sore throats, and the like to be a case of polio. Who is going to disprove it? It is easy then to see how statistics can be very misleading.

Here in the United States the subject of polio has produced a state of hysteria. People do not know which way to turn. Mothers and fathers are worried about "will I or won't I submit my children to the vaccine shots?"

One *should* be safe in relying on his doctor, but unfortunately history has proved beyond a shadow of doubt that this is *not* so. Fifty years ago all so-called authorities stated that polio occurred in the first four, five or six years of life. That is why it has been referred to as Infantile Paralysis. Today, fifty years later, it seems that it may be developed by anyone regardless of age. Why? There must be a reason, if it is true. Perhaps the statistics are wrong. Perhaps some "eager-beaver" family doctors made a wrong diagnosis here and there.

The political health authorities are almost insisting that all persons up to forty years of age get their shots of Salk vaccine. It is publicly announced that there is plenty of the vaccine for everyone. The family doctors are told to urge their patients to submit.

The furor and hysteria produced by the most outrageous actions of those who gave vent to their ideas about polio, Salk vaccine — good, bad, or indifferent — in the newspapers, on radio, television, made people fear polio as they would a plague of Black Death.

If you and I give no opposition, then one day in the not too distant future, the Salk vaccine will be instituted as a compulsory procedure like the smallpox vaccination measure is right now. It may come to the point that every man, woman and child in the United States will be *compelled* by *Law* to submit to this wholesale poisoning.

The same hysterical action was prevalent years ago in regard to smallpox vaccination. It is just a case of Jenner's having come to life again to repeat with polio vaccine what was done with smallpox vaccine.

No wonder cancer at long last has become the No. 1 killer of our little ones. Do you think it is fair to jeopardize our helpless little ones while they are too young to defend themselves, when grown-ups do not have to submit to it?

What evidence is there anywhere in the world that polio can be prevented by vaccine? Why should it be the only sickness that can be wiped off the map by any such measure?

If paralysis in varying degrees did not so often obtain in polio, it would pass with very little notice. Seeing innocent children and grown-ups too, but especially children, forever crippled is what people dread. The pull on this human sympathy is what made possible the contribution (over a period) of some $400,000,000.00 in the hope of preventing the horror. Those who received this vast sum are still asking for more. This is now big business. It spawns "specialists," "experts," and "authorities." People at large take their pronouncements almost as if they were words of God. Yet the National Foundation for Infantile Paralysis, when it was offered an opportunity to look into Homœopathy and to test it, declined. Here is a broad field of medicine arbitrarily passed up. Before a man or woman qualifies as an expert or an authority, he or she must be familiar with all branches of science bearing on the subject in hand. I submit that until the people of the National Foundation for Infantile Paralysis have become conversant with Homœopathy and know its capabilities none of them is expert or carries authority.

All during the past summer, experts surfeited the public with pronouncements: it was a good vaccine; it was doubtful or bad; it was a dead vaccine; it had live virus in it; it was safe; it was harmful; it was perfected; it was not yet finished; boards of health disagreed among themselves and often with the experts.

In widely separated areas, experts are now in accord as to certain aspects of the matter. For example, they agree that they were aware that Massachusetts was in for a heavy dose of polio in 1955. They were in fact expecting it in 1954. Of course the precise date is not so important. The important thing is that they knew it was coming. How did they know? It seems Massachusetts had so few cases over the several years preceding that the population had grown "non-immune" and on top of this there had been an "enormous baby crop in communities where people live and play close to each other" which "opened the way for spread of the disease once it got a start." Hence, "if it had been possible to give two shots of Salk vaccine to all the 203,000 first and second graders in Massachusetts and if it had been just as effective as claimed, it would not have materially affected the course of the 1955 epidemic." Thus it is that no blame attaches to the experts, either those who were for giving the shots or those who were against or whoever may have caused a shortage of the vaccine.

Now, there is a lot that can be done by way of clothing and food and precaution against careless chilling exposure, if an epidemic is predicted by the so-called experts. The experts, who announced in December that they knew it all along, might have sounded the warning in March, before hot weather set in and the polio season started, with advice about safe, sound and appropriate precautions, well in advance. If they had actually known and were actually expert, why were they so silent?

It is a strange philosophy indeed which accepts the alleged wonderful claims of a preventive measure such as the Salk vaccine, that it is necessary to prevent polio and then negates its value by stating that it is useless in a non-immune population. It would seem that an immune population does not need any vaccine, but should be given it anyway, and that in a non-immune population it is useless. It does not make sense to me. The real reason 1956 had comparatively few cases of polio was because it had a cold, damp summer which discouraged the usual vacations, and so fewer children were subjected to the adverse environment that so often goes with vacations. This alone should be proof to any thinking person that no germ or virus (except the child's own virus) is responsible for polio.

According to the experts, if a community is comparatively free from sickness for a matter of a few years, it must pay the price in the form of an epidemic afterward. Health, they tell us, does not breed health. Instead, it is dangerous! What the community must have is plenty of experts and a lot of vaccine to be safe against the *consequences of health*.

If medicine be the true healing art, then the treatment administered in sickness leaves the patient in a better condition to remain well. This is the approach to health. Health is not a precarious state. Health is a power. The person is healthy in direct proportion to his power to remain well. The only thing that can deny such power and make health a menace is an "expert."

Several years ago I had the opportunity to observe in a little boy of 12 the beginning and development of a sickness that according to ordinary medicine is called cerebrospinal meningitis, closely akin to what ordinary medicine calls poliomyelitis. It was a warm, sunny day late in March. The little fellow went with me to my farm. He decided to dig a "fox hole" such as soldiers dig for themselves on a battlefield. He dug and dug. He got too warm and shed his coat. He dug some more and shed his shirt. He was still digging and did not notice the sun gradually sinking and the March air getting chilly. Leaving his coat and shirt off, he next decided to go down to the pond and see if there were any fish. Soon he did feel cold. He got his shirt and coat back on and we went home. That night, he suffered severe headache, high temperature and vomiting. By actual count during the night he vomited forty times. I put him in a tub of hot water twice. (This might just as likely have been polio.)

His early symptoms called unmistakably for *Aconite*. I gave him several doses. Later on, his symptoms changed and *Belladonna* was indicated. I gave him this. When morning came I took him to the hospital and called in men of ordinary medicine as well as some Homœopaths. They agreed the diagnosis was cerebrospinal meningitis. The doctors of ordinary medicine advised serum and sulfa drugs. Of course I did not give these to the little boy. By this time the symptoms had changed again. The slightest jar on the bed caused the little fellow to cry out wih pain in the head. A dog barking in the neighborhood caused severe aggravation. Very definitely *Bryonia* was indicated. This he received and in a few hours improvement was marked. To shorten the story, he was back in school in six days, perfectly well.

The Orthodox doctors, though amazed by this incident, could not perceive or even concede the cure. We of the new school took it in our stride. I know that any deviation from the treatment which the boy received would have resulted differently, but you cannot undo what has been done and try something else to see how it will come out.

A successful case here and there does not prove very much, but when you apply remedies according to a definite rule, a law of Nature, and secure the results that are expected and promised, and get them consistently in case after case, year after year, that is as near proof of the correctness of the method as medicine can possibly show.

As a contrast to this case I offer the following: Years before a little boy of exactly the same age did almost exactly what this little boy had done at almost exactly the same time of year. The diagnosis that time also was cerebrospinal meningitis. He was treated under ordinary medicine with the regulation treatment and in six days was dead and buried. The second case was a brother of the first little boy's mother.

Here then were two boys, similar in inheritance, similar in adverse environment (chilly March evening, after getting overheated in insufficient clothing) who developed as a consequence a similar illness diagnosed identically. One received the prevailing ordinary type of treatment and died. The other received scientifically chosen remedies according to Nature's Law of Similars and lived. Either one or both of these children could have developed symptoms that might have been diagnosed as polio. One condition is as deadly as the other. Different children exposed to that same adverse environment would develop different symptoms warranting, by the standards of ordinary medicine, diagnoses of tonsillitis, pneumonia, grippe, or any one of many other cousins of the common cold, all from the same exciting cause, yet evoking symptoms according to the make-up, nature and general condition of the individual child, thus requiring for each child the *one remedy that fits that one sick individual*.

As to those two small boys, both with cerebrospinal meningitis, no germ or virus was responsible. It was their own deadly poisons, normally and naturally excreted through the skin, but stopped when chilly evening air closed up their pores at a time when they were overheated and discharging poisons through the skin at an unusually high rate. Now, when the skin is blocked as an avenue of excretion, the detour or alternate route is through the internal skin, that is, the mucous membranes lining the nose, throat, bronchi and lungs, and next after that the kidneys. This is how stoppage at the skin leads to deeper ills and dangerous sickness.

It is worth noticing right here that the polio season coincides with the vacation season. This is the time when outdoor sports under a hot sun call the signals, everybody strips to expose the skin and perspiration flows in rivers. The soft drink business booms at the watering places and vacationers dive in for a swim in water thirty or forty degrees colder than the body. One minute the body pours out sweat to cool it off against a broiling sun and panting exercise, tearing down body cells at a glorious rate and sending out the poisons freely through the pores; the next minute the body is in reverse, sweating halted, pores closed and turned to goose pimples, and instead of seeking to discharge heat the body now has to generate it and do it fast. The nervous system governing these functions sustains a violent shock, and poisons that ought to be flowing outward are suddenly locked in.

If a child shows signs of sickness in the summertime, turn to the Pointers to the Common Remedies which you'll find in the back of this book, probably under the heading of Colds, Influenza, Sore Throats, etc., because, as I have stated before, polio is just a form of the common cold. From the list of remedies you will find there, choose the one which corresponds to the symptoms of your child. The proper remedy then given will take care of the whole situation and the child will get well in a very short time.

The difficulty will be in getting the remedy if you have no homœopathic doctor in your town and unless you have a case of homœopathic medicines in the house. The only recourse then would be to send away to a homœopathic pharmacy and ask for the remedy. In case you cannot do any of these things, put the child to bed, give it good nursing and the child will be well in time — but I do warn you against the strong drugs that are given today which will only make the child worse.

A few years ago a young man of twenty-one, an only son, was brought to the hospital with cerebrospinal meningitis. It was the most severe case I had ever seen, temperature 106°, delirium, head and heels drawn backwards until they almost touched. I saw at once the homœopathic remedy that should be used and gave several small doses. The next morning the temperature had fallen to 101°, and the patient was free from delirium. His symptoms had changed somewhat so that a complementary remedy was given in small doses — one millionth of a grain at a dose. He was making remarkable progress toward recovery. I had called in a specialist, a well-known brain man, and he confirmed the diagnosis. He found the "pure germ" of meningitis by lumbar puncture, and, according to his opinion, the patient needed a shot of serum in the spinal cord. This was the fashionable Orthodox procedure at the time.

"No!" I said, "he is getting well."

The specialist replied, "*Serum* is what *everyone* is using, and I must give it."

Again I said, "No, if you insist, I will withdraw from the case."

The parents did not wish it. They were satisfied that their boy was getting well, and so he was. However, the specialist's large fee apparently impressed and won over the parents, and their consent was finally, though reluctantly, given. The serum was injected, the boy died almost instantly. Again no one can *prove* that the serum in his spinal cord killed him. I am convinced that it did. I will tell you my reason in this case.

I knew the first remedy, Belladonna, was indicated by the symptoms he presented then. Every scientific Homœopath in the world would have prescribed this remedy. The results which followed were expected and would have been expected by every Homœopathic doctor.

The changed symptoms consisted of a great drop in temperature, mind back to normal, the patient relaxed and comfortable.

Some new symptoms appeared which were significant. His face and lips broke out in a profuse rash of cold sores. This was definite proof that the poison was being expelled and that recovery was on its way. The second remedy was Rhus Tox as indicated by his symptoms, especially the eruptions.

It would have been a beautiful cure had *not* this young man been killed by measures that upset Nature's efforts and the good effect of the proper remedies which were prescribed.

What kind of treatment have the ordinary doctors been giving to the thousands of victims of polio in the last epidemic? Have you ever thought of that? How many deaths were due to the current anti-biotic craze? How many became paralyzed because of lack of the Homœopathic remedy? Think it over. Then think how fortunate it is for suffering humanity that there does exist a permanent, never-changing, natural law to guide the physician to choose the proper remedy for any kind of sickness.

In 1904 there were in Boston alone, 645 Homœopathic physicians. There were many thousands throughout the United States. Today there are but a few hundred in the whole United States, and only several in Boston. Is there not some connection between the great increase in chronic cases and the disappearance of Homœopathic doctors?

CHAPTER 13

Arthritis

Arthritis is a common ailment — so much so that a so-called research foundation has been formed by some private individuals ostensibly for the purpose of attempting to find the cause and cure for this very disturbing ailment.

Again, as this is not an entity — not a disease all by itself — being symptomatic of some disturbance in the health of the individual, it does not appear under the name arthritis (rheumatism) in the Pointers in the Materia Medica.

For those who may be interested, the following are some of the remedies most frequently indicated for this complaint:

Aconite	Dulcamara
Bryonia	Ledum Palustrum
Cimicifuga	Mercurius
Colchicum	Rhus. Tox.

The two remedies which are most frequently indicated in New England are Rhus Tox and Bryonia. When Bryonia is indicated, the patient has painful joints, sometimes red and inflamed. Motion in the slightest degree causes pain. Patient must lie or sit still; seeks cold applications and cold drinks.

The Rhus Tox patient, on the other hand, is extremely restless, worse at night. He must move about in bed trying to find a comfortable position. Pain on beginning to move, like getting up from a chair, but much relief after he gets going. He seeks heat and warm applications, which relieve.

As arthritis and rheumatism are caused basically by too much food and/or unsuitable food, careful consideration must be given to diet. Exposure to cold is the immediate cause in some cases, because of the suppression of perspiration by cold — but it must always be remembered that the kind and amount of food one eats determines what kind and amount of poisons are produced in the body, and if the elimination of them is in any way hindered, then it is that circumstance which sets off the symptoms which we call arthritis or rheumatism.

Therefore, it would be a very foolish move to add insult to injury by taking any of the much advertised pain-killing agents. The Homœopathic remedy helps Nature in her eliminating process in just the way she wants to be helped, and it is almost miraculous the way Rhus Tox, especially, will cure this condition almost overnight.

Too much citrus fruit is responsible for this condition in many people, particularly in the New England climate. If one eats the proper food in the proper quantity, and wears adequate clothing to keep his body warm at *all* times, one will never be plagued with arthritis or rheumatism.

The following article, entitled "Creaking Legions," appeared in *Time*,[1] May 8, 1950.

A year had passed since the Mayo Clinic first announced the dramatic effects of treating rheumatoid arthritis sufferers with the hormone ACTH and cortisone (*Time*, May 2, 1949). In that year, millions of pain-racked arthritics had clamored for the "new cure," or begged their doctors to tell them how soon they could expect relief and how much. Last week the answer was plain: they could expect nothing certain for a long, long time.

Much of the raising of false hope could be laid to the *showmanship* which marked the first news. Patients who had been crippled were photographed dancing a jig after a few shots of either hormone. But the research team headed by Drs. Philip S. Hench and Edward C. Kendall, which touched off the foofaraw, ends a solemn, 120-page report in the Archives of Internal Medicine with these sobering words:

". . . The use of these hormones should be considered an investigative procedure, not a treatment . . . It is hoped and believed that (further) studies will in time lead to an improved and practical method of treatment . . ."

This was a far cry from the optimism still being voiced in less-informed quarters. The truth is, when the hormone injections are stopped, the rheumatic miseries usually come back promptly in full force. Drs. Hench and Kendall saw one patient win relief for ten months and another for twelve. But in such an erratic disease as arthritis, the same things might happen *without* hormones.

[1]Courtesy *TIME*, The Weekly Newsmagazine, copyright Time, Inc., 1950.

There are also *irksome side-effects*. Both hormones are apt to cause acne, hair-growth, rounding of the face, irritability and depression. The side-effects usually disappear when the injections are stopped, but some do not show up until afterward.

The doctors are still deep in argument over possible substitutes for the wonder hormones ACTH and cortisone. A few Swedish, British and U. S. investigators claim wondrous results with desoxycorticosterone acetate ('DOCA', an adrenal hormone) and vitamin C injections given within a few minutes of each other. Others in the U. S. sing the praises of such hormones as 21-acetoxy-pregnenolone. None of these, said Drs. Hench and Kendall, have stood up under proper testing.

In fact, the uncounted, creaking legions of rheumatoid arthritis victims had nothing last week that they did not have last year — except more hope. They were not likely ever to get ACTH or cortisone for routine treatment. Now, as for years past, they would get bed rest, exercises and aspirin to ease the pain."

These people are suffering from chronic arthritis because of the inefficiencies of the Orthodox medical profession.

Some years ago I needed a publicity man for one of my enterprises. I found one who had the qualifications, but every third week he was "laid low" by arthritis. Under such circumstances, I deemed it best not to employ him unless he would allow me to cure his ailment. After a careful review of the history of the case, I decided on a remedy, but he had a doctor who promised him a cure, so he did not want to try anything else just then. A couple of weeks later he called on me all enthused because he was elected as head of the Arthritis Fund which was being established. I said, "How interesting." I asked him who the men were behind the foundation. He said his own physician was one of them. I asked him if this doctor attended his own case of arthritis from its beginning and my friend said that he did. Then I asked him, "If he couldn't cure you in the beginning of your case when it could have been cured almost overnight, and hasn't been able to cure you in all these years (five or six), how in the world can he be expected to aid any one of the two million chronic arthritic victims?"

He replied, "Gee, I never thought of that." Well, I'll give him credit — he refused the job.

Arthritis is a condition which slowly and gradually progresses from a very simple beginning. If the doctors who are mentioned in the above article could not help the sufferers when the ailment first started, how can you expect help from them after the disease has progressed far enough to be called arthritis?

Arthritis can be a terrible disease, eventually becoming incurable in many cases, yet it is easily prevented by doctors who know their business. Each person suffering from arthritis manifests the condition in his own way, by his *own* symptoms. The symptoms in their totality indicate the remedy in each and every case. There is no specific for this ailment any more than there is for any kind of illness.

At this point I should like to offer the case of Dr. D. F., who came limping down the corridor of my hospital and into my office. He had been shored up in iron braces by his orthopedic specialist, so that he was able to get around to attend some of his duties. The first thing he said was, "Well, Shad, I have finally come to you for help. I have exhausted everything in Orthodox medicine, to no avail. Can you help me?"

I said, "You have been knocking Homœopathy for years and now you want its help. I should tell you to go plumb to the hot spot down below, but I won't."

I took his history, prescribed a remedy and he went home. Next morning, just twenty-four hours later, he came briskly down the corridor to my office, *without his brace*. He almost shouted with joy. He said, "My God, Shad, is it possible that those little white pills did all this to me? I slept soundly last night, the first time in months. I have absolutely no pain. I just can't believe it! Is it going to last?"

That was more than ten years ago and so far it has lasted. He only needed five or six doses. The medicine cost me about one-tenth of a penny. He was grateful and he did say, "If I were not exclusively a surgeon I would leave no stone unturned until I became able to do such a wonderful job of curing."

An old friend of mine and I were out for a ride one day and he complained about the trouble he was having with his back. Upon questioning he said that he had been released from the Navy because they had made a diagnosis of arthritis and that they had absolutely no cure for it, especially for a man of his age (between forty and fifty). I went into his symptoms quite carefully, and as I had my medicine case in the car, I gave him a remedy which he took immediately. I had already noticed that this friend of mine had a difficult time getting into the car, and that he was uneasy and uncomfortable in sitting still. But when we reached our destination he seemed to be able to get out of the car more easily.

When, a couple of hours later, we headed for home, he got into the car much more easily than before and began to be very cheerful. When we got home he said, "My gosh, Doc, don't tell me those little pills can be working already!"

I said, "Yes, they can and they do when they suit the case."

Now, this man, an intelligent insurance executive, was discharged from the Navy as *incurable*. He had been X-rayed and calcareous deposits were found in his backbone, and therefore nothing could be done for him — nothing, that is, by Orthodox medicine.

Well, that medicine I gave him cured him completely. He went to see the Navy doctors and had more X-rays taken and the calcareous deposits had absolutely, completely disappeared. The doctors were amazed and said they would not have believed it if they had not seen it with their own eyes. I have had personal experience in hundreds of such cases and the proper remedy has always produced the results I looked for.

That, my friends, is scientific medicine. The medicine cost him nothing. It cost me a penny or two. That is all. Remember, *that remedy will not cure every case of arthritis or rheumatism*. Each remedy is chosen by matching it to the patient's *totality* of symptoms.

The true science of medicine is one of the most wonderful blessings that man can enjoy, if and when he can find it in this day and age when there is so much advertising to lead him astray.

Four years ago, I went into a hardware store and was attended by a tall, nice-looking clerk who limped around evidently in pain. He asked my opinion on a drug currently being advertised under a new name. I told him it was not only absolutely worthless but could be dangerous if used too frequently. I took his symptoms and decided on a remedy and advised how it was to be taken. Recently, after four years, I saw him again and was pleased to learn that the remedy cured him immediately and that he had had no return of the symptoms.

A young patient of mine called me on the telephone and said, "Do you think you could help my mother? She has arthritis in both arms and hands. The pain is so severe, especially at night, that she cannot sleep. She tosses from side to side of the bed, but cannot find a comfortable position. She feels better from heat and worse from cold."

To the Homœopathic physician those symptoms called for Rhus Tox. I asked, "Have you any Rhus. in the house among the other remedies that you have there?"

The answer was, "Yes — the 30th potency."

I advised her to give her mother two pills, one grain size. That night the pain all left and she had a fine sleep. She has been free of all pain and sleeplessness since. The mother was amazed; "dumbfounded" was her word. She had had no particular faith in such little pills, but she has now. That is how simple it can be. Now compare that kind of medicine with the great "to-do" of Orthodox measures with their strong, killing drugs that have *never yet cured* a case of arthritis. What a wonderful satisfaction it is to a physician who is able to relieve suffering in such an apparently easy manner.

Several years ago I met a friend I had not seen for thirty years. We talked of old times, and then he told me he was "pulling up stakes" and going to Florida to live. When I asked the reason for the move he said, "My wife is sick and the doctors say she must go South as they can do nothing for her in this climate. She has arthritis."

I suggested that he bring her over to see me, which he did several days later. I found her to be in a pitiable condition. She could hardly get in or out of the car. In fact, I took her symptoms while she sat in the car.

Her face was all broken out in a distressing rash. She could hardly walk, she could not raise her arms high enough to comb her hair or wash her face. She hadn't had a good night's sleep for months on end. She had all the symptoms of a certain remedy which I gave her then and there and told her how it was to be taken. Fifteen minutes after the first dose she fell asleep in the car on the way home. The husband was frightened, thinking maybe I had given her a strong narcotic, and he was about to turn around and come back when she opened her eyes and said, "Oh, what a wonderful day." She immediately began to get better and has remained well ever since. I know this to be a fact because only recently my old friend drove out to my farm to see me. I was delighted because I had been thinking a lot about him lately and was wondering what he was doing. Then, of course I asked about his wife. He said, "Doc, it is absolutely fantastic. She is cured absolutely."

Well, my friend's wife looked like a young girl. Her skin was as smooth as satin. She looked wonderful. My friend told me they had spent thousands of dollars on her, all to no avail, and to top it all had been advised to move to Florida. He had made all arrangements to do so before he met me that day several years ago. He had sold his house and had even sent some of their belongings to Florida. They moved back again, and re-established in his old business of drilling water wells.

The remedies which cured all of the cases of arthritis and rheumatism mentioned in this book are available to Orthodox doctors if they want to use them, and not one of the patients I just mentioned had to pay one cent for the medicine that cured him.

There are about 80 different Homoeopathic remedies that may be indicated in Rheumatism or Arthritis, according to the symptoms in each case. To enumerate them all would occupy too much space here. Inasmuch as all sickness is usually due to faulty living (except in babies, as mentioned elsewhere) it is quite possible, after one has learned what faulty living actually is, that prevention will turn out to be the best cure.

CHAPTER 14

Food and Drink

All parts and organs of the digestive tract are provided solely for the acceptance, treatment, digestion and absorption of vitamins and minerals and final expulsion of whatever we have eaten. The food, which is gratefully accepted into the mouth, would cause distress in any other part of the system if put there without being properly prepared by each preceding part or organ.

Food thoroughly prepared by the mouth is received by the stomach. There it is further processed to prepare it for the intestines, and from there it is prepared for the colon, where it is then prepared for expulsion. Food after it is swallowed should reveal no sensation whatever until it is felt leaving the body — unless something has interfered with its orderly progress or unless too much food or unsuitable food was eaten.

The following ailments are caused by mistakes in diet. Proper food (and temperance in its use) is vital to life and health. If careful consideration is given to proper nourishment, these sicknesses will seldom occur:

Indigestion (dyspepsia)	Kidney stones
Eructation (belching)	Lassitude (weakness)
Fainting	Mental depression
Flatulence	Nausea
Gall bladder	Vomiting
Gall stones	Pain
Headaches	Palpitation
Heartburn	Pressure as from a stone
Hiccoughs	Pulsation
Regurgitation of food	Vertigo (dizziness)
Salivation	Rheumatism
Sweating	Arthritis
Toothache	High blood pressure

and almost all skin manifestations such as: acne, eczema, psoriasis, itching, etc.

Man, having long since lost his natural instinct to choose the right food, has to use the trial and error method. In this day of highly centralized and mechanized food processing it is almost impossible to get perfect food. There are still plenty of suitable foods, but even more unsuitable. A good many people get into the habit of eating food which, even though they like it, is not suitable to them. That is why it is a good idea to vary your menu frequently. Eat mainly those things which come from your own environment. If you can hit on the proper diet you can live on it in health for years, but long-continued errors in diet eventually lead to sickness. These errors are: (1) too much food, (2) improper food, (3) improper preparation, (4) insufficient mastication (chewing), and (5) condiments, etc.

Overeating is deadly! If you are too fat and heavy, it is because you have eaten too much. Food costs a lot of money nowadays, so don't spend your money putting on extra weight. Remember, fat people don't last as long.

There was a time when man ate all his food raw, but that was long ago. Now, most cookbooks seem to vie with each other in concocting recipes overloaded with harmful ingredients and spices to tickle the already gluttonous appetite of America.

There are a host of foods on the market with artificial flavoring, preservatives and other synthetic ingredients which ought to be avoided. Among the articles of customary and ordinary diet to be found in all markets are white sugar, white flour, pasteurized milk, coffee, tea, cola drinks and other varieties of tonic, cheap candies, synthetic gelatine, chocolate, polished rice — none of which are good for man.

Some of these foods are useless but others are actually harmful. None will kill immediately, but if they become the diet daily for years, the accumulated effects will lead to a long list of symptoms, diagnosed as many diseases. Food must be pure, natural, and varied enough to supply all the required vitamins and minerals. Too much food goes either to fat or produces poisons, both of which are productive of poor health. No two people are affected exactly alike from errors in diet, either in kind or amount of food taken. Eating is practically a continuous performance — we eat every day of our entire lives. Slight errors produce a delayed result; gross errors result in quicker penalties.

It is unfortunate indeed that it is almost impossible for many millions
of city dwellers to get an adequate supply of good organically grown
vegetables,[1] especially green ones, and good, natural whole grain cereals.
It would be a great help if one could get these grains and then use a small,
grinder to grind them as needed. Everyone should subscribe to *Organic
Gardening* by Rodale, Emmaus, Pennsylvania, and *Natural Food and
Farming*, official publication of Natural Food Associates, Inc., Atlanta,
Texas.

Pies, pastries, cookies, etc., are no better than the ingredients from which
they are made. The effect of white flour is, shall we say, negative in these
items except where alum has been added. Eggs and milk help take off
the curse, but the white sugar is very deleterious. It is an almost pure
carbon and steals important calcium from the body, uniting with it to form
useless calcium carbonate. That is why white sugar, cheap candies, cola
drinks, etc., are so damaging to children's teeth.

Generally speaking, too much meat is not good for most people. There
are those who cannot take any. After all, when one eats meat, he is relying
on second-hand material for nourishment. The steer eats only grass and
corn — a pure vegetarian diet. Besides, animals manufacture their own
poisons in their process of living and these poisons aren't necessarily
completely eliminated during slaughter. Then too, who knows if possibly
the fear of death when slaughter time nears causes secretions which are
retained in the animal about to be slaughtered — secretions which would
be deleterious to those people eating the meat. Many cases of cancer have
been cured by removing all meat from the diet.

A person who engages in hard outdoor labor or exercise of any kind
naturally needs more food than one of more sedentary habits. If a man
works hard he must have enough food to supply the needed energy.
Others must eat accordingly, but the food must be proper.

The great intemperance in eating that prevails today has produced many
forms of indigestion. "Acid indigestion" is continually dinned in the

[1] If you wish to explore further the dangers which exist not only from improper nutrition,
but from various "interests" which inhibit the dissemination of the true facts pertaining
to devitalized foods and deleterious substances which are used as preservatives in the
coloring of foodstuffs, read the series of five open letters from the Boston Nutrition Society,
Inc., John D. Pearmain, Chairman, Educational Committee, to Dr. Nathan M. Pusey,
President of Harvard University, on the Matter of "Standards of Research under Dr. Frederick J. Stare, Head of the Department of Nutrition, Harvard School of Public Health,
Re: Our National Health."

ears of everyone who listens to radio and television, for the sole purpose of selling some patented anti-acid drug. As long as people over-eat and then try to palliate the results of it by drugs, just so long will they not only continue to produce the distressing symptoms, but surely pave the way for ulcers and cancer. Besides, never have such drugs been known to *cure* indigestion.

Man should enjoy a long, healthy life, but remember: you cannot eat at forty the way you did at twenty. It is up to the individual whether he dies at 70, or 60, or 50, or whether he lives to 100 or more, which it is possible to do. It is also up to man whether he lives *healthy* years. Man cannot *get old* because every cell as it is worn out is replaced by a new one, if this process is left undisturbed. Man may, however, make himself *decrepit,* which is usually called old age. Age should have nothing to do with it except as it gives one time to produce decrepitude. That would be foolish when by proper living, man can live quite indefinitely, healthfully, and happily too. It is up to you, folks.

It must be thoroughly understood that the aforementioned ailments are absolutely self-produced, consciously or through ignorance and self-indulgence. What and how you eat, combined with what kind of care is taken to maintain necessary body temperature, determines whether you get sick or stay well. This is the general rule, but there are always some exceptions — such as inherited weaknesses, susceptibilities, idiosyncrasies. In such cases where the greatest care in living habits falls short, then search must be made for the constitutional remedy. This cannot be done by any doctor who does not have a profound knowledge of *Materia Medica* and does not know how to prescribe the proper remedy.

The stomach is a very important part of the digestive tract, probably the most important. It is an impassive organ and can do only the work intended for it. It is involuntary, it has no inherent volition. It is, however, so intimately connected with the entire man — mind and body — that any and every part may be beneficially or adversely affected by it and accompanied by pleasurable or distressing symptoms.

As the stomach is the involuntary "receiving station" for the food we eat, it is of the utmost importance that proper consideration be given to that which it is forced to receive. It is the duty and function of this organ then to process, mix, dilute, and prepare this mass of material to the point where it is safe to pass on to the small intestines where it is further prepared to enable the absorbing villi (roots) to appropriate any and all acceptable material which the system needs. Unfortunately, the system is also forced to absorb poisons too.

Excessive fatigue, great mental excitement, long and continued watchfulness, the depressing passions of fear and anger, all take their toll. Men who overstrain the intellect in the pursuit of wealth, or those whose labors are mental rather than physical, are liable to dyspepsia, even when their general habits of life are not the worst. Victorious on every field where they encountered only physical tasks, votaries of literature and business are vanquished by that sterner enemy, *care*.

Sickness may come in spite of eating food proper both in quality and quantity, if you indulge in the almost universal habit of daily poisoning by nicotine, alcohol, tea, large quantities of white sugar, gallons of coffee, plus an almost unbelievable amount of all kinds of drugs. Is it any wonder that cancer, heart disease, arthritis and all kindred diseases are allowed, yes, even forced, to occur? Verily, man is the producer of his own miseries.

Nature is kind, Nature is patient, but she cannot do the impossible. It is too bad that man is so indifferent to the preservation of health. Just a little care and intelligence would prevent most human illnesses.

The May, 1957 issue of *The Layman Speaks* has an interesting item regarding the coloring of foods.

The New York Times, August 11, 1956, ran a news report quoted in part in Bulletin No. 486 of Citizens Medical Reference Bureau, Inc., Setauket, Long Island, N. Y. It seems to be a milestone on the rough road toward that democratic freedom which will make the citizen the captain of his own body — provided enough citizens care enough. So we present passages here:

"Coal tar coloring commonly used in a wide variety of foods was condemned by the United States Court of Appeals here yesterday. The court's decision was unanimous.

"Federal Judge Thomas F. Murphy wrote an opinion upholding an order of Marion B. Folsom, Secretary of Health, Education and Public Welfare. The order removed certain coal tar colorings from the list of harmless ingredients approved for use in foodstuffs, drugs and certain cosmetics. Judge Harold Medina and Sterry R. Waterman concurred with Judge Murphy. Secretary Folsom issued his order on November 10, 1955, to be effective last February. The court's decision was based on an appeal made by an industry committee. The committee included the Allied Chemical and Dye Corporation, the American Cyanamid Company, the Bates Chemical Corporation, Dyestuffs and Chemicals, Inc., H. Kohn-Stamm & Co.,

William J. Strange Company, Sterwin Chemicals, Inc., and the Warner Jenkinson Manufacturing Company."

The named companies, according to the *Times,* make coal tar colors designated as FD and C Orange No. 2 and Red No. 32.

Touching on the proper relation between the three parties most concerned, the public, the Government and the manufacturers, Judge Murphy's written comment is quoted in part by the *Times:*

"The Government need not prove that these colors are in fact injurious. It is enough if it shows that their use might render an article of food harmful. This it has done by an overwhelming weight of the evidence.

"The colors here involved have been shown to be alarmingly toxic. It would be unconscionable for any court to require the secretary to permit their use without the clearest and most uncompromising evidence that usage at certain levels was absolutely safe.

"Public contact with the colors occurs in cakes, cookies, pies, bread, cheese, ice cream, frankfurters, bolognas, spreads, oranges, canned and frozen vegetables, candy, desserts, puddings, soft drinks, condiments, soups and in drugs and cosmetics."

For a signal public service, Citizens Medical Reference Bureau, Inc., suggests that everyone interested in medical liberty write to the Secretary with congratulations and praise . . .

There was a time when a lot of cooking was done in copper. It was stopped because of copper poisoning. Today a large percentage of our cooking utensils are made of aluminum and are used almost universally, from which practice much sickness is caused.

According to the *United States Dispensatory,* aluminum "combines in an easily ionizable salt, such as sulphate or chloride and acts as an astringent and as a detergent."

Small quantities of soluble salts of aluminum, when introduced into the circulation, it says, produce a slow form of poisoning characterized by areas of local anesthesia, motor paralysis, fatty degeneration of the kidney and liver. Nervous symptoms are presumably due to anatomic changes in the nerve centers. Another symptom is gastro-intestinal inflammation, possibly resulting from the effort of the glands in the digestive tract to eliminate the poison.

Aluminum chloride and aluminum acetate combined would make an ideal disinfectant or embalming fluid, and this combination can easily be obtained by adding salt to pickles as they cook in aluminum. The addition of salt to any vegetable cooking in aluminum results in the formation of aluminum chloride compounds. Since many waters contain salt, anyway, aluminum chloride forms as a matter of course when vegetables are cooked in aluminum ware using that water.

It is known that compounds of aluminum destroy pepsin. Many vegetables containing soda, potash, or sulphur, could, when cooked in aluminum, combine with it to form aluminum sulphate. For example, sauerkraut, when cooked in aluminum, will produce aluminum chloride.

My good friend, Dr. LeHunte Cooper of London, England, has this to say about aluminum:[2]

When my eyes were first opened to the importance of this matter in 1930, I saw at once how great an asset I had in Hahnemann's provings in the first place, augmented as they were by the wide general use of this metal in connection with food, together with the efficacy of Homœopathy in countering its deleterious effects.

For proving whether any particular case was due to, or aggravated by, Aluminum, I had three means at my disposal, viz:

1. The effect of stopping the intake of Aluminum, alone, on various maladies and derangements of health,

2. The effect of specifically (homœopathically) antidoting its influence.

3. The resemblance of the symptoms observed in human beings, and those produced in Hahnemann's provings, thus having an enormous advantage over researchers in this field of the usual type.

It seemed strange at first that the dangerous properties of this metal should have remained unsuspected so long, but I found *its universal use, and the insidious and varied effects produced by it,* sufficient explanation; this being well exemplified at my interview, in 1931, with the late editor of one of our chief medical journals, after I had worked at the matter for over a year.

When I explained to him that I had come to see him on account of the effects suffered by the public from its culinary use, he leaned back in his chair, and widely extending his arms, exclaimed, "But it is used in all these houses, restaurants, and public buildings round us." "Yes," I said, "also in my own house, and in yours also, no doubt, and it is this very universality of use which has obscured its responsibility for a very great many of the diverse disabilities with which we are afflicted."

"And," he replied, "you say its use is dangerous to health; how can you

[2] From "Aluminum and the World's Health" in *The Layman Speaks,* April, 1957, reprinted from the *Journal of the American Institute of Homœopathy,* Vol. 49, No. 9, October, 1956.

prove this?" I said, "I only ask you to read the results of my researches in my paper here, and publish them in your journal, if you think fit."

"But," he said, "you may not be aware that we have already tested this matter." "Yes," I replied, "in 1913, as published in your journal when you found that it came off in all foods." "But," he remarked, "an insoluble form of the oxide, Alumina." "I know," I said, "but you overlooked the fact that this becomes united with the hydrochloric acid naturally existing in the stomach, forming Aluminum Chloride, which is both soluble and toxic."

"Well," he said, apparently reluctantly, "I will give it to my expert, and communicate with you later."

Two days after this, he wrote to say, "This matter is too much against generally accepted opinion to be put in a responsible journal," so I took the matter in my own hands and sent out 30,000 copies of my paper to medical men in England. This resulted in many acknowledgements, and confirmation of my opinions; one doctor in particular informing me that he and his family had recovered from ill health, which had previously resisted all remedial measures, and adding that he had been able to resume his practice, because *his memory had come back*.

This last statement was of the greatest importance, as indicating an action on the brain, which I subsequently confirmed to my own satisfaction (I, and others, being susceptible in this regard).

In my own case, I found that the *difficulty in finding my own words* which had greatly hampered me when speaking in public in the past, had been definitely influenced by this metal, which we had used in our family for many years, being completely unaware of its possible dangerous effect. Needless to say, it was an enormous relief to me when I recovered from this disability, by discontinuing and antidoting this metal.

Surprise, amounting almost to disbelief, brought a metallic expert from the North to inform me that his wife, incurable before, had not only recovered her general health, and resumed speaking in public, but that *she now was able to speak without notes* (an impossibility before); her recovery being due simply to stopping the intake of the metal, without any remedies whatsoever. He came to see me to confirm the fact that this metal alone could have such an effect. I gave him other cases to reassure him.

Needless to say, some individuals are far more susceptible to the Aluminum influence than others, and, fortunately for my investigations, this applied to myself and my wife, but before I became aware of this, I had been suffering from grave symptoms affecting *my knees,* pointing to a low form of arthritis, suggestive of commencing rheumatoid arthritis.

Besides pains when ascending and descending the stairs, my knees were beginning to give way and *"lock"* — especially when I was walking over rough country, or when I caught my foot in a carpet, or when descending from a motor-car. When locked, the leg had to be pulled out to free it.

I had not, at that time, suspected Aluminum as being in any way associated with these symptoms, but as I was investigating the action of that metal, I decided to take a high potency to watch its effects on myself. This I did, in the form of Alumina 200. in a single dose, subsequently forgetting that I had done so; but as nothing had occurred, I took another dose in about a fortnight, and again forgot the fact.

Then one evening, when having dinner, I had a sudden attack of severe pain in both semilunar cartilages, it being sufficiently intense to necessitate my going upstairs to lie down till the paroxysm passed, which it did in about ¼ of an hour. No further symptoms were experienced till about 3 a.m., when red-hot pokers seemed to be piercing these same cartilages, lasting some minutes till I could get off to sleep again.

Similar attacks followed on other nights, at about the same time, and I began waking later in the morning, with stiffness and aching in the back of the neck and shoulders. Still later, I became conscious of sore tenderness affecting the roots of my teeth, with tenderness of the gums. The sensation was as if the roots of the teeth rested on a soft pulp substance, and the continuance of this directed my attention to its effects on the gums as a whole, it being of significance that I found that a Dr. C. T. Betts (a Dental Surgeon) in America had, some months before, published a treatise on the constitutional effect of Aluminum as a cause of pyorrhœa.

When it is remembered how many varieties of ill-health have been shown to be caused by pyorrhœa, all these may be added to the indictment against this metal.

When on the subject of the "mouth," a most interesting case of extensive aphthous stomatitis [3] came to me many years ago complaining that for years she had suffered from this, in an intractable form. All treatment by ordinary medicine had proved completely unavailing as to "cure," and with very little mitigation at any time. The doctors who had seen her throat had declared that they had never seen this particular disability in such a severe or extensively diffuse form, for it involved the mouth and pharynx and extended some way down the throat.

Stopping and antidoting Aluminum resulted in almost immediate and dramatic improvement, with subsequent complete cure, and only trivial relapses at long intervals.

That its influence on the mucous membrane of the mouth does not stop there,

[3] Inflammation of the mouth characterized by the appearance of small white vesicles, occurring chiefly in children under 3.

in individuals susceptible to nasal irritability, was well shown in a case of severe chronic nasal catarrh in a middle-aged lady with a remarkable talent for painting (her "forte" being the illustrating of children's books). Constant nasal discharge distressed her to an intense degree, interfering with her work, which necessitated her leaning forward for long periods of time, it being only possible for her to do so by constantly holding a large handkerchief before her face, and changing this when it became saturated. This rendered her existence miserable in the extreme, for she could obtain no relief in any way, it being imperative that she should continue her work.

Imagine her joy when the stopping of the use of Aluminum and the anti-doting of it homœopathically soon began to give her relief, and in a few months completely cured her.

No one need have any difficulty in proving that this metal is toxic. All that is necessary is to seek for a case of gastro-enteric derangement (for this is the system specially susceptible to Aluminum influence), especially if the duode-num [4] is involved. Tell him to stop cooking in this metal, while taking every precaution to avoid jams and fruit likely to have been in contact with the metal. Then tell him not to change his diet, or habitat, or take any remedies and watch the effect!

The following will serve to illustrate the above suggestions: I noticed that the proprietor of a garage which supplied me with petrol was becoming more and more depressed and listless. One day I asked him the cause of his trouble. "Oh," he answered, "it is my wife's grave state of health which has been de-teriorating for years, and now seems beyond hope, and the despair of her medical attendant." The main symptoms were gastric pain and discomfort, which careful questioning proved to be worse when digestion was complete, or nearly so, being relieved for a time by taking more food into the stomach.

He admitted to the free use of Aluminum cooking at home, and I told him to ask his doctor whether he did not think this might be the cause of the trouble. He did so, but the suggestion was received with contempt, as being ridiculous in the extreme! I therefore advised his taking the matter into his own hands, and adopting the measures I have outlined above.

When I next saw him, he hesitatingly admitted his wife had been slightly better . . . when I saw him in about two weeks' time his depression had changed to hope. After this she made a rapid recovery. . . .

Cases like this abound; and one can imagine the millions of them needlessly suffering similar digestive troubles. They are, of course, cases of "Duodenitis" [5] which, if left untreated, go on to ulceration. It is a well known fact that the

[4] First part of the small intestine, beginning at the outlet of the stomach and extending 8 or 10 inches.
[5] Inflammation of the duodenum.

incidence of "duodenal ulceration" mounts every year, with corresponding loss of time to the nation's workers.

We all vary in our reaction to Aluminum, it being easier for some to throw it off from the system than others. This power gradually weakens with advancing age. Hence it is comparatively rare for the young to show any signs of it; but it is from about 40 to 50 years of age onwards that symptoms begin to appear.

This article contained many examples of aluminum poisoning, too numerous to mention. At this point, as a conclusion, perhaps the remarks of the Editor of *The Layman Speaks* which appeared beneath Dr. Le Hunt Cooper's article, will suffice.

Often the robust have a little sneer for the weaklings who think they must be so very careful about their food and cooking. True, the robust generally get by better than the sickly, for the person in flowing health can withstand conditions that make the less robust sick; but it is also true that periodic exposure to a morbid influence will break through and bring down the most hearty if continued long enough. This is the importance of ridding the kitchen of that soft and medically active metal, aluminum.

Generally the authorities in ordinary medicine and the political officers who are guided by them dismiss all apprehension about aluminum because by their training they expect to find the effects of aluminum distinctly aluminum effects and quite uniform for all, or most individuals, whereas different individuals have different consequences from aluminum according to their individual susceptibilities. The authorities in ordinary medicine fail to consider sufficiently the differences among people and tend to think of people in the mass. That can blind any physician to what is most important.

Water (H_2O) is just as necessary to a living organism as oxygen. People give a lot of thought to fresh air. How much do they exert themselves to get pure water?

Water is a component part of every cell in the body. It is also used as a solvent and a diluent. To serve these purposes it must be pure, just H_2O. As such it is the greatest solvent there is. It comes down from the sky as H_2O except perhaps over a smoky city where the first showers will wash out and dissolve a lot of the impurities in such air.

Generally it comes down as distilled water. That is what people should drink. If everyone did so, I believe there would be few if any cases of kidney stones, calcareous deposits such as occur in arthritis, gouty deposits in finger joints, a reduction in the incidence of hardening of the arteries, etc. In fact I have seen great improvement in such cases from the use of pure water (distilled) as an exclusive beverage. I have heard my claims disputed by people who think that as distilled water contains no minerals, it is not good. I have heard otherwise very intelligent people express such ideas.

They are wrong, nevertheless. All raw water contains various minerals in varying amounts in different parts of the world. But — they are inorganic, and as such are of no use to the body. They may be deleterious. Our body needs vital minerals but they must be organic. They must go through plants and even animals to be processed into the organic form which can be utilized.

So be sure the water you drink is pure. Who knows how much vital force is used up in the process of purifying the liquid concoctions that people drink today?

It is a well-known fact among Homœopaths that nearly a century ago calcium fluoride and hydrofluoric acid were proved homœopathically and to this very day are useful in curing the sick *when indicated* by the patient's totality of symptoms. But, as soon as action starts the remedy must be stopped. There are numerous dangers in fluoridating public water supplies. Fluorides are not only deleterious, even in the small doses permitted, but cause different reactions in different people. I have had patients who had backaches precipitated by the intake of fluorides in the drinking water. Many symptoms (such as undue anxiety over money matters, loss of memory, discontent, mottled teeth, fragility of bones) brought about by the fluorides are not ordinarily connected with fluorides unless one studies the scientific provings Homœopathy has made on the subject. To determine the effect of this poison on human life, very careful and painstaking provings have been made on people by eminent physicians, resulting in the compilation[6] of some fifteen full pages of symptoms showing its effects on every part of the body with special emphasis on the *Mind,* heart, veins, sex organs and bones, for no part of the body escapes its malignant influence. These provings were made with repeated doses of an even *smaller* amount than is proposed to put in our drinking water. And remember, the form of the poison to be used in fluoridation is a salt of fluorine, Sodium Fluoride, readily soluble in water and much more deadly in effect.

[6]In the authentic Homœopathic *Materia Medica.*

The U. S. Public Health Service may recommend fluoridation, but this organization is not infallible as may be shown by the fact that, according to Claude M. Palmer's testimony at the hearings before the Committee on Interstate and Foreign Commerce, in the House of Representatives, the Public Health Service once advocated iodine in the drinking water as a preventive of goiter. Iodine was introduced into the drinking water some 20 or so years ago in several communities, Rochester, New York, being the first one. Hardly had the campaign started, however, when the medical profession discovered that the addition of iodine, instead of preventing goiter or curing goiter, encouraged the development of goiter. The process was stopped and those who had proposed it were discredited.

The body does not require fluorine. According to the aforementioned hearings, "Fluorine in water is a deadly poison, inorganic, and cannot be properly assimilated by the human organism."

As a matter of fact, Nature seems to try in many ways to protect man from the little natural fluoride he does get, storing fluorides in small deposits in baby teeth which are expendable, or giving it off in the placenta of a woman after childbirth. Fluorine plays no important part in the body metabolism and is not necessary in the development of the human organism. It is there as an invader. It has a very strong affinity for calcium, and for that reason the excess of fluorine that we may get from our food or our drinking water may be stored up in the bones.

Sodium fluoride is a by-product of aluminum and fertilizer industries. Until recently, its only commercial uses were for rat and cockroach poisons but these two items used up very little of the available supply. Those who back fluoridation paint a rosy picture of its attributes but seem to be unaware of the possibility of chronic fluorine poisoning. Claims that dosage is controllable must be challenged when it is realized that fluorine, unlike chlorine which boils out, gets more concentrated when boiled.

In Charlotte, North Carolina, monthly analyses of fluorine concentration in the water supply showed variations from 14 per cent to 35 per cent below prescribed amount. Many operating difficulties have been noted such as the clogging of piping. Severe erosion necessitates weekly replacement of fittings. We cannot replace our own internal fittings quite so simply! Read further into those Hearings for a good liberal education!

Prescribing the same pill to everyone, regardless of age, health, or ability to withstand its cumulative effect and telling the patient to take as much or as

little of the drug as he pleased would hardly be considered acceptable procedure on the part of a practising physician. Yet men who are not practising
physicians assume the prerogative of prescribing the same amount on fluorine
to every person in every community on a life-long basis, despite individual
tolerance or needs. (Page 32-33 of the Hearings.)

The Hearings go on to say it is important to realise that substances have
been used for many years on the assumption that they were completely
safe because it had not been established in advance that they were toxic,
and yet it was subsequently determined that a hazard to health did in
fact exist, and some of these toxic substances were listed.

With the growing number of chronic sick, it is hardly safe to put a
potentially dangerous substance into the drinking water for consumption
of all *without regard* to each person's state of health, his individual susceptibilities, the medicines being taken by him and, of equal importance,
his freedom of choice. If a man wants a medicine he can always get it
from a drugstore, or from his doctor. Besides, the purpose of fluoridating
the drinking water is to reduce tooth decay, but Toronto reduced its tooth
decay 45.3% during a six-year period by plying its children with information on proper diet, exercising and other aids to good health and good
teeth. The teeth, remember, are a part of a human being just as other
portions of the body are, and healthy teeth are the result of a person's
habits, inheritances and environment. You can hardly expect fluorine to
effect just the teeth and by-pass the rest of the human economy.

In treating a patient homœopathically, there is one individual remedy
at one time for the *whole person* — mind, soul and body — one that gets
at the *cause* of the trouble instead of working on end results. Of course,
all the medicine in the world is not going to help you if you continue to
inflict on yourself the very cause of your trouble. White sugar products,
cola drinks, and the like play an important role in tooth decay. Poisoning
the water supply will not alter the poor eating habits which help to bring
about dental decay.

CHAPTER 15

Constipation

There are probably more people in the U.S. today who think they are constipated than in any country in the world, yet there is no such disease entity as constipation. Constipation is the great American bugaboo. Most people today are obsessed with the fallacious idea that dire results will happen and that their health will be threatened if, by hook or crook, the bowels cannot be induced to move daily.

This erroneous, silly idea makes people "pushovers" for alluring advertisements of many and various laxatives. Many millions of dollars are spent yearly for these drugs and all that can be said for the best of them is that they do produce a temporary, artificial bowel action. What people do not seem to understand is that these very drugs which give temporary action, in reality produce an artificial constipation which is very difficult to cure. This is all quite unnecessary as well as expensive and leads to a lot of complications in health.

In all my years of active practice, I have never prescribed a cathartic and I have never seen a patient die for lack of one. Many of you have been taught from childhood by your own family doctor or your parents that it was of the greatest importance to keep the bowels open at all costs. You are the ones who will be hard to convince that you have been sold a bill of goods. You have been misinformed from the beginning, and so to you the makers of laxatives are the friends of man.

There are many ailments among people, the symptoms of which *include* an interruption of the functions of the lower bowel. Many people only too often think, "I am constipated and it is making me sick," when in reality it is just the reverse — you are sick and it is making you constipated. That being the case, how foolish it is to add to the misery of a sick body the poisons of a physic. How much damage has been done to people of all ages down through the centuries by physicians' almost universal habit of prescribing a laxative for every case of sickness, no one will ever know.

In order for you to intelligently comprehend the nature of constipation, I will present some facts for your consideration.

The large bowel, which is a continuation of the general intestinal tract, begins just where the small one ends at the iliocecal junction. A valve is there which is supposed to prevent the material from going back the other way once it has arrived at the junction. The large bowel is one continuous organ and is divided arbitrarily into ascending colon, transverse colon, descending colon and can contain, when fully distended, about eight quarts. This organ, in its entirety, serves as a receptacle and storage room for the remains of what was once the food we ate, and for which the system has no further use. When this material first enters from the small gut, it is in the form of brownish fluids. It is injected by the small intestine in frequent small jets, being activated by the peristaltic wave of the gut. The first function of the large intestine then is one of dehydrating this material. When it reaches the rectum, it is quite solid in consistency, but still fairly soft. The fluid which the system has reclaimed in this dehydrating process is used over again in various capacities to be eventually excreted by the kidneys, skin and respiratory system. It is a very wonderful provision of Nature that instead of being obliged to have a small liquid evacuation at frequent intervals, the large bowel, as a storage receptacle, allows infrequent movements, thereby providing ample opportunities for business, personal and social diversions. It is entirely automatic. When the material has been sufficiently dehydrated and has been projected into the rectum for final expulsion, it passes a plexus of nerves which gives the signal. If the signal is obeyed by the individual, everything is well. If not, then Nature says, "O.K., I'll wait until later on." How much later depends on many factors, but in the meantime, should the individual become anxious or scared and trust to the pill bottle, then he will become artificially constipated, and that is not so easily corrected. And so a wonderful automatic process, arranged for our good, may be upset by our own stupidity.

Contrary to general opinion that immediate danger follows from failure of a daily evacuation, the fact is, no harm at all will result. A regular, daily movement, at a time that is convenient, is of course desirable and should be accomplished. It is the ideal arrangement, but if it is found inconvenient or impossible to respond to Nature's signal, at the moment, just be patient, another day is coming. Nature will eventually give the signal again, but don't neglect the signal too often.

The normal, rhythmic, onward, wave-like motion of the bowels, any part of them, is determined by the general well-being of the individual. Anything that upsets the system may also affect the normal action of any particular organ and the bowels are not immune by any means. As the system recovers its equilibrium, all organs again carry on their normal functions. Because the action of the large bowel is easily influenced by neglect of timing in regular habit, by the emotions, by various kinds of foods, by the general state of health, by not sufficient intake of water, etc., many millions of people fall easy prey to the laxative habit.

This constipation panic has made many a manufacturer of patent medicines rich, and, as a result, they have immense sums of money with which to drum their products into the tired ears of TV viewers. Of course you know that advertising is a deductible item of expense and doesn't hurt the drug makers very much. So we have the vicious circle. Drug makers advertise and sell millions of dollars worth of physics yearly to you, the people. Now you become really constipated, so you continue to buy more and more as time goes on, and all the while if you'd let the bowels alone they would function perfectly well. Don't take physics! It is not necessary. It is dangerous. Remember that any substance that causes an artificial bowel movement does so because it is a poison and the system is only trying to get rid of it. After this is accomplished, you are right back where you started, with the added burden to your system of reaction to poison, and you are then more constipated.

Colonic irrigation, so prevalent in some places, is not good, and may lead to trouble later. Look at the list of remedies which are useful for this ailment, and if you have a case of Homœopathic remedies in the house, you may be able to choose the proper ones and cure will result.

Diarrhea is another condition which plagues many people. It is the opposite of constipation and is usually due to a disturbance of the vital force caused by improper eating or sometimes by emotional disturbance. Quite often it can be the result of a "cold."

The usual method of treatment by doctors is the prescribing of some sort of astringent like Bismuth, etc. This treatment is just as unjustifiable as giving physics to constipated patients. At best it is only temporarily palliative but may lead to serious trouble. It does not cure or remove the

primary cause. Generally speaking one may say that anything that increases the normal *peristaltic action* of the gut will produce this condition
whether it be laxatives, emotional disturbances, ptomaine poisoning,
wrong foods, or colds.

Whatever the cause, the first remedy is to remove any obvious cause,
then choose the proper Homœopathic remedy — but *never stop Nature
in her endeavor to expel deleterious material* from the intestinal tract. To
do so is a form of suppression which may lead to more serious trouble.

I have had many cases of chronic diarrhea which were caused by irritation of adhesions at the site of the appendix, and which yielded to operation. I hesitate to mention this because too many doctors and laymen
alike are only too willing to accept any excuse for an appendix operation.

There are cases of diarrhea caused by the presence of an amœba which
got into the system accidentally, usually through contaminated or impure
drinking water. There are cases caused by drugs. Search for the cause,
remove it, if possible, apply the proper Homœopathic remedy and recovery
will be prompt. Chronic diarrhea can be very trying and very dangerous
in more ways than one.

When Orthodox doctors fail to help an ordinary case they finally make
a diagnosis of colitis, or even ulcerative colitis. A few years back, colitis
was quite the rage, in fact, quite the rage for some doctors to operate for
it. Their theory was that the tired, overworked colon should have a
complete rest to allow the ulcers to heal. They thought it would take
about two years before the colon would get good and rested and able to
resume its function. They took the trusting patient (only too often young
people) and opened the abdomen and cut the small intestine off from
the large one. Then they closed the end of the large bowel and brought
the end of the small one outside the body and closed the abdominal incision around it. The contents of the bowel then discharged into some
receptacle provided for the purpose.

For two long years the patient suffered the torment of this wicked
piece of surgery. After the two-year period was up, the same surgeons
were determined to make the colon get back on the job, so they operated
again. The closed end of the colon (large intestine) was opened, the
end of the small intestine was dissected away from the abdominal wall
and the two open ends were united again. This all sounds easy, but it is
not. It is fraught with difficulties and is very dangerous. Many have died

as the result. I do not hear so much about the procedure nowadays. I think it has been largely abandoned. But how about all the experimental victims!

This operation was first brought to my attention at a meeting of the Massachusetts Medical Society, which was held at the Children's Hospital in a nearby city. It was there that a paper was read by the head of the hospital which described this "wonderful" new operation as performed at a famous Western clinic. At the finish, the doctor was generously applauded by all but me. In the question period which followed, I arose and condemned the procedure as a most ridiculous, stupid, wicked and meddlesome practice, especially as all cases of so-called ulcerative colitis were readily cured by medicine. The essayist turned a nice red and retorted, "If such cases can be cured by medicine, I wish to God you would tell me how," and stalked off the platform. When I started to tell him the treatment was Homœopathic, he wouldn't listen.

My friends were aghast at my temerity, but I never was a conformist. Well, as fate would have it, just a week later a little boy was brought to see me. He had just been taken home from that very same hospital where he went to be treated for diarrhea. Everything he ate went right through him, undigested. If he ate an apple, it came out apple, etc. At the hospital they proposed this operation, but the father said, "No," so they sent the boy home. He came to see me on a Friday and stayed till Monday. I prescribed the proper Homœopathic remedy and Monday he went home practically well. Just recently I was at church when a young man and his mother came up to me and shook hands. He was the same little boy now grown up, and he told me he has not had a sick day since.

CHAPTER 16

Eczema

I had in my office one day about 8 years ago, two young allopathic physicians to whom I was trying to teach Homœopathy, when a patient came in suffering from a very severe and extensive skin manifestation which doctors call "eczema." I proceeded to put the two doctors "on the spot."

"Gentlemen," I said, "here is a patient who might have come to your office instead of mine seeking relief and cure of a very distressing ailment. What are you going to do for her?"

This patient had been to almost every hospital and clinic in Boston without relief. The last doctor she had consulted put on a goodly amount of sulfa drugs in powder form. Well, that did it. It nearly killed her; so she thought she should at last consult a Homœopath. She was a nurse of the allopathic persuasion, and it was quite a condescension for her to employ a Homœopath, but it was done in sheer desperation.

The two young men were really on the spot. They had not as yet had much Homœopathic training. They suggested ointments and salves, etc., all of which she had tried, and they finally gave up and admitted they wouldn't really know what to do. This poor woman's arms from her neck to her fingertips were covered with moist, itching, scabby eruptions. Scabs on some spots were thick and green. It was all over the back of her neck, behind the ears and even on both legs down to the feet.

I said, "Here is a woman who is sick. We call it eczema, but never mind the diagnosis for the moment, as it has no value in making a prescription. We are treating a sick human being. Let us analyze her. She is obese, blonde, blue-eyed, chronically constipated, thirstless, does not perspire, and is chilly. This physical make-up taken together with the skin eruption itself adds up to just one remedy. What is it?"

They didn't know. No one would know unless he had studied the

Homœopathic *Materia Medica* and could recall a substance which had its *most marked effects* on a person of the patient's physical make-up, and which was *capable of producing on a well person* of such description the symptoms from which this patient suffered. There was such a substance which did just that on various provers. I knew the remedy, of course. I opened the *Materia Medica,* turned to the remedy, and read its pathogenesis to the two young doctors. It fitted her case to perfection. She was given a dose of moderate high potency once a week, and in six weeks when she came in again, I had the young doctors called into my office.

They did not recognize the patient. She was entirely cured, her skin as smooth as a baby's. This case was so unusual that the nurses and office girls were invited to look at it before and after treatment, and everyone, including the patient, was amazed at such a dramatic cure. *That type of patient* suffering from *that kind* of skin disease will always be cured by *that same remedy.* I purposely do not name the remedy because there are lots of people who may have the same *diagnosis* that this remedy wouldn't cure at all.

The amount of medicine needed for the cure cost less than one cent.

There are many conditions that plague many people which are not specifically mentioned in the list of "Pointers to the Common Remedies." That is because they are just *symptoms* produced by error in living and which clear up under the remedy given to cure the original condition. Eczema is one of these conditions.

It sometimes becomes a very distressing ailment and may become chronic simply because under Orthodox regime the patient is treated usually with one of the local applications in vogue, when in reality no medication should ever be applied to a skin eruption of any kind. (A burn, however, is not a skin eruption.) Skin eruptions, as previously mentioned, are the result of Nature's effort to cure some internal disorder by pushing it out through the skin and away from vital organs. When the original ailment is cured, the skin manifestation disappears.

Among the many remedies for this condition — rather, people who have this condition — there are several outstanding ones, but success in curing is due to the fact that the remedy suits the individual. In other words, cure the sick person; cure the original trouble and all skin symptoms disappear. The *patient* is cured. The following remedies, and their matching symptoms, are the outstanding cures for those sick people complaining of these symptoms:

Arsenicum Alb.

Itching, burning, smarting, swelling. Oedema, eruption; papular, dry, rough, scaly, worse from cold and scratching; malignant pustules. Ulcers with offensive discharge. Urticaria (hives) with burning and restlessness. Psoriasis. Patient seeks warmth. Restless and worse at night, with great anguish. Fears death, fears being left alone.

Anacardium

Intensely itching eczema with mental irritability with inclination to swear, worse from hot water, better from eating. Easily offended, impaired memory, sensation of a plug in varying parts — eyes, rectum, bladder, head, etc.

Antimonium Crudum

Child cannot bear to be touched or looked at. Eczema with stomach disturbance, pimples, vesicles and pustules. Thick, hard, honey-colored scabs. Hives. Itching when warm in bed. Dry skin. Warts. Horny patches on soles of feet. Feet very tender. Generally thick-white coat on tongue.

Graphites

Fat, chilly, costive people. Music makes them weep. Lack of disposition to work. Despondent, worse warmth, at night, better in the dark from wrapping up. Rough, hard, dryness of skin where not affected by eczema. Eruption oozing out, a sticky exudation. Rawness in bends of limbs, groin, neck, between fingers and toes and behind ears. Unhealthy skin, very little injury suppurates. Feelings of cobwebs on face. Thick, various colored scabs from head to foot.

Mezerium

Useful in eczema intolerably itchy. Worse in motion and at night. Pain and burning in skin and long bones. Legs and feet go to sleep. Patient is very sensitive to cold air.

A case: Mrs. C., age 42, eczema of twenty years standing. Eruption on backs of hands and wrists half way up to the elbows, itching made worse by scratching. Small burning vesicles drying down with crusts, itching and burning after scratching and becoming worse again. Much worse from application of water. In less than four weeks skin became soft and normal and remained healthy.

Rhus Tox.   Skin red, swollen, itching intense. Burning eczematous eruptions with tendency to scale formation. Worse during sleep and cold, wet, rainy weather. During rest, extreme restlessness, must change position often whether sitting or lying. Better warm dry weather, motion, walking, rubbing, warm applications and from stretching out limbs.

Sepia   Predominantly a woman's remedy, but not exclusively. Brunette type. Indifferent to those loved best. Dreads to be alone. Very sad, weeps when relating symptoms. Skin: cold sores on isolated spots. Itching, *not* relieved by scratching, worse in bends of elbows and knees. Almost any skin eruption may occur on scalp, face, lips, nose. The patient is generally thin rather than fat. Strong odor of perspiration in arm pits. Sweat on feet, worse on toes, bad odor.

Sulphur   Skin: dry, scaly, unhealthy. Every little injury suppurates. Itching, burning, worse scratching and washing. Pimply eruption, pustules, hangnails. Excoriation, especially in folds. Skin affections following local medicines. Whole skin itches, especially at night and in bed.

Petroleum   Especially for dark-type people who suffer from catarrhal conditions of the mucous membranes, gastric acidity and skin eruptions.
Skin: itching at night, chilblains moist, itch and burn. Red sores, skin dry, constricted, very sensitive, rough, cracked and leathery. Slightest scratch makes skin suppurate. Psoriasis of hands. Thick, greenish crusts, burning and itching; redness, raw, cracks and bleeds easily. Skin darkens and thickens after much scratching.

Again, we do not treat diseases but people who are sick, and they must be treated as a whole with the one individual remedy which matches the symptoms satisfactorily. This remedy is called the similimum and is based on The Law of Similars.

People who manifest their sickness by symptoms of such a nature that arbitrary names, such as multiple sclerosis, muscular dystrophy, cystic fibrosis, etc., are applied must receive treatment by remedies which may be indicated by the *symptoms* and not by any so-called diagnosis. It is not a disease entity which is to be cured, but a disturbed condition of the vital force — a purely personal affair. For such cases it usually takes the best of homœopathic physicians to choose the proper remedy in each case.

Such ultimate conditions with these fearsome diagnoses for which Orthodox doctors have no cure should have and could have been prevented if properly chosen remedies were given in the beginning of the illness which might very well have had a resemblance to the common cold.

One day an allopathic doctor came in suffering with a pain in his back and legs. He had had it for a long time and everything the allopaths had was tried without benefit. He came in for an X-ray. I said, "Why do you want an X-ray?"

He replied, "To see what's wrong with my back."

I asked, "Did you have an injury of any kind?"

He said, "No."

Then I said, "Don't you know that the X-ray will reveal nothing? Come into my office, I'll prescribe for you on your symptoms."

I gave him a Homœopathic remedy and he got well promptly. He was so surprised that he asked me if I could cure eczema with my Homœopathy, and I said yes. He then sent in one of his patients who had had eczema for years and nothing he could do for it helped at all. I called the same two young doctors in the office again and said, "Here is another case of eczema. What would you do for her?"

"Ah!" they said, "We would give her x—, the remedy that cured the other case."

Wrong! That remedy, of course, would not have given her the slightest bit of help. Why? Because, although the diagnosis was the same — eczema — the patient was entirely different. This patient was dark skinned, brown-eyed, skinny, quick in action and perspired freely with a strong odor. She was indifferent to her family and her husband, and was in striking physical contrast to the first one. Her remedy had to be something that fitted her as a person. There was just such a remedy, a few doses of which cured her completely. I again referred to the *Materia Medica* and pointed out the pathogenesis of the remedy which fitted this woman and her symptoms perfectly.

Later on I met the doctor and asked about the patient. He said, "She is all cured, but she doesn't know what did it."

That is the way Homœopathy works, and to one who has been used to heavy doses of strong drugs and local applications of all kinds, it is hard to believe that a cure could come about in such a mild, simple manner. Most people think that if a little medicine is good, a lot would be better. But such is not the case.

I could go on and on and give thousands of such examples to illustrate what Homœopathy can and will do, but by now it should not be necessary. Besides, it would take up too much valuable space which I wish to use to tell you how you may preserve your health and not need a doctor many times during your lifetime.

However, I must yield to temptation and tell you about a case that came to my office just a few months ago. This happened to be another case of skin disease. The patient was an elderly man of about seventy years. He was accompanied by three friends who helped him in. He carried his arms straight out in front of him and walked very feebly. His legs pained him, and his forearms, hands and fingers were covered with thick greenish cracked scabs from which oozed a thin fluid. His hands were swollen and he could not move his fingers. He had suffered from this condition for many months, for which he had been treated by several doctors who had prescribed an almost unlimited number of salves, ointments, etc. He had also been given sulfa and penicillin, all of which only made him worse. My secretary and two business associates were in the office when this patient came in. From their facial expressions I gathered that they were all of the opinion that "well, at last here is a case that is hopeless. The doctor is surely up against it this time. What can anyone do for this poor old man?" They admitted later that I surely had their sympathy.

Well, as a matter of fact, such cases do not present much difficulty to an experienced Homœopath — one who knows his *Materia Medica*. I knew what he needed immediately and gave him three doses of a remedy in an almost infinitesimal dose the first week. At the end of the week he came back. His hands showed no improvement, but his eyes were brighter and he walked with a brisker step, he had hope and a general feeling of well being.

I said, "O.K., go home — take no more medicine, and come in again in a week."

You see, the three doses of medicine (two small pills at a dose) were working; so it must have no interference.

At the end of the week he returned feeling much better generally, and exclaimed almost joyously, "Doctor, I can move my fingers!"

I replied, "That's fine," and gave him two more doses to be taken two days apart. He was to report at the end of another week. When he came in he kissed the hand of his friend who advised his coming to me. He proudly showed his hands, which were completely cured. The skin was clean and healthy and the patient said he felt better than he had for years. He brought with him the original three, along with several others who had various ailments.

Can you imagine the wonderful thrill of satisfaction which comes to all Homœopathic doctors when such success crowns their efforts? The commercial aspect never intrudes. The one and only desire is to choose the proper remedy and then watch the action of the immutable law as it unfolds and blossoms out in the form of a beautiful cure, the re-establishment of health to some human being.

That is the kind of service one is willing to pay for without being asked. This man would have given me his last cent. I was delighted to have restored his health. I thought it would make him feel better to pay something; so I allowed him to pay me $10 — just in case you are interested.

I did not treat him for his diagnosis — eczema. I treated a sick man, the totality of his symptoms leading to the choice of a remedy, the action of which removed all of his symptoms, including the skin condition.

CHAPTER 17

Injuries and Burns

A young doctor brought to my hospital a boy with a "green stick" fracture of the right forearm. X-ray revealed the condition and I said, "I will straighten it out and apply a cast."

But the young doctor wanted all the credit for caring for the patient and applied the cast himself. The boy was his patient, so I had to step out. The cast was applied and the patient went home. A week later the boy's arm was amputated at the elbow because of gangrene due to improper cast. A carpenter could have done a better job than this "doctor" who, in his lack of experience, had made the cast for the arm in a straight-down position and then put the arm in a sling. With the arm thus bent at the elbow, the circulation was cut off and gangrene set in.

Thousands of accidents happen every day ranging from the simple to the serious. I have seen disastrous results follow improper handling of all kinds of injuries. On the other hand, with proper handling, I have seen miraculous results. My long experience in surgery has taught me the proper way to treat such conditions, and it is very important that you should receive this information.

It is neither necessary nor expedient to describe the many kinds of *injuries* to which man is liable, because basically the treatment is the same. Some will cut or break the skin, some the bones, others will be in the form of bruises of the flesh in varying degree. There are often injuries to the head which may affect the brain, ranging from rupture of brain substance to mere concussion.

First aid remedies and instructions for their use are available at Homœopathic pharmacies. It is mighty handy to have such remedies on hand as Arnica for bruises and charley horse; rhus. tox. for torn ligaments or sprains; calendula for cuts and knife wounds; and all the other wonderful first aid remedies which are of great value in emergencies.

Theoretically and almost actually, germs are to be found everywhere. The fear of what these germs will or might do to people through injuries which cut the skin has led to wrong and dangerous treatment, which has been practiced ever since the microscope disclosed these little vegetative growths. Where an injury occurs which cuts or tears the skin, germs are introduced into the cut either from the object that made the injury or from the patient's own skin, or both. If bleeding is fairly active, these germs are usually washed out immediately and the ensuing clot fills the cut and prevents the further entry of germs. That being the case, the wound itself is the cleanest spot in the vicinity. Nothing should be done to change it. Bleeding from such injuries will stop of itself usually, as soon as the clot forms. Then nothing but a dry, sterile dressing should be applied, and in a very few days the injury will heal with no delay or complications.

If, however, as is too often the case, someone, perhaps the doctor, comes in and proceeds to wash the wound and its vicinity, and then applies some fancied antiseptic material, then the damage is done. Germs are washed *into* the wound, the protective clot having been also washed away, and there the germs find dead cells, dead blood and serum and it becomes their "happy hunting ground." They multiply and increase just as long as there is something there for them to eat, and so with an infected wound and its accompanying soreness, pus, and temperature, if not something even more serious, the final healing is greatly delayed.

Germicides are a delusion and a snare. Fire is the only sure destroyer of these pestiferous trouble-makers that I know — that is, if you provide the chance for them to make themselves obnoxious.

Even in cases where bleeding is severe, do try to stop it — but avoid touching the wound itself. It is clean. Do nothing to infect it. Scalp wounds often bleed freely. Stop the bleeding by hard, firm pressure on the cut, with a thick piece of sterile cotton or gauze. *Do not ever wash the wound,* and it will heal in twenty-four hours. In cases which are brought to the hospital, the usual routine of the doctors and especially the insurance doctors is to shave the scalp to a varying degree, wash and "sterilize" and then apply the germicides. This is Orthodox routine.

I have seen literally hundreds of such cases and the results of such treatment were a long, hard, expensive convalescence.

Not one of my personal cases got any such treatment, never had to go to a hospital, never once in over fifty years have I ever used an antiseptic, nor have I ever shaved the head or messed around with the actual wound, and furthermore, every last one of those cases cured itself within twenty-four hours. I mean that by that time the bleeding had stopped, the clot, protected against invasion of germs, was underlaid by the healing serum, and no more attention was needed except to avoid carelessness that could open the wound. In several days the healing was complete.

I could write a whole book describing the miserable results of meddle-some interference.

A woman brought her daughter to see me because of a badly lacerated forearm. The cut reached from wrist to elbow on the palm side of the arm. It seemed that this young lady put too much weight on a glass-topped serving table. It broke and her arm went through it. They were frightened, fearing blood poison. I asked and they replied that they had not touched the wound in any way. The wound looked clean. The bleeding had almost ceased. I approximated the edges of the wound with adhesive plaster in half dozen or more strips, being careful not to touch the wound. I then wrapped it in sterile dressing and sent them home, advising them to return in a week if the arm did not become painful. The mother then very indignantly wanted to know what kind of a doctor I was, that would not, or at least did not, apply some sort of germicide. I counted to ten. I finally convinced her that I knew what I was doing. The next time they came in they were very humble. In ten days the arm had entirely and beautifully healed. I removed the adhesive strips and the scar was very slight, and so at last everyone was happy.

Now, I know absolutely that if I had used disinfectants and germicides, and by so doing, destroyed the healing serum of Nature, the injury would have been a long time in healing, with what complications no one will ever know.

One summer day a fourteen-year-old boy came to my office with his right index finger severed diagonally between the first and second joint. He had been working with another boy, cutting the hedge in my own yard. I saw him a moment or two after the accident, the blood was still spurting. I was about to throw the severed end away when I got an idea. Instead of throwing it away, I applied splints to the hand and stump in such a manner as to allow the end of the finger to be placed back in its proper place and bound firmly. Blood still flowed profusely. I then packed the whole hand in sterile gauze and cotton in such a manner that the end of the finger would remain in position. In a few minutes the blood began to seep through the dressing. I let it alone. In half an hour all dripping ceased. I told the boy to be most careful not to disturb the dressing, not under any condition to get it wet, to keep it outside on top of bedclothes at night and to see me in three days.

He came and I smelt the dressing. It was all right. I told him he was doing a good job and that he was to come back in a week. I again smelt it and it was still all right. At the end of the second week I removed all dressing and splints and his finger was as good as new. One must look carefully to see the scar today, ten years later.

The usual treatment would have been to stop the bleeding by various methods, sterilize the stump, find skin enough to cover it and hope for clean healing. Had I applied antiseptics, stopped the bleeding and then put the finger in place, the first time I smelt it there would have been the odor of gangrene and no saving of the finger. Nature will do wonders if given a chance.

Many times large arteries and veins are severed and the wounds are large enough to require stitching. Sometimes ligatures [1] are necessary. Great care then is necessary in tying off the bleeding so as not to introduce infection. It would be advisable to have a reliable doctor or surgeon tie off arteries. The edges of extensive cuts often require approximation. Do it carefully, either by stitching or by adhesive tape. Never use antiseptics.

In cases where infection does take place, the remedy which I invariably use is the aqueous tincture of Calendula diluted with water ten parts and medicine one part. It is almost unbelievable, until one sees it, how quickly soreness and pus disappear and how quickly reparative granulation tissue begins.

A young man was changing a tire in the darkness of early morning when he was struck and dragged eighty feet by another car. Among his many injuries, which included broken bones, were those of both his lower legs where all the flesh of the shin side (front) was destroyed and torn off. A physician had sewed up the gaping wounds to cover the bones and at the end of twenty-four hours he was brought to me at my hospital. He was in a very critical condition. He had gangrene bacillus infection and the odor was almost unbearable.

Two surgeons who saw the case with me advised immediate amputation above the knees. I said, "No, there is a better way." I cut out all of the stitches which freed a lot of pus, debris, etc. I wiped the wounds out with

[1] A thread tied around a blood vessel to arrest bleeding.

dry sterile gauze and poured into the deep gouges of the wounds Calendula tincture diluted 10-1, and let it stay there. The wounds being long and deep could contain almost a pint of this medicine in each leg. I let the legs lie bare on the bed. In an hour the odor had absolutely disappeared. The patient felt much revived. Shortly the deep trenches of the wound began to fill with granulation tissue. In two days it had entirely covered the bare bones, and to make a long story short, within three weeks the patient left for home. That was many years ago. He has two good legs; scars, yes, but that is all. This patient had no blood transfusions, no "miracle" or "wonder" drugs, no antibiotics — and, no bills for medicine!

A young man was brought by ambulance to my hospital with his head literally half severed from his body, caused by being thrown head first through the windshield of his car. This boy was almost bloodless and almost lifeless. His jugular vein and all superficial veins and arteries were cut. Open to plain view were his larynx, esophagus, base of tongue and all tissues in one half of his neck.

The first thing I did was to pack tightly the entire depth and breadth of the wound with sterile gauze. I then gave him an intravenous injection of normal saline and put him to bed. In twenty-four hours I carefully removed the packing and was pleased to note that there was no infection. I then took four strong, four-pronged, grasping forceps and after getting the boy's head on his neck in a normal position, I clamped it into place with those heavy clamps. No sewing was done. If infection did develop it would be a simple matter to remove one or two clamps to allow drainage. To make another long story short, he healed by "first intention" and had no bad effects from the injury.

This patient was bloodless when he arrived. To give the heart fluid to pump, normal saline was given — *no blood transfusion, no drugs* of any kind. Nature wants *no* interference. She sometimes welcomes help. If infection had occurred, Calendula would have been the required help.

Bones will heal just as readily as bruises and cuts. If the blood is clean, it won't take long. Simplicity in treatment is the magic word in all cases of sickness or accident. Nature likes it and so does your purse.

In numerous cases of bone fracture in tobacco addicts, I have found it necessary to stop their smoking because the fracture refused to heal. After the smoking was eliminated, the healing took place. I have seen the same deleterious effects of tobacco in cases of abdominal incision which refused to heal until the tobacco poisoning was stopped. So you see clean blood is necessary at all times.

In 1942, the great Coconut Grove fire in Boston which killed 491 people supplied a large number of burn cases on which the doctors of Orthodox medicine experimented. They got absolutely nowhere. In fact, a doctor from the staff of one of Boston's largest hospitals read a paper before a medical gathering at my hospital on the subject of Treatment of Burns. He presented gruesome pictures of some of the victims of this fire. He described all the experimental procedures that were used. He stated that the number of patients on which the previous Orthodox methods were used was sufficient to prove that none of these methods were of any value. He then said that so far, in spite of the hundreds of cases in which new experiments were made, the conclusions were that nothing of value was discovered, and the final decision was to apply a coating of vaseline. That was the best they could offer. In the discussion that followed I tried to show what a wonderfully curative medicine Calendula was. As soon as he learned that Calendula was of Homœopathic origin, he turned and closed the discussion.

Such an ostrich-like attitude, my friends, is not indicative of a very scientific approach to the art of healing.

Fourteen years later, in *Time*,[2] August 20, 1956, there appeared an article entitled "Home Remedy for Burns." It confirms Orthodoxy's ever-present lack of know-how and also confirms something of what I have said about blood transfusions. Here is the item:

To fight severe burns, modern medicine has experimented with all kinds of remedies — tannic acid (now in some disrepute), bandaging, baths, skin grafting, diet, even hypnosis. But the victim of an extensive burn (more than 10% of the skin) is in most critical danger from loss of fluid and shock. The standard treatment for this has long been to administer either whole blood or blood plasma intravenously. Since plasma is often not available and since it often contins hepatitis virus, doctors have been looking for a simpler remedy. Last week a team of U. S. Public Health Service scientists announced that they had found it. Their remedy: a solution of simple table salt and baking soda, taken orally.

Although salt and baking soda has been a remedy for burns for many years,

[2]Courtesy TIME, The Weekly Newsmagazine, copyright Time Inc., 1956.

nobody has suggested that it could be substituted for plasma injections. The present findings are based on a four-year study of burn victims conducted by U. S. and Peruvian researchers in Lima. If administered within three hours after injury, the scientists found, the *saline solution*[3] (two teaspoons of table salt to one of baking soda in two quarts of water) acts just as effectively as plasma in warding off shock. The victim may drink as many as seven quarts of the solution in the first twelve hours. Later, the patient gets standard hospital burn treatment.

Everyone should have a bottle of Calendula in the house. I personally have a gallon of it always on hand. Burns, cuts, infected injuries, sores, and the like, are cured by it in an unbelievably short time.

Calendula should not be applied full strength, however — a dilution of one part medicine to ten parts water, as before stated, is about right. In the case of burns, soak a piece of clean linen or gauze or cotton in this solution and apply. The dressing must be well soaked so that the liquid gets on the burn, and, in the case of burns, it must be applied *hot*. Not hot enough to burn, but as hot as the hands can stand.

I have seen scald burns cured overnight. For sunburn it has no equal.

A woman brought her little boy to the hospital one Friday afternoon suffering from sunburn. His little face was deeply blistered. The skin was all off his nose and his neck had numerous sores. He was a pitiful sight. I asked the mother to let me keep him till Monday morning and then she could come and get him. She agreed. I applied the remedy as described. All pain disappeared after the first sharp pain of the hot application and when Monday came the little fellow was absolutely cured. His mother was amazed but delightedly thankful.

This remedy is no secret. It has been used by the Homœopathic doctors for a hundred years, but so far it has been ignored by so-called orthodox doctors. Why? Calendula is the common marigold which is so extensively grown in New England flower gardens.

---

[3] Saline solution instead of blood transfusion has been used for over a hundred years by good Homœopaths all over the world.

CHAPTER 18

The Heart

Every living organism has a circulatory system, a system which makes possible a supply of vital fluid — sap — blood — to every cell in the organism — plants, animals, microbes, man included. The circulatory system means life itself.

Watching the development of the embryo chick, one may observe the beginning of this marvelous system of arteries, veins, etc. At an appointed time there will commence the pulsating rhythm of a node or enlarged spot in this network, which has been named the heart. This wonderful system is dependent on each and every component in order to function. One part is as important as any other and each part functions automatically and involuntarily, according to the plan of its Creator. The starting of the heartbeat is as mysterious as life itself.

This system will function faithfully so long as the vital spark remains in the organism. The part which we call the heart, constructed of strong, involuntary muscle tissue, mysteriously receives at the appointed moment the Word to pulsate — beat — and that Order is obeyed so long as the breath of life remains. And this wonderful and faithful organ has been termed the No. 1 killer of man. For shame! How can man be so stupid as to think such a thing! He, through his ignorance, stupidity, carelessness and greed (aided and abetted by a host of self-acclaimed "heart specialists") has conducted himself in such a fashion that he, Man, has become the No. 1 Killer of the Heart. No other animal in its natural habitat has heart trouble.

Today, heart disease has become an entity in the eyes of the public and profession as well, and as a result we have an army of 20,000 so-called "heart specialists," who, knowing very little about the subject, have saved their collective reputations by proclaiming the heart the No. 1 Killer. Heart specialists are not the answer to this problem. Proper living is the answer. Proper living makes possible the clean bloodstream Nature intended us to have. Since every cell in man's body depends on blood, does it not follow that when the supply is reduced or is of inferior quality, the cells suffer? When the blood is polluted with poison, anything may happen. The organs which need the most blood are the ones to suffer first. They are the vital organs — heart, kidney, lungs, liver, brain and especially all parts of the circulatory system itself. The heart is helpless under these conditions. It is not the sinner. It is sinned against.

So why don't these great heart specialists tell the people right out in plain English why there are so many heart failures in ever increasing numbers? Do they know, or don't they?

Reams of words have been written by writers quoting these same sacrosanct heart specialists, but has one word been given the public as to the cause? There is a cause (or causes), of course. What is it? Is not the public entitled to information on this matter? If heart disease is an entity, and the heart actually is a killer, then there must be a definite, single cause. But such is not the case. No two people ever react exactly alike under adverse environment nor to any poison that may enter the body or be produced by the living body. In each individual case of sickness there may be one or a dozen contributory causes. A careful study of the *individual as a whole* — mind, body and soul — should reveal the cause or causes in each case.

Studying the sick organ alone will reveal nothing as to the cause. Only the results will be found, leaving the cause a mystery. The cause is what we want revealed so we can make prevention possible. The heart is a long-suffering and patient organ. It was intended by the Creator that it should pump the vital fluid to the uttermost parts of the body as its sole duty. This it will faithfully do till the very end of life. It will do so in spite of faulty valves, in spite of the surgeon's invasion with the scalpel. There have been some dramatic surgical successes in this field, and I feel that lately the heart specialist is giving his attention to that phase of it at the expense of the less dramatic search for cause and prevention in the non-surgical field. The surgical manipulations that have been imposed on the heart of late years prove what a tough and robust organ it really is. It is a shame that it is so woefully abused by careless errors in everyday living.

Earth's environment provides air, water and food, all of which are essential to life. Life is impossible without water, but a man can lose his life by drowning in it if he is careless or unfortunate. Proper food is essential, but man can lose his health and perhaps life if he eats improperly both in quantity and quality. Nature never intended man to drink any such stuff as tea, coffee, alcohol and a host of other commercial drinks available everywhere today. In short, nothing but pure water and proper food should enter the stomach.

Besides the errors in diet, we as a nation consume fourteen thousand million dollars worth of drugs per year — none of which in my estimation have any curative value but all of which cause an untold number of various kinds of ailments. It is almost impossible to point an accusing finger at the particular drug or combinations of drugs in any individual case. The amount of alcoholic beverages and coffee consumed today staggers the imagination and contributes to all kinds of sickness including heart ailments. The addiction to the drug nicotine is a universal disgrace and is destroying the health of more people than any other single cause. It causes more deaths by *killing the heart* than any other single cause.

Does any man in his right mind fail to realize that the daily, yes, hourly, introduction into the vital bloodstream of a deadly drug like nicotine constitutes a deadly peril to his life? Should there be any logical ground for debate where such transgression is so obvious? Have you ever heard of a heart specialist coming right out flat-footed without double talk and telling the public the unvarnished truth about the dangers of cigarette smoking? Why don't they tell what caused the President to develop heart trouble despite the fact he had just had a clean bill of health a couple of months prior to the attack, so that others may avoid such a condition? Their job as heart specialists is to inform and warn the public. What a wonderful chance they have at the moment to do just such a service. Why don't they do it?

The specialists talk a lot nowadays about cholesterol and other fatty accumulations in the circulatory system, revealed by the microscope. They don't explain the situation which allows this circumstance to occur.

"Best Advice: Don't Overeat. Calories — Not Fat — Called Coronary Key." The aforementioned advice heads up a newspaper item by Louis Cassels (Excerpt from U.P. dispatch) in *The Boston Globe* of May 20, 1957, which states:

You can eat your way into a coronary, a leading heart specialist said today, with "any kind of diet that contains too many calories."

"It's getting fat, and not merely making fat, that builds up the cholesterol deposits on the walls of your arteries and invites coronary heart disease," said Dr. Simond Dack, retiring president of the American College of Cardiology.

Dack, a cardiologist at New York's Mount Sinai Hospital and editor of the *American Journal of Cardiology*, acknowledged in an interview that laymen have every right to be "confused" by the conflicting statements that have emanated from medical researchers recently about the relation between diet and heart trouble.

"Doctors get confused too," he said. "We are in a situation where knowledge is advancing and interpretations are changing so rapidly that it is difficult to make dogmatic statements about the precise effects of various kinds of foods."

"But you don't have to wait until medical scientists reach 100 percent agreement before you start eating sensibly," he said.

"There is definite evidence that plain overeating — taking in too many calories of all types and gaining weight — is a very important factor in increasing your chances of coronary heart disease."

Thousands of autopsies have confirmed the presence of thick cholesterol deposits in the arteries of heart attack victims.

Epidemiological studies also have shown that the incidence of heart disease is much higher in countries where the diet is rich in cholesterol-laden fats.

Dack said that while medical scientists generally agree that these findings are highly significant there still is much controversy over their precise meaning.

His strongest conviction, however, is that these scientific arguments are no excuse for the average person to shrug off the whole problem of diet and heart disease as something on which "the doctors can't make up their minds."

"From a purely practical point of view," he said, "the important thing to keep in mind is that the body can manufacture cholesterol out of any type of food, not merely out of fats.

"If you eat too much sugar, proteins and carbohydrates, you are asking for trouble even if you are consciously avoiding what you consider to be fatty foods."

What is the specific advice he would give to a patient who came to him for guidance about diet?

"I would tell him to beware of excess calories, regardless of the type. A little undernourishment would do overfed Americans a lot of good.

"I would tell him to go ahead and eat a balanced diet — but use a little common sense about cutting out extra-rich foods from which we get 'empty calories' that we don't need for nutrition.

"I would tell him to broil his food instead of frying it, to trim all the fat from his meat before he eats it; to lay off rich desserts; to go easy on pure fats, such as butter, margarine and salad oils, to substitute fish or other seafoods (which are low in cholesterol) for meat at some meals; to eat a few eggs a week, which he needs for nutrition, but not to have two fried in butter every morning."

Dack paused for a moment, then added:

"If this patient was overweight, I would advise him to reduce. But I would also tell him that it doesn't do much good to lose 20 or 30 pounds, and then gradually gain it all back.

"Experiments have shown that cholesterol builds up in your arteries while you are gaining weight. Some of the deposits are removed when you lose weight — but part of the damage is irreversible.

"Thus it is very important to keep your weight stable at a proper level, instead of losing and gaining, losing and gaining."

Up until recently the experts have been claiming cholesterol as the cause of heart trouble, not explaining what *made* the cholesterol in the first place, and the only suggestion they could make was to stop eating fat, such as butter, fried foods, etc. But now some seem to have given it more thought and the above clipping suggests they have come to the conclusion that *too much food* — what I have been cautioning throughout this book — is the primary factor. However, too much food not only produces an over-abundance of cholesterol, but various other manifestations of sickness.

No particular organ can be sick, alone, by itself. The entire body is involved. Therefore, it is the entire sick man that must be treated. Such method of treatment is termed psychosomatic medicine. I am encouraged to find that some of the thinkers in Orthodox medicine are beginning to realize that there is too much so-called specialization — that it is not rational, desirable or sensible. If these same thinkers would turn to scientific medicine (Homœopathy) and put their potential mentality to work along the proper line, some great and wonderful results might come to pass, not only in heart sickness but in every kind of ailment that mankind has brought upon itself.

Bear in mind that there are no single organ or organs collectively in the body guilty of anything. This includes the heart. All organs are passive, obedient to the laws of Nature, and they function only as they were intended to. When any of them fail in their functions the fault seldom lies in them. The organ affected is determined by the makeup of the individual, his heredity, and his own peculiar reaction to the specific cause or causes. Nicotine causes coronary disease of the heart, Buerger's disease,

cancer of the lung, kidney disease, etc., along with many other manifestations of sickness. Whenever I hear of anyone dying of "coronary," I know
without asking that nicotine probably did it.

I have seen many patients in my many years of practice that were
diagnosed by other doctors as having heart conditions when the heart
was absolutely sound and normal. One cold winter night I was called
to see a new patient. I was called because the family doctor, who had
been treating this patient for several years for a heart condition, was out
of town. I found a woman of middle life lying in bed, her heart beating
so violently that the bedclothes were going up and down with the heart
beats. She was anguished and frightened. I examined the heart and found
it to be organically normal. On further study I found the abdomen
distended with gas, especially in the upper left quadrant. I stayed there
about an hour and then told them that the patient *did not* have anything
wrong with the heart. That, of course, was a reflection on their own much-
loved family doctor, so I was not too politely shown the door. I was very
young and felt badly but I knew I was right. I had told them that gas in a
certain portion of the gut was responsible for the heart action and that I
believed the gas was caused by a chronic condition of the appendix. I
went home sadly dejected.

Imagine, then, my surprise when the family phoned me next morning
and asked if I would come back. They apologized for their treatment of
me the night before, and said, on thinking things over, I had seemed
confident of my opinion and gradually they too began to wonder if, after
all, their own doctor had not been wrong. To make this story as short
as possible, I took the patient to the hospital, took out the appendix, and
found it to be in the condition I had suspected. She made a fine recovery
and had no further sign of heart trouble — and that was forty years ago.
Before the operation this patient was confined largely to her home. Her
family did manage to get her out to church once a week, but that was
the only place she did go. After the operation, she went everywhere.

Case number two was an old friend of mine, a Methodist minister.
One day while playing golf, he felt a sudden pain go down his left arm.
He was then living quite a distance from my home and so rather than
bother me, he got a local doctor who said, "You have a coronary and it is
very serious. You must go to bed for quite a while and I'll treat you."

Not having heard from this friend for weeks, which was unusual, I
telephoned him. His wife told me what the other doctor had said and so

I went right over to their home. Rosie, the wife, met me at the door. She put her fingers to her lips and said, "Sh!" and whispered that Frank had had a heart attack and that they had a wonderful doctor who was absorbing the heart clot and that I mustn't say anything that would disturb Frank. I looked at her and said, "Rosie, what the heck are you talking about? Frank has no more heart trouble than I have. Where is he?"

When I saw him I said, "Frank, what are you doing here in bed?"

He said, "Shad, I have a bad heart and the doctor won't let me up."

I said, "Get up, now!"

I had had him up and walking around town for two weeks before the doctor said one day, "You are looking better, I guess you may sit up for a while." The doctor had been calling every day or so, but Frank always saw him coming and was dutifully in bed on his arrival. Well, strange as it may seem, his symptoms were due also to a chronic appendix. I had been after him for years to let me remove it. I finally convinced him after this experience. I removed the appendix, separated the adhesions. In two weeks he was out at my farm helping me build a bull pen. That was fifteen years ago and he has never had any more "heart trouble." He is now around eighty-five. But — he has not yet gotten over the *fear* of heart trouble engendered by the doctor who told him he had a "coronary."

Dr. Goldwater remarks on this very phase of heart conditions. This quotation is taken from *Time*,[1] January 28, 1952:

Many people whose doctors tell them that they have something the matter with their hearts have nothing of the sort. That is the conclusion of three Manhattan physicians, headed by Dr. Leonard J. Goldwater, after a ten-year study of hundreds of "heart cases" sent to them by the New York State Employment Service, which wanted to find out what kind of work was suitable for its "handicapped" clients.

The three doctors worked in a special clinic set up at Bellevue Hospital. They took their time — unlike many of the doctors who had diagnosed the patients originally. Among 631 cases, 175 (or 28%) were found to have no heart disease at all. (All but 19 had been told that they had; the 19 had misdiagnosed themselves.) The biggest group of wrong diagnoses (38) had been made by draft doctors at induction centers, but private and school physicians, hospital clinics, insurance examiners and industrial physicians all contributed to the total of bad guesses.

[1]Courtesy *TIME*, The Weekly Newsmagazine, copyright Time, 1952.

How did the doctors come to err so often? Their commonest stumble was a "functional" (i.e., not organic) heart murmur, of a type which Dr. Goldwater describes as "transitory, innocent." Sometimes they were misled by high blood pressure. Other errors were more surprising: tuberculosis, cancer of the stomach and latent syphilis were all mistaken for heart trouble.

In 56 cases, doctors had advised the patients to take it easy; in some instances they had gone so far as to recommend quitting a job or turning down a new one. But the perversity of human nature is evident in the Goldwater report: only 19 of the 56 took the doctor's advice, while seven who had not been told to cut down their activities did so anyway.

"When non-cardiac patients are advised to limit their activities, as a result of incorrect diagnosis, the result is calamitous," say Dr. Goldwater and his colleagues. "Not only needless disability has been created, but irreparable psychic trauma also is often produced. . . . Large numbers of young men are again being examined in connection with military service. It seems particularly timely to point out again that what is designed to serve as a preventive measure may prove to be just the opposite."

The heart muscle, like any other muscle, is strong or weak according to the amount of work it is called upon to do. When a racehorse is being prepared for a season of racing there is a gradual strengthening of legs, wind, and heart, all at the same time.

I have often been asked, "How about exercise in heart cases?" Basically, exercise (bodily activity) is absolutely necessary to health in normal people. Children could not develop properly without constant muscular exercise. If it is so essential to well people, how much more necessary is it to sick people!

Normally, a healthy body and a healthy heart go hand in hand. A weak body makes a weak heart and vice versa. Many people go through a lifetime with leaking valves in the heart. If they exercise to a point of exertion, Nature comes to the rescue with a safeguard in the form of loss of wind, a shortness of breath in other words, so that a continuance of such strenuous activity is automatically stopped. In such chronic cases, a person learns not to overstep the bounds. Those heart defects are anatomical and not a state of systemic illness.

With an absolutely sound heart, organically, but with a sedentary, lazy, overeating existence, where the heart muscle is, like the body muscles, out of condition, one runs up against the same loss of wind under undue exercise. That warning people should *heed* immediately and their sloth-ful way of living be corrected. But how many will do it?

The most universal condition is when the whole system is poisoned by impure blood due to the individual's own habits of indulgence in such poisons as nicotine, alcohol, coffee, tea, etc. The heart then may be right on the verge of failure if any undue strain is put on it. In such cases the vessels which supply blood to the heart muscle itself are usually constricted or clogged and cannot supply the amount of blood needed. In case of constriction, the cause is usually nicotine and don't let anyone convince you otherwise. If the vessels are clogged, then this is due to overeating and/or coffee, tea and alcohol — and don't forget it either. It may mean your life and it will be your own doing. So there are heart conditions which demand much care in the kind and amount of exercise to be allowed, but what horrible conditions for a thinking human being to *bring upon himself!*

Verily, I repeat what I have said before — man is the No. 1 killer of the heart.

If one should find himself out of wind from what would be normal exercise, then he should immediately check himself and discover what he is doing that is wrong. Of course, if one prefers his self-indulgences more than good health, no advice that I, or anyone else, can give will be heeded, and so in a short while another death from "coronary" is recorded and the victim of his own carelessness is buried and forgotten. Don't let it happen to you, my good readers.

Much advice is handed out to people who have reached three score years or more about shoveling snow, for instance. Age should have nothing to do with it. I know a man who is in his eighty-first year and he shoveled out his driveway last winter eleven times, and the driveway is 150 feet long and 20 feet wide — and he always felt better after doing it! This man was in good condition and so was his heart, and that is the way everyone should be and could be too.

Walking is man's best form of exercise. The almost universal habit of riding even short distances in automobiles, of course, reduces one's chance of getting the benefit of such exercise. People who are obliged to stand a lot are prone to flat feet, mountain climbers, never. The reason for this is that the heart drives the blood to all parts of the body, but not *back* again. That is accomplished by the combined action of all the muscles in the body. Walking gets the blood back from the feet and into the lungs and heart again for redistribution. And don't be afraid to take a deep breath now and then. It will do you good.

If the heart shows prominent symptoms, such as pronounced variation in beats, palpitations, missing of beats, weakness of function, etc., then the symptoms would indicate certain remedies which may be classified in the *Materia Medica* as Heart Remedies. There are more than eighty remedies presently recorded. But remember that any heart symptoms must be tied in with any and all other symptoms which the patient presents in order to choose a proper remody.

Digitalis, invaluable when properly used, may be more deadly than the ailment it is meant to cure when it is improperly used. This is a drug which is used (and misused) almost universally by Orthodoxy.

The almost universal habit of Orthodoxy of drugging children suffering with rheumatic fever with heavy doses of salycilate of soda and later with sulfa and antibiotics is deplorable. Almost invariably this causes heart complications and permanent damage. Vaccinations of all kinds likewise contribute to heart disease.

Let's see to it that legislation is enacted to prevent the use of radio and television to induce our children to indulge in drugging, overmedication, and especially smoking and alcoholism. Let's see to it that the other side of the picture is given. For every inane postured advertisement of young couples enjoying life because of the cigarettes in their hands, let's show a picture of an old couple enjoying life because they never had cigarettes in their hands. Let's give the heart a chance to live.

CHAPTER 19

Cancer

I wish everybody in the world could read the December, 1956, issue of *The Reader's Digest* and give his soul-searching consideration to an article describing the sickness and death of a nine-year-old girl named Gabrielle. This article was poignantly written in the heart-blood of the anguished mother.

We read only too frequently of the misfortunes of many children, such as that of the two little boys who were blinded for life when their eyes were removed by surgery because of alleged malignancy.

Now the crowning touch — the story of this little girl's sickness and death, together with the additional suffering she was forced to bear at the hands of her doctors, was the most harrowing one I have ever read. It affected all my friends who read it the same way. This little girl died from a condition that should never have occurred. She died of an alleged cancerous growth. No child ever should have cancer. It has only been of late years that children suffer from this dread illness. It has always been heretofore a disease of middle life or old age. Today cancer in its various manifestations is the No. 1 killer of children. Why? Why? Why?

Below is the therapeutic sequence of treatment given Gabrielle as taken from an article by Dr. Eugene Underhill, Jr.

Bed rest and an aspirin every three hours.
Codeine prescribed by phone.
Possibility of Infectious Hepatitis or Catarrhal Jaundice.
More codeine but it didn't help.
Liver found to be enlarged.
Doctor thought patient seemed deranged but this was disproven.
Patient hospitalized in one of the best medical centers in the world.
Tests made but never dreamed there would be so many.

Took blood from arm twice, finger pricked several times.
Stuck with needle 17 times during first week, then lost count.
Finally decided it was Infectious Hepatitis.
Case was brought before weekly staff conference.
Doctors had many different opinions about what was wrong.
One doctor began to talk about an exploratory operation.
Mentioned possibility of a small tumor.
X-rays showed shadowy indentation in part of stomach.
Operation ordered.
Blood transfusion in preparation for operation.
Found tumor from spine invading everything.
Kind of tumor that does not respond to radiotherapy.
No drugs benefit this kind of cancer.
Tumor malignant and completely untreatable.
Patient in "best possible hospital with best possible doctors."
Prescription filled for demerol.
Codeine injected, then another injection, then demerol.
More demerol, then phenobarbital.
Effect of demerol worn off, had to switch to morphine.
Flesh black and blue and very sore from so many injections.
Had frequent shots of Vitamin K.
Shots of penicillin occasionally.
Gamma globulin twice because of measles in hospital.
Blood transfusion every few days, a long and exhausting procedure.
Symptoms shifted. Doctors could only guess at what was going on.
Even the patient observed the doctors don't know everything.
Luminol injection.
Paraldehyde for convulsions, repeated as necessary.
NOTE: *The patient died.*

It usually takes a lifetime of repeated errors in living to develop the insidious growth of cancer, and this has been an accepted fact for centuries; but suddenly, some sinister influence has begun its deadly work and forced upon innocent little children the development of this malignancy. Cancer never comes to a person from the outside. It comes from within man; of himself and by himself. Children have not lived long enough to develop a cancerous condition on their own through improper living. Cancer is forced on them by others, not consciously or purposely, but through ignorance, bigotry and greed.

I have practiced homœopathic, scientific, curative medicine very successfully for 53 years. I had my own hospital of 165 beds. On the courtesy staff were 500 or more orthodox physicians. I thus had an unprecedented opportunity to compare the methods of the treatment of the two schools — allopathy and Homœopathy. Whether or not this little girl could have been helped by scientific, Homœopathic treatment, I do not know. The kind of treatment she did get certainly could not be expected to effect a cure. Such treatment has often killed stronger patients than she was. I know, because I have seen it with my own eyes.

To form an opinion about this little girl's sickness, I should have to know the habits of her parents, what illnesses they had had and when, what was the state of their health at the time of her conception, was the mother exposed to X-ray in any way while carrying the child? The importance of avoiding the danger of X-ray is shown by a study of its effects in the following reference:

Among the foreign letters in the AMA Journal of November 3, 1956, is an article from Great Britain entitled, "Cancer and Leukemia in Children," which states, "A recent extensive survey has been made of children under 16 years of age who have died of leukemia or cancer. From this survey it would appear that the number of mothers of leukemic children who had a radiological examination of their abdomens during pregnancy was twice that of the mothers who did not. This was also true of the mothers of children dying from cancer."

Was the seed from which Gabrielle came healthy or sick? Was it tainted with blood disease, alcohol, nicotine, drugs, serum, X-ray? What previous illness did the little girl suffer, what drugs were given her, what kind and how many immunization shots, was she vaccinated against smallpox, when, how many times? If research were made along these lines — the study of the patient — success would soon crown the effort. To my knowledge, there was never a vaccine or serum that prevented, mitigated or cured any sickness known to man.

The thought goes through my mind that perhaps God in His inscrutable and infinite wisdom is using the case of this little girl and the inspired recording of it by her mother to shock the people out of their complacent acceptance of prevailing Orthodox medicine and into the realization that there is something better.

As the condition called cancer is developed by and within the individual, it becomes one's own personal affair, and it is the individual himself who needs treatment and not an entity called cancer. Therefore, there never will be a *cure* for *cancer*. The *patient* may be cured by proper treatment and the growth disappear. That is not only theoretical but actual and quite possible.

Cutting out the growth has no effect whatever on the original cause or causes. Many ways of wrong living, which include drugs, vaccines and an inherited tendency, are just such causes. Attempts to suppress the growth by X-ray and radium only make it worse. In fact, some people with cancer recover spontaneously when their living habits are corrected.

If, when a surgeon removes a growth, he knows its original cause and corrects it, then he renders a service to the patient.

One has but to consider the ability of Nature to automatically mend broken bones, heal cuts, bruises, burns, to realize the wonderful power of the vital force which can accomplish all those things as well as to produce new cells for old, worn-out ones. In order to make a perfect job of it, health must prevail at the time. When a person is in a chronic, unhealthy condition with poisoned blood, one may look for failure of one kind or another. Remember the reference on another page where bones refused to knit and wounds refused to heal until the blood was cleaned of the poisons of tobacco? This does not apply to everyone, of course, but to some it does. No two people react exactly alike to adverse environment. Everyone does not get cancerous growths from the same broken laws of health or the same kinds of poison in the bloodstream. Others pay the price of wrong living in various ways. It is not difficult to imagine then the production of abnormal cells, both in quantity and quality, when an abnormal vital force is unable to guide, direct and/or stop cell reproduction. These cells accumulate and become what are known as cancer cells. Not only are the cells themselves abnormal (malignant), but the same disturbed vitality lacks the power to *stop* their production. They grow because the individual has made the soil suitable for their growth.

A surgeon may make a large incision in the flesh, and a healthy, normal vital force automatically starts a process of repair, and when the repair is completed, stops the process. Proliferation of cells, unguided by a healthy vital force, will keep on proliferating just as long as nutriment and proper temperature is supplied.

As an example, just recall how many years a piece of chicken heart kept on producing cells blindly and to no purpose, just because no healthy vital force guided it. The cells were not malignant cancer cells, they were just unguided cells. Cancer cells keep on proliferating without definite purpose because the automatic, normal, healthy vital force has been unbalanced by years of wrong living with its accumulation of poisons so that it is unable to control cell proliferation when it started in some hit or miss location in the body.

Incidentally, just why and how can anyone qualify as a cancer expert when he knows absolutely nothing about it? (He is so busy with end results instead of causes, which vary with the individual.) One claims he is an expert and talks long and loud enough about cancer and he heads, maybe, a society of his own making and then asks for a lot of money — and gets it — and then he is an expert. No wonder cancer is increasing. It will continue to increase just so long as the environment is to its liking. If health can be restored to the body, the cancer cells just stop growing because they cannot grow on healthy tissue. I often think of cancer as I do of weeds which grow lushly in a garden of vegetables or flowers, crowding them out and finally destroying them, all because the soil is suitable to that peculiar kind of weed and not so suitable for vegetables and flowers. Sour grass will not thrive on sweet soil. Timothy will not thrive or even grow on sour, wet soil.

Cancer is cell growth which thrives on sick soil. Make the soil well and healthy and cancer cells will have no use for it. The cure of cancer, once it is developed, is not so easy as its prevention.

So long as people continue to eat too much, eat wrong food, make themselves sick and *then* drug themselves until they are *sicker,* then consume more drugs, and if they have been vaccinated and "immunized" in childhood and/or have had X-ray examinations and a lot of nicotine, alcohol, coffee, white flour, white sugar, food additives, so-called carcinogenic substances, food cooked in aluminum, and then if through their inherited tendencies get cancer — who is to blame? And if all this doesn't do it, then the cancer societies will do it by scaring people to death.

So it is up to you, folks. You do not have to develop cancer, even if both parents died of it. You have to do a lot of wrong living to accomplish it. Little children who come from sick seed and who have had all kinds of serums needled into them are forced to have cancer. They are the one about whom I am especially concerned. Children cannot help themselves. Grown-ups should know better than to *abuse* themselves and thereby develop all kinds of ailments.

I have seen many cases of cancer. I have operated on many — mostly in my earlier years of practice. Operative cases do better if no radium or X-ray treatments follow. If no medical care is given to *correct* the *results* of wrong living, the cancer usually recurs. I have had cases that lived many years after operations, with no recurrence, but in all such cases the indicated constitutional remedy was given and mistakes in living habits were corrected. I have seen cases of cancer of the breast which came to a head, broke open and discharged, and the patient remained otherwise well for many years, dying eventually of old age. It would seem that this discharge (which continued for years) relieved the body of the poisons which allowed the cancer to grow in the first place. Now I believe that if any of these patients had had the breast removed, the growth would have occurred somewhere else, trying to find an exit for the poison that caused it.

I remember one case where the breast was removed and the X-ray treatment which followed (as is so often the case) caused a very serious, deep burn that persisted for years. It was hard to determine whether it was burn or cancer. I prescribed a Homœopathic remedy internally but without apparent effect over a period of two years. The remedy was so plainly indicated that I wouldn't change it for something else. It then occurred to me that the potency of the remedy was wrong. It was too low — the 6X. I changed it to the 200th and in a very few weeks the sore was completely healed. The patient eventually died of old age.

I might add that I have seen men, somewhat advanced in life, who were apparently healthy, suddenly develop cancer at a time when serious financial reverses were forced upon them. This then naturally imposes the advice — never worry. Easier said than done, but worth attention.

See what Samuel Hahnemann, the greatest physician of them all, has to say about worry and overwork in a letter to one of his patients, a prominent clothier:

Man (the delicate human machine) is not constituted for overwork. If he does so from ambition, love of gain, or other praiseworthy or blameworthy motive, he sets himself in opposition to the order of nature, and his body suffers injury or destruction. The more so if his body is already in a weakened condition; then what you cannot accomplish in a week you can do in two weeks. Your customers may not be willing to wait, but they cannot reasonably expect that you will make yourself ill and work yourself to the grave for their sake, leaving your wife a widow and your children orphans. It is not only the greater bodily exertion that injures you, but even more the attendant strain on the mind; the overwrought mind in its turn affects the body injuriously. If you do not assume an attitude of calm indifference, adopting the principle of living first for yourself and only secondly for others, then there is small chance of your recovery. When you are in your grave, men will still be clothed, perhaps not so tastefully, but still tolerably well.

If you are a philosopher you may become healthy, you may even attain to old age.

If anything annoys you, ignore it; if anything is too much for you, have nothing to do with it; if others seek to drive you, go slowly and laugh at the fools who wish to worry you. What you can do comfortably, that do; what you cannot accomplish do not bother yourself about, for our temporal circumstances are not improved by over-pressure of work. You only spend proportionately more on your domestic affairs, and so nothing is gained. Economy, limitation of superfluities (of which the hard worker has often very few) place us in a position to live with greater comfort — that is to say, more rationally, more intelligently, more in accordance with nature, more cheerfully, more quietly and more healthily. Thus we shall act more commendably, more wisely and more prudently than by working in a breathless hurry, with our nerves constantly overstrung, to the destruction of the most precious treasures of life, a peaceful mind and good health. Be more prudent, consider yourself first, let everything else be only of secondary importance to you; and should they venture to assert that you are in honour bound to do more, that it is good for your mental and physical powers, even then do not, for God's sake, allow yourself to be driven to do what is contrary to your own welfare. Remain deaf to the bribery of praise, remain cold and pursue your own course slowly and quietly like a wise and sensible man. To enjoy with tranquil mind and body, that is what man is in the world for, and to do only as much work as will procure him the means of enjoyment — certainly not to let himself be harassed and worn out with work.

The everlasting pushing and striving of short-sighted mortals in order to gain so and so much, to secure some honour or other, to do a service to this or that great personage — this is generally fatal to our welfare, this is a common cause of young people aging and dying before their time.

The calm cool-headed man, who lets things glide softly, attains the same object, lives more tranquilly and healthily, and reaches a good old age; and this leisurely man sometimes lights upon a lucky idea, the fruit of serious original thought, which will give much more profitable impetus to his temporal affairs than can ever be gained by the overwrought man who can never find time to collect his thoughts.

In order to win the race, speed alone will not suffice. Strive to remain a little indifferent, to be cool and calm, then you will be what I wish you to be. You will see marvelous things; you will see how healthy you will become by follow-ing my advice. Then shall your blood course through your veins calmly and sedately, without effort and without heat. No horrible dreams disturb the sleep of him who lies down to rest with calm nerves, and the man who is free from care wakes in the morning without anxiety about the multifarious occu-pations of the day. What does he care? The happiness of life concerns him more than anything else. With fresh vigour he sets about his moderate work, and at his meals nothing, no ebullitions of blood, no cares, no solicitude of mind, hinders him from relishing what the beneficent Preserver of Life sets before him; and so one day follows another in quiet succession, until finally advanced age brings him to the termination of a well-spent life, and he rests serenely in another world, as he has calmly lived in this one.

Is not that more rational, more sensible? Let restless self-destroying men act as irrationally, as injuriously towards themselves as they please; let them be fools, but do you be wiser. Do not let me preach this wisdom of life in vain. I mean well by you.

Farewell, follow my advice, and when all goes well with you, remember.

DR. S. HAHNEMANN

P.S.—Even should you be reduced to your last sixpence, remain cheerful and happy. Providence watches over us, and a lucky chance puts things right again. How much do we need in order to live, to restore our powers by food and drink, to shield ourselves from cold and heat? Little more than courage; when we possess that, we can find the minor essentials without much trouble. The wise man needs but little. Conserved strength does not need to be renewed by medicine.

I was discussing this subject today with a man who is a little above the average in intelligence and he said, "You have not fully convinced me that cancer is developed by and within the individual." He went on to say, "I still believe it is caused by infection or a virus."

How familiar that kind of thinking has become to me. I think it would be better described by calling it non-thinking — the result of propaganda and gross misinformation so prevalent today. Then I told him about the experiments in 1956 which were made on inmates of prisons who volun-teered to have cancer cells implanted in their bodies. It was found that no cancer would grow in a non-cancerous person. The implants were destroyed in *every* case. Not so, however, with those who already had de-veloped it. When my friend finally sensed the fact that cancer cells themselves would not live in a non-cancerous person's body, he began to suspect that any germ or virus would find pretty hard going to produce the cancer itself in unsuitable soil, and so he now admits that after all man produces his own cancer. Our job is to find out just what the patient does to produce the cancer in himself. Work along these lines should finally prevent this disease and besides, this sort of research would be relatively inexpensive.

Even though man has, by devious and cruel methods, produced in dumb animals growths which have the appearance of malignancy, cancer is a disease of the human race.

Therefore, it seems to me that untold tortures on 2½ million animals (currently, although increasing every year) is not only useless but wicked indeed and should *not* be allowed. It breeds sadism and cruelty in men and women, uses up, needlessly, millions of dollars yearly that could and should be put to a better use, and finally, and most important of all, delays the kind of research that would lead to success in preventing not only cancer but any and all kinds of sickness in the human race.

I believe that the great Creator frowns on such actions, regardless of what some of the clergy and some college heads say in favor of so-called vivisection. Why *any* clergyman should be in favor of it I cannot understand. There are better ways to learn how to prevent and cure human ills.

There is a lot of controversy going on now about *a* cure for *cancer*. The American Cancer Society is looking for *a* *cure* for cancer. The surgeons usually claim that cutting it out is the only cure, but X-ray men say their treatment is the best. The radium men are likely to say radium is the thing. The Independent Cancer Research Committee says Krebiozen is the cure.

Now I will leave it to your own good common sense and judgment. Can there possibly be a cure for cancer itself when it is only a *condition* in the individual who produced the growth or allowed it to develop? The cure must come through the counteracting of the disturbances of the patient's vital force which produced the cancer. The individual must be studied and treated and no attention need be given to the growth itself because if the treatment is successful, the growth will disappear. In fact, if more attention were given to the individual at all times for all kinds of sickness instead of to a fancied diagnosis of a disease entity, the precancerous symptoms in certain individuals who may be headed eventually for this malignant growth could be analyzed, treated and cancer *prevented*. Prevention is what we want.

Cancer is the end result, the ultimate, of years of wrong living in those who have inherited the susceptibility to it.

That is the whole story. So you can readily see that money donated for today's kind of research just goes down the drain. One may study the cancer growth from now to doomsday and nothing will come of it. There are as many kinds of cancerous growths as there are people who develop them. Cure the sick individual. That is our goal.

CHAPTER 20

Smoking

I have not taken the time to fully discuss the dangers of tobacco, although I have mentioned the subject from time to time in various chapters. But if anybody has any question in his mind or any hope that he will escape the penalties of nicotine, then I offer the following article which was taken from *Time,*[1] June 17, 1957. This is an unbiased opinion of men who made it their business — not as practicing physicians, mind you, but as painstaking researchers — to investigate the subject, and this is what they have to say about nicotine and its dangers to people's health.

SMOKING AND HEALTH

After a massive study of 188,000 American men observed for almost four years, two American Cancer Society researchers last week reported their final figures on the connection between smoking habits and premature death — especially from cancer and heart disease. With a total of 11,870 deaths among the men (ages 50 to 70 when the study began in 1952), Drs. E. Cuyler Hammond and Daniel Horn were able to go far beyond the findings they had earlier reported (*Time,* July 5, 1954 et seq.). From a mountain of cross-checked statistics submitted to the A.M.A. last week, they concluded: 1) all smoking shortens life; 2) cigarette smoking is by far the worst offender, and the risk goes up with the amount smoked.

Especially startling was the finding that, although the increased death rate from lung cancer was the most dramatic (*Time,* March 7, 1949 et seq.), smoking may cause a far greater loss of life by speeding up the process of heart disease — where a relatively modest increase in the mortality rate means many more deaths because the disease is so much commoner.

Death rates from all causes combined are 68% higher for cigarette smokers than for nonsmokers. The rates rise with the number of cigarettes smoked

[1]Courtesy *TIME*, The Weekly Newsmagazine, copyright Time Inc., 1957.

daily, the A.C.S. statisticians reported. As compared with the rates for those who have never smoked, they are:

Up 34% for those smoking less than half a pack a day.
Up 70% on half a pack to a pack a day.
Up 96% on one to two packs.
Up 123% on two packs or more.

For those who smoke only cigars the rate goes up 22%, and for pipe smokers only 12%. Mixed smokers, e.g., pipe and cigarettes, have intermediate rates.

The researchers' findings on the association between cigarette smoking and various causes of death:

Lung Cancer. "A spectacular relationship." Among 32,392 men who had never smoked, only four died of microscopically proved cancer originating in the lung, but among 108,000 cigarette smokers there were 265 similarly proved cases (of 397 reported). Even men who smoked less than half a pack a day ran a risk of lung cancer 15 times as great as that of nonsmokers; between one and two packs 43 times as great; on two packs or more 64 times as great.

Other Cancers. For the first time Drs. Hammond and Horn found a significant tie between cigarette smoking and cancer in other sites; the pancreas, where the death rate goes up 50%; the kidneys, up 58%; the stomach, up 61%; the prostate, up 75%; the bladder, up 117%; liver and gall bladder, up 352%. Cancer at some such sites might have been caused either by direct action of substances in cigarette tar, or by spread from an undetected tumor in the lung. No relationship was found between smoking and leukemia, or cancer of the brain, colon or rectum.

Other Lung Diseases. Smokers' death rate was almost twice as high as that of nonsmokers; almost four times as high for deaths from pneumonia and influenza.

Peptic Ulcers. Smokers' death rate was 116% higher for duodenal ulcers. When they got to the comparison for stomach-ulcer deaths, Hammond and Horn's bar graph ran off the chart; there was not a single such death among the nonsmokers, but there were 46 among cigarette smokers (five among other smokers).

Cirrhosis of the Liver. Smokers' rate 93% higher.

Heart & Artery Disease. Deaths attributed to disease of the coronary arteries went up step-fashion according to the amount smoked: less than half a pack a day, up 29%; half a pack to a pack, up 89%; one to two packs, up 115%; two packs or more, up 141%. (Pipe smokers' rates were up only 3%; cigar smokers' rates were up 28%.) Cigarette smokers' death rate from strokes was 30% higher than among nonsmokers; from general arteriosclerosis, 46% higher.

Accidents & Suicide. Smokers' death rate lower than nonsmokers' by 6% — which, Researchers Hammond and Horn say, is too small to be significant.

If cigarette smokers had died at the same rate as nonsmokers, the researchers would have expected 4,651 deaths among the men studied; actually, they recorded 7,316. Of the 2,665 "excess deaths," no fewer than 1,338 (52%) were attributed to coronary artery disease, 1,670 (64%) to all diseases of the heart and arteries combined. This compared with 360 deaths caused by lung cancer and 359 by all other cancers.

Quit Smoking? Even after a man has been a heavy cigarette smoker for many years, he can still reduce his risk of premature death by kicking the habit, declared Hammond and Horn. After a man had been off the weed for a year or more, his prospects improved; among men who had quit light smoking (less than a pack a day) ten or more years previously, the death rate from most causes was scarcely greater than among lifetime nonsmokers; ten years after heavier smoking, it was 50% greater — and markedly higher from lung cancer.

City v. Country. Cigarette smoking increases with a movement from rural areas to bigger towns and large cities; so does the incidence of lung cancer. When Hammond and Horn adjusted their figures to allow for the smoking difference (50% of rural men smoke cigarettes, 62½% of big-city men), they found that the lung-cancer death rate was still one-third higher in the cities. This might be a reflection of better diagnosis in major medical centers, or a result of big-city air pollution.

Researchers Hammond and Horn are not physicians, but practitioners of biometrics — the study of diseases by analyzing the medical who, what, when and how-many of people in health and illness. Baltimore-born Hammond, 45, has an Sc.D. in biology; Horn, 41, native of Rochester. N. Y., has a Ph.D. in psychology. Both were heavy cigarette smokers when their first findings came in four years ago; now they smoke pipes.

I could write a whole book based on personal experiences showing the deadliness of nicotine, but it seems to me that there is evidence enough to be seen by everybody in every walk of life to make unnecessary any argument against this deadly drug. I have personally seen many thousands of highly educated people, people from the highest to the lowest walk of life, die horrible deaths from the effects of nicotine, long before their allotted time, so to speak. So don't smoke. Whatever its imagined pleasure, it's not worth even a minute of your life, much less ten or twenty years.

CHAPTER 21

Having a Baby

Lately this simple and natural procedure has been presented to the public as a serious matter by many doctors. The young prospective mothers are induced into believing that bringing a child into the world is a deep, dark, mysterious and dangerous ordeal, and that one must have *pre-natal* care and a lot of hocus-pocus — and of course at a price.

Now, my friend, just remember this: Having a baby is a wonderful experience, and it is the most important act that a woman can perform. A woman is at her best when she is pregnant. It brings out all that is good and healthy. In fact, it makes good health and happiness. That is what Nature intended.

After a young woman has conceived and she is in the process of producing what should be a beautiful, healthy human baby, she should exercise all care in living a normal, healthy life. She should be subjected to no emotional strain, she should rid herself of any and all bad habits such as smoking, drinking alcoholic beverages, coffee, tea and any deleterious articles of food such as white sugar, too much white flour, too much chocolate, etc.

In fact, to get right down to the basic principles, such as I have impressed upon you so many times — one must have a clean, healthy bloodstream in order to produce a normal, healthy baby and a following flow of good milk for some months after the baby is born.

To do all this, one has but to use one's own common sense and intelligence. There is no advantage whatever in the prevailing pre-natal ritual. It in itself can become bothersome and annoying.

Anyone who through wrong living has produced sickness of any kind should not try to have a baby. Get well first. That is very easy to do because, as I have said so many times elsewhere in this book, health is normal, sickness abnormal. Nature is always trying to cure the ills that are made by the individual, and will do so if given a chance.

Each mother must contribute her part. The occasional complication which may arise in childbirth is usually because of some illness in the mother. It may be slight and it may be serious. So it is important to keep well.

This is *not* hard to do. You, yourself, will be your worst enemy. So watch your step! No woman should *ever* smoke, not even one cigarette, while carrying a baby. No woman should ever plan on having a baby if she is a victim of the smoking habit, until she has stopped long enough to allow a clean bloodstream and a healthy seed. An unhealthy seed produces an unhealthy baby. Everything I have said before about health and sickness applies doubly where a baby is contemplated.

Some time ago a series of autopsies was done on stillborn babies, the mothers of whom were cigarette smokers, and large amounts of nicotine were found in the liver of these unfortunate little bodies. So think it over very carefully. If one wants a baby, one wants a healthy baby, and above all, a live one. The first question a young mother asks is, "Doctor, is my baby all right?" That is a natural question, born of instinctive mother love. Let each young woman who decides to have a baby, and those who have one whether planned or not, see to it that the baby will have every possible chance for good health. Remember, a healthy child is a jewel beyond price. A sickly child is a trial and disappointment, however well loved.

These admonitions so far have applied to conditions of ill health in the mother due to every-day errors in living habits, especially in the line of self-indulgences.

There are other conditions which are more or less chronic and which are constitutional. Such conditions as latent or active venereal diseases, T. B., anemia, diabetes, chronic kidney ailments, and today, unfortunately, cancer as it is now appearing in women of childbearing age — such conditions are relatively rare and require definite, scientific, Homœopathic treatment.

No young pregnant woman should ever be subjected to hypodermic injections of any substance which include vaccines and serums. Neither should she be subjected to X-ray examination, especially in the early months (see previous references).

The question will arise sooner or later — "Will I have my baby at home or at a hospital?" That is a good question. I hope I can give you some good advice.

As I have stated, I owned and conducted my own hospital for many years. It contained a very large and active maternity department. I was most unusually busy during those years and I asked my personal patients to come to the hospital to have their babies. I just simply did not have the time to go their homes, so you see it was of personal advantage to me in that respect. However, I delivered hundreds of babies in the homes of my patients.

Most doctors will advise the hospital and, in fact, many will *not* deliver at home. However, there are some things in hospital routine which are not all that could be desired, and when I point them out, you may make your own choice as to whether you go or stay at home.

There was a time when it was really dangerous to be delivered in a hospital. That was when doctors delivered one case after another, going from patient to patient and never even washing their hands between cases; where unsterile dressings were used and when instruments went uncleaned and so-called childbed fever was rife. Today nothing like that happens in well-regulated hospitals. Theoretically, the modern hospital is the place to have a baby. But, once there a patient must submit to routine, ritual and all measures that facilitate the service given by the hospital. If you have as your physician a man who is always in a hurry, it is often expedient for him to hurry things along. As you are in a hospital where it is an easy matter for you to be anæsthetized and delivered by forceps hours before you are ready, often the baby's head will be injured. This results in arm or leg paralysis (usually arm, to a more or less degree) and is the usual cause of the so-called cerebral palsy which one hears about today.

When the child is still in its mother's womb, its head is almost round. During the normal process of being born, Nature, by the intermittent womb contractions, gradually fits and shapes the round head into an oblong one so that it can emerge without damage to the brain. It is a slow process — about twenty hours — and any force applied to the skull sufficient to deliver the baby to suit the doctor's time may and does do damage — but after all, the doctor kept his golf appointment.

I have seen such incidents many times. If one were home, the doctor would be more likely to wait for Nature to do its part, and he would find that he had indeed little to do to earn his money.

I have often said that a young woman would be far better, and it would be safer, if on a nice summer day she could go off by herself and lie down on nice clean grass in the shade of a tree and have her baby as Nature intended, not meddled with by anyone — that is, of course, if she were a normal, healthy young woman.

I am not advising this, of course. I merely give food for thought. It could be done and it has been done from time immemorial. I just want you to realize that it is *not* always necessary to submit to expensive, routine hospital care for so simple a matter. Do not let any doctor or hospital lure you into thinking that having a baby is a mysterious, complicated or dangerous affair.

At many hospitals the invariable advice is to bottle-feed the baby and dry up the mother's milk as soon as possible. This, my friends, is wrong — absolutely wrong as routine practice. It is bad for the baby and bad for the mother.

Nursing the baby if you have good milk (and you will have if you are healthy and intelligent) is what the baby needs most. It also helps the pelvic organs of the mother to get back to normal, thus minimizing the chance of prolapsed and/or tipped uterus, for which operations are only too frequently advised.

Also, *routine hospital medications* should be avoided. Having a baby is natural. Medicines are needed only rarely. *Drugs* are *never* needed.

The ordinary family doctor is not an expert on obstetrics. Once in a while a patient will need expert advice and treatment, because of some inherent anatomical and/or physical condition.

Valvular heart trouble does not preclude having a baby, but in such cases properly selected remedies may be needed. Above all someone must be in attendance who may recognize danger signs as the time for delivery nears and who should be able to determine when to bring about safe delivery. There are times when a Caesarean operation offers the least risk for mother and baby. A flat or contracted pelvis is relatively easy to determine by one who knows how to do it, and in such conditions Caesarean birth must be considered.

A test of labor to determine, in such cases, whether or not the baby can come through the bony pelvis, should not be prolonged beyond twenty hours from onset of contraction pains. Also under expert observance, the time may be shortened if normal progress has not taken place. The position of the baby may be such as to complicate easy and normal delivery. These faulty positions are easily corrected by experts.

Placenta Previa (where the placenta or afterbirth is implanted at or near the cervix, i.e., outlet of the womb) is really one serious condition which calls for rapid delivery and Caesarean section may be the choice.

The above-cited complications are relatively rare, but can be successfully handled by dotors who are qualified. In these cases the ordinary family doctor is useless and may be a menace. Thousands of babies are sacrificed every year on account of the inability of ordinary doctors to cope with such cases.

Let me quote from a paper which I wrote forty-two years ago:

Last year a woman was brought to the Forest Hills Hospital in a very exsanguinated condition, having been in labor but an hour with her first pregnancy. On examination, a condition of placenta previa centralis was found, and a Caesarean operation was advised and accepted with results which we expected — recovery of mother and a living child.

The physician who brought the case then went back for another case and found that in his absence another physician had been called who attempted to deliver from below a woman who also had placenta previa, and the result was that the mother bled to death and the child was killed during extraction.

The article from which the above was quoted was presented to the Seventh Annual Meeting of the American Association of Clinical Research, September 25, 1915, at Philadelphia, and was the report of a series of 66 cases of Caesarean operations performed by me, with no mortality to mother or child.

I recite the possible complications of childbirth not to frighten anyone but to point out two important facts: (1) giving birth to a baby is in a normal, healthy young woman natural and entirely devoid of danger if no meddling doctor improperly interferes; most doctors today feel so insecure because of their lack of knowledge of curative medicine and because of their fear of losing a patient that they try to impress the patient by a lot of advice as to tonics, diets, exercises, drugs, etc., which is mostly all nonsense but can be dangerous; (2) if there should be any suggestion, suspicion or knowledge that childbirth in an individual might be complicated *at the time of delivery,* then an expert must be employed for the occasion.

If a person has some constitutional ailment, then competent prescribing — not of drugs — but of scientific medicine will be beneficial. If bleeding occurs in any amount at or near the time for delivery, then one should consult an expert because that is usually a sign of placenta previa, and can be dangerous. Do not let your family doctor convince you that he is an expert at this kind of work.

Before I leave the subject of having a baby, I should like to relate the remarkable and unusual case I was called in to treat many years ago. A prominent physician in Brookline telephoned me and said, "I have a patient in collapse. I can't understand it. She is almost ready for delivery. Today, without warning, she collapsed and her abdomen seems to have flattened out to a noticeable degree."

I went over immediately, examined the patient, and found a normal-sized, non-pregnant uterus (womb). On further examination, I decided that she had the very rare condition of abdominal pregnancy. She was taken to my hospital immediately. On opening the abdomen, I found it contained a large amount of amniotic fluid, which is the fluid contained in the sac in which the baby floats protected from jars and bruises which might occur during the nine months of pregnancy. At the mysterious appointed time, this sac ruptured even as it does in normal delivery. The sudden flooding of the abdominal cavity with this fluid in itself should not have caused the woman to collapse. However, as the situation was serious and called for immediate help, Nature apparently used that method in sending out the alarm, and is another example of Nature's cry for help which she uses by various symptoms in various forms of sickness. I knew that an immediate operation was absolutely necessary.

On opening the abdomen, I discovered a beautiful, full-term, healthy, normal baby. His little hands and feet were poking around the intestines of the mother. I tied the cord immediately in two places, severed it between the ties and gave the baby to the nurse. Then my next job was to safely remove the placenta (afterbirth) from its attachment to the broad ligament of the uterus and several loops of intestines. As there was a collateral circulation of sufficient magnitude to produce the baby and keep it alive till full term, great care and patience were necessary to get the placenta away without damaging the organs to which it was attached. This was done finally and successfully, and so mother and child lived.

Now this case illustrates the relentlessness of Nature in its determination to reproduce its kind. In order for a pregnancy to be normal, the sperm and the ovum must meet at the desired location, namely the fundus (body) of the uterus, where the tissues are prepared to allow the

growth of a normal placenta, after which all goes well. In this case the
energetic sperm wiggled its way up through the cervical canal into the
uterus and not finding the object of its search there, kept on going up
through the fallopian tube and out through the opening and found itself
in strange territory — the abdominal cavity. By good luck, fate and/or
accident, he met face to face with the ovum which had just left the ovary,
waiting to be carried down through the tube into the uterus. They stood
on no ceremony but embraced and merged and decided to build their nest
right on the spot. Kindly Nature then saw to it that the object of the
meeting culminated in a beautiful living child.

CHAPTER 22

It's Up to You

Who is your doctor and why? After reading this book, does he still measure up? Did you have any basis other than the fact that he had the title "doctor" for selecting him? I hope you can answer these questions in a way that is satisfactory to you and the rest of your family.

If he is a Homœopath you are indeed fortunate. If he is not, and you are devoted to him, ask him to read my book. Encourage him to study Homœopathy. He will then be infinitely more serviceable to you as a physician.

Anyone who wishes to study this marvelous system will be able to get help and assistance by writing to the American Foundation for Homœopathy, 1726 Eye Street, Northwest, Washington 6, D. C. Wouldn't it be wonderful if everyone could find and employ a good Homœopath when and if sickness comes.

Bad health and its resultant shortening of your life come generally from two directions: from doctors and drug makers and from another party. This other party is particularly vicious because he has no profit to be gained from murdering you. All he wants is for you to eat wrong, drink wrong, and smoke. Do you recognize him? He's none other than a part of yourself.

Is it worth living to an old age? "Whom the gods love dies young," say the Greeks. But Shadman says, "You don't really begin to get a bang out of life 'til you're eighty." I think most people would prefer to live to a ripe old age. There is absolutely no reason why they shouldn't if they are willing to live right, keep warm, and stay away from drugs. So don't get sick. This book has told you how to maintain your health. Good luck to you all.

POINTERS TO THE COMMON REMEDIES

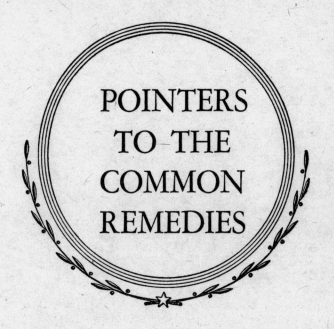

POINTERS
TO THE
COMMON
REMEDIES

by

M. L. TYLER
L. R. C. P. & S. (Brux.)

Revised by

D. M. BORLAND
M.B., Ch.B. (Glas.)

PREFACE

SET FORTH in this Appendix are extracts from a series of pamphlets entitled "Pointers to the Common Remedies" reprinted under the auspices of the British Homœopathic Association from the magazine *Homœopathy* and containing a compilation of homœopathic remedies prepared by two eminent British Homœopathic doctors, Dr. Margaret L. Tyler and Dr. Douglas M. Borland, to whom full credit is hereby given.

The author includes the list of remedies set forth below to provide what the author has found to be a useful compilation of homœopathic remedies available and to illustrate to the non-professional reader the type of remedies applied in homœopathic medicine.

As explained earlier in this book and as is apparent from the paragraph "On Prescribing" quoted below, which is also taken from one of Dr. Tyler's and Dr. Borland's pamphlets, selection of the proper remedy in any particular instance depends on the patient's total symptoms and is an art requiring a degree of training and skill. Various climates produce symptoms of varying kinds and medicines are chosen accordingly. These medicines are in the form of small grain size tablets and should be put up in small glass vials carefully labeled and contained in a suitable box or case.

The usual method of giving the medicine is in doses of one or two pills every 2 or 3 hours, dry on tongue, to be dissolved in the mouth. The medicine is to be discontinued as soon as improvement is apparent. Doses repeated too often may be harmful. The rule is the single remedy, the minimum dose, and only as often as is absolutely necessary — which is best learned by experience.

I suggest that a family should have a case of Homœopathic medicine; owing to the fact that the indications for the prescribing of Homœopathic remedies never change, people of average intelligence may learn how to prescribe for their own *simple* ailments.

In the past all Homœopathic pharmacists made cases of various sizes to hold the little bottles of remedies. At present, due to a dwindling demand for Homœopathy, due to causes which have been previously mentioned, one may be obliged to make his own little box to hold the bottles.

No home should be without the Aqueous Tincture of Calendula, because its effect on burns, including sunburns and septic wounds is most magical. This medicine comes in the tincture form with just enough alcohol to preserve it, but it should not be used full strength. The dilution is one part medicine to ten parts water, and only diluted as it is used because it will not keep after it has been diluted.

POINTERS TO THE COMMON REMEDIES

DIGESTIVE DISORDERS (Continued)

CHILDREN

COMMON DISEASES

COMMON DISEASES (Continued)

HEAD, NERVES, SHOCK

INJURIES AND BURNS

CONCERNING THE REMEDIES

The remedies are put up as medicated granules; their most convenient form for carrying, and for keeping in good condition.

A DOSE consists of half a dozen granules — less or more.

It may be given dry on the tongue, to be dissolved before swallowing.

Or, where quick effect is wanted in acute conditions, dissolve half a dozen granules in half a tumbler of water, stir, and administer in doses of a dessertspoonful six hours apart; or, in very urgent conditions, every hour, or half hour for a few doses, till reaction sets in; *then stop, so long as improvement is maintained.*

CAMPHOR ANTIDOTES MOST OF THE MEDICINES. So the camphor bottle must be kept away from the medicine chest.

POTENCIES. — The best potencies for intial experiments in Homœopathy are the 12th and the 30th.

ON PRESCRIBING

MANY drugs have produced the symptoms of, and can therefore cure the common cold: but, alas! only the one that has evoked the exact conditions of the individual patient will CURE that patient: i.e. not merely palliate while he recovers, but CURE.

Why? Because there is Law behind cure; and if we desire to evoke Power, we must conform to its conditions. The only known Law of Healing is Hahnemann's *similia similibus curentur*. In acute work, if you can get exact correspondence between the symptoms of the patient and the symptoms evoked in healthy persons by some drug, it is a mathematical certainty that you will cure — *because of the Law of Similars*. If you do not get the correspondence it is equally certain that you will NOT cure — *because of the Law of Similars*. Law does not fail. It is we who fail in our attempts to put it in action. We may do bad work and call it Homœopathy, discrediting it in the patient's eyes and in our own: only it did not happen to *be* Homœopathy! When an aeroplane crashes no one says, "The laws of gravitation — motion — physics — have failed in *this* case!" — the fault is sought in faulty adaptation. Law is inexorable.

At times the question of an epidemic has to be reckoned with, Hahnemann says that by taking the symptoms of a number of cases you can select a drug that covers the lot, and cure, practically, every case of THAT epidemic. We have all found that the medicine that was so widely curative one year, was useless the next. One has often heard, "This is a *Bryonia* year!" "*Mercurius* is curing all the colds just now. . . ." Then, wind and weather change, and another set of remedies *for another set of patients* crops up.

If the blighting influence that bowled over people of a certain temperament was a cold, *dry*, East wind, such drugs as *Aconite, Bryonia, Hepar, Nux* will suggest themselves. Whereas a sudden cold *wet* spell would play havoc with the people who cannot stand *cold wet* conditions,

and here *Dulcamara, Natrum sulph.,* or *Rhus* would come up for consideration. Why is it that good prescribers will find that they are suddenly
getting quite a number of *Lycopodium* cases? It is not that they are
framing their questions to lead up to that drug, but because conditions —
perhaps social — economic — or even meteoric are putting a severe strain
on persons of the *Lycopodium* make-up.

Among the remedies of the Common Cold, then, some suit the illness
brought on by dry cold, some by damp cold, some even by warm wet.
The affected mucous membranes may be dry — or they may pour.
Relief may come in cold, open air, or there may be utter intolerance of
cold air, of open air, of draughts, of uncovering, and so on. Without
precision, results are poor.

COMMON REMEDIES OF THE COMMON COLD*

Camphor ..	A person who has been chilled, and cannot get warm. For the cold stage, before catarrhal symptoms have ultimated, to prevent.

A couple of drops of *Camphor* (strong tincture) on a lump of sugar, repeat till warm.

But "as *Camphor* antidotes most of our drugs, the *Camphor* bottle should be put away in the other end of the house." *Kent.*

Aconite ..	Sudden onset from exposure to COLD; TO COLD DRY WINDS.

NOSE. Coryza dry, with headache, roaring in ears, fever, thirst, sleeplessness.

Checked coryza, better open air, worse talking.

Fluent coryza, frequent sneezing; dropping of a clear hot water: fluent mornings.

THROAT. Acute inflammation of the throat with high fever, dark redness of the parts, burning and stinging in fauces.

Larynx sensitive to touch and inspired air, as if denuded.

Laryngitis with inflammatory fever; also with suffocative spasms (spasm of glottis).

CROUP: child in agony, tosses about: dry short cough, not much wheezing . . .

After exposure to dry, cold winds.

CHEST. Tightness and oppression. Stitches when breathing.

Cough clear ringing and whistling, caused by burning, pricking in larynx and trachea.

Cough hoarse, dry, loud: spasmodic. Breath hot.

Cough wakes him from sleep, is dry, croupy, suffocating: *Great anxiety.*

Sputum absent — scanty: bloody or blood-streaked: bright red blood.

Early stages of pneumonia, bronchitis, croup.

Aconite is RESTLESS, ANXIOUS, FRIGHTENED:

Onset sudden. Worse at night.

* These drugs are arranged, more or less, for acuteness, and for comparison.

Allium cepa .. Coryza, streaming eyes and nose, with headache; frequent sneezing, profuse *acrid* discharge from nose, corroding lip and nose.

Lachrymation also profuse, but *bland* (reverse of *Euphrasia*).

Hot and thirsty: worse evenings: indoors: warm room. Better open air.

Violent catarrhallaryngitis. Tickling in larynx.

Cough seems to split and tear larynx: grasps larynx, feels as if cough will tear it.

Cough from inhaling cold air.

Belladonna .. Suppressed catarrh with maddening headache.

Throat raw and sore: very red and shining.

Hoarseness with painful dryness of larynx.

As if larynx inflamed and swollen, with snoring breathing and danger of suffocation.

Acute catarrhal laryngitis.

Cough with red, injected throat.

Dry, tearing cough, which scrapes throat.

Belladonna is red, and hot, and dry.

Bryonia .. Often begins in the nose, sneezing, coryza, running at nose, lachrymation, aching eyes, nose and head the first day: then trouble goes down to posterior nares, throat, larynx, with hoarseness, and a bronchitis comes on: may end in pleurisy and pneumonia.

Trouble travels down from the beginning of respiratory tract. (Reverse of *Lyc.*)

Dry, spasmodic cough, worse at night; after eating and drinking; on entering a warm room; on taking a deep inspiration.

Cough with *stitches in chest,* with headache as if the *head would fly to pieces.*

Cough shaking the whole body.

Stitches in chest and pleura: worse breathing and coughing.

Cough dry, hard, racking, expectoration scanty.

Bryonia is irritable: thirsty for long drinks: wants to lie still and be let alone. Dryness of mucous membranes. (*Bell.*)

Bryonia (cont.)   Lips parched and dry.
                      Worse cold, dry weather.

Euphrasia   ..   Nasal catarrh bland, with lachrymation which is excoriating (exact opposite of *Allium cepa*).
Severe fluent coryza, apt to extend down to larynx with
hard cough.
Coryza worse by night; lying down: cough worse
by day, and better lying down.

Hepar   ..   From cold, dry weather (*Acon., Nux*). Catarrh of
nose, ears, throat, larynx and chest.
Cold in nose, with much discharge: with *sneezing
every time he goes into a cold wind.*
Sneezing and running from nose, first watery; then
thick, yellow, *offensive.*
Every time he goes into *dry, cold wind,* gets hoarse,
and coughs: worse inspiring cold air: or putting
hand or foot out of bed.
Sweating all night without relief (*Merc.*).
Hypersensitive, to touch, pain, draughts, cold air.
Wants to hit anybody who makes a draught in
room.
Better moist, wet weather (reverse of *Gels.*).
(Farrington (only) says, *Hepar* is not indicated in
the early stages of a cold; apt to stop it in the nose,
while it goes down to chest: "here *Phos.* follows
and cures.")

Nux   ..   Colds from DRY COLD WEATHER (*Acon.*) (reverse of
Dulc.). *Acon.* is anxious; *Nux* irritable.
Nose stuffed and dry, initial stage: throat rough as
if scraped; raw, sore.
Sneezing, nose stuffed up at night and in open air.
Fluent coryza in warm room and by day.
Coldness of whole body, not better by warmth of
stove, or by any amount of covering.
Chills, back, limbs, or whole body, not relieved by
warmth.
Can't stir from fire.
Shivering after drinking: from slightest contact with
open air; *from slightest motion.*

Nux (cont.) — Chill as soon as he moves the bed clothes.

Chill alternating with heat. Heat with internal chilliness.

Nux is oversensitive: irritable; touchy; sensitive to least draught. (*Hepar.*)

Dulcamara .. Colds from COLD WET WEATHER (*Rhus*) and snow.

From getting wet, or chilled when heated.

Worse sudden changes from hot to cold.

Dry coryza, sore throat, stiff neck.

Coryza worse in open air.

More fluent in house, in warmth; less fluent in cold air — cold room. (*Nux.*)

Starts sneezing in a cold room.

Eyes become red and sore with every cold.

Nose stuffs up when there is cold rain.

Profuse discharge of water from nose and eyes, worse in the open air.

Stiff neck: sore throat, back and limbs painful.

Mercurius sol. .. *Creeping chilliness* in the beginning of a cold.

Much sneezing, fluent discharge, *corrosive*.

Acrid, offensive matter flows from nose: greenish, fetid pus.

Nose red, swollen, shining.

Catarrhal inflammation of frontal sinuses, etc.

Hoarse voice; dry, rough, tickling cough.

Feels bad in a warm room, yet cannot bear the cold.

Taste sweet, salty, metallic, putrid.

Creeping chilliness.

Profuse offensive sweats, and worse from sweating. (Reverse of *Nat. sul.*)

Swollen, flabby tongue, tooth-notched.

Offensive breath: offensive salivation.

Gelsemium .. Catarrhs of *warm, moist, relaxing weather* (*Carbo veg.*), (reverse of *Hepar* and *Dulc.*).

Discharge excoriating: nostrils sore.

As if red-hot water passing through nostrils.

Gels. colds "develop several days after exposure: the *Acon.* cold comes on in a few hours."

Suits the colds and fevers of mild winters.

Gelsemium (cont.) Teasing, tickling cough, better near the fire.
Great weight and tiredness of the whole body.
Chills up and down the back.
Headache.
(One of the greatest of 'flu medicines.)

Iodium   .. Loss of smell. Nose dry and stuffed up.
Dry coryza, fluent in open air.
Severe coryza, with fever, severe headache, excessive
    secretion and much sneezing.
Catarrh, thin, excoriating. Hot water drops out.
The *Iodine* patient is lean and hungry and can't stand
    heat.

Kali iod   .. Colds from every exposure — from DAMP.
Nose red, swollen, ACRID watery discharge.
Eyes smart and lachrymate.
Catarrhal headaches with inflammation of mucous
    membranes of FRONTAL SINUSES, eyes, throat and
    chest.
Forehead heavy; dull and stupid.
Violent sneezing, eyes bloated, profuse lachrymation.
    Violent acrid coryza.
Nose tender, face red. Uneasy. Tongue white.
Nasal voice; violent thirst.
Catarrhal inflammation of frontal sinuses, antra and
    fauces.
Hot and dry, then, alternately drenched with sweat.
    Alternate heat and chill.
Heat with intermittent shuddering.

Arsenicum   .. *Thin watery discharge from nose which excoriates
    upper lip: while nose is stuffed up all the time.*
"Sneezing no joke!" — and affords no relief.
Sneezing from irritation in one spot (like a tickling
    feather), after sneeze, irritation as before.
Always taking colds in the nose, and sneezes from
    every change of weather.
Colds begin in the nose and go down to the chest.
Always chilly, suffers from draughts (*Hep.*).
Always freezing: hovers round fire: can't get enough
    clothes to keep warm. (*Nux.*)

Arsenicum (cont.) *Ars.* is chilly: with *burnings, relieved by heat*:

Is restless: anxious: morbidly fastidious.

During rigors and chills feels as if blood flowing through vessels were ice-cold water: a rushing through body of ice-cold waves.

With fever, intensely hot, with feeling of boiling water going through blood vessels.

Natrum mur. . . Catarrhs watery, or thick whitish, like white of egg "raw or cooked."

Catarrhs with abnormal quantity of secretion.

Paroxysms of sneezing.

Fluent alternating with dry catarrh.

Worse exposure to fresh air.

Watery vesicles about lips and wings of nose.

Cough with bursting headache (*Bry.*).

Hoarseness.

Urine spurts when coughing (*Caust., Scilla.*).

Nat. mur. loves salt: hates fuss: weepy, but no one to see. Depressed.

Pulsatilla . . "One of our sheet anchors in old catarrhs with loss of smell, thick yellow discharge, and amelioration in the open air (in the nervous, timid, yielding). Discharge NOT excoriating.

Stuffing up of the nose at night and copious flow in the morning."

Fluent in open air: stopped up in house. (Reverse of *Nux.*)

Well in open air, but violent catarrh as soon as he enters a room, and in the evening.

Lips chapped and peel.

Stuffed coryza, with blowing of blood from nose.

A weepy patient: craves sympathy. Craves air: cool air; better motion.

Rhus tox. . . From COLD DAMP weather: exposure to cold damp when perspiring. (*Dulc.*)

Violent coryza: redness and oedema of throat.

Nose stopped up with every cold.

Worse cold: better warmth.

Thick yellow offensive mucus.

Fear and restlessness at night.

Rhus tox. (cont.)   Hoarseness, rawness, roughness: worse first beginning to sing or to talk: wears off after singing a few notes or talking a little while.

Thirst for cold drinks especially at night: but cold drinks bring on chilliness and cough.

Worse uncovering.

Bones ache: sneezing and coughing: worse evening and night: tickling behind upper part of sternum.

Ipecacuanha .. Simple common colds: settle in nose: blowing of blood from nose with excessive sneezing.

Bronchitis of infancy: to break it up. (Later stages *Ant. tart.*)

Colds begin in nose, spread very rapidly to chest.

Stopping of nose.

Violent chill: frame shakes and teeth chatter.

No thirst: overwhelming nausea.

NAUSEA is a guide to *Ipecac.* in most sicknesses.

Carbo veg. .. Worse *warm moist weather.*

Worse evening.

Aphonia every evening (*Phos.*).

Dry tickling cough.

Rawness larynx and pharynx.

Natrum c. .. Fluent catarrh, provoked by the least draught.

With a periodical aggravation *every other day.*

Entirely relieved by sweating. (Reverse of *Merc.*)

Phosphorus .. Frequent alternations of fluent and stopped coryza (*Nux, Puls.*).

Sore throat: head dull: Feverish.

Secretion dries to crusts which adhere tightly. Hoarseness and bronchial catarrh.

Discharge from one nostril and stoppage of the other.

Sneezing causes pain in throat or head.

Blowing blood from nose.

Nose red, shiny, painful.

Chest tight.

Cough hard, tight, dry, racks the patient: worse open air.

Phos. colds generally begin in chest or larynx.

Kali bichr.   ..   Catarrh with thick yellow or greenish, ropy, stringy
                    mucous discharges, or tough and jelly-like.
                    Discharge offensive.
                    Adherent mucus, which can be drawn out into long
                        strings.
                    Plugs in nostrils.
                    Dryness nose with pressive pain at root of nose.

ESPECIALLY IN LATER STAGES OR TO CLEAR UP

Sulphur   ..   Subject to coryza: constant sneezing, stoppage of nose,
                    Fluent, like water trickling from nose.
                    Nasal discharges acrid and burning.
                    Cannot take a bath, cannot become overheated, can-
                        not get into a cold place, cannot over-exert with-
                        out getting this cold in the nose.
                    The typical *Sulphur* patient likes fat: gets hungry
                        about 11 a.m.: feels the heat.

Calcarea   ..   Lingering catarrhs; thick yellow discharge.
                    Great crusts from nose.
                    Breathes part of night through nose, then it clogs up,
                        and has to breathe through mouth.
                    Chilly: perspires much.
                    So sensitive to cold he finds it difficult to dress to
                        protect himself.

Tuberculinum ..   Persons with a family history of T.B.
                    Always catching cold.
                    Always tired.
                    Worse in warm room.

*   *   *

Drugs produce peculiar symptoms. Where these agree in drug and
patient, the ailment is cancelled, and health results. (This is most
strikingly seen in acute and uncomplicated sickness.)

When you give to a patient a remedy that can produce his symptoms,
you must give it in the small dose to which his sensitive condition will
respond without undue aggravation and suffering.

THE COMMONER INFLUENZA REMEDIES

Aconite   ..   Sudden onset of fever, with chilliness, throbbing pulses, and great restlessness — *from anxiety.*
A remedy of cold, dry weather, bitter winds (opp. to *Gels.*).

Gelsemium   ..   Heaviness and tiredness of body and limbs.
Head heavy; eyelids heavy; limbs heavy.
Colds and fevers of mild winters (opp. to *Acon.*).
Chills in back. "Chills and heats chase one another."
Bursting headache, from neck, over head to eyes and forehead; relieved by copious urination.
No thirst.

Eupatorium perf.   Intense aching limbs and back, as if BONES were broken.
Dare not move for pain (opp. of *Pyrogen*).
Aching in all bones, with soreness of flesh.
Bones feel broken: dislocated: as if would break.
Bursting headache: dare not move for pain.
Shivering; chills in back. (*Gels., Pyrog.*)
Chill begins 7 to 9 a.m.
Eyeballs sore. (*Bry., Gels.*)
There may be vomiting of bile.
Like the "break-bone fever" (Dengue).

Pyrogen   ..   *For the fever of violent pulsations and intense restlessness.*
Pulse very rapid: ratio between pulse and temperature disturbed. High temperature with slow pulse, or the reverse.
Chilliness no fire can warm. (*Nux, Gels.*)
Creeping chills in back, with thumping heart.
Bursting headache, with intense restlessness.
Hard bed sensation: feels beaten, bruised (*Arn.*).
Better beginning to move (opp. to *Rhus*), has to keep on moving, rocking, wriggling, for momentary relief.*
Copious urination of clear water, with fever.

* *One very bad 'flu year, all the cases one came across cleared up in twenty-four to forty-eight hours with* Pyrogen 6 *six-hourly. The symptoms, besides the thumping heart and the fever, were agonizing pain in lumbar and upper thigh muscles that made it impossible to keep still one moment.*

Baptisia ..	Rapid onset. Sinks rapidly into a stupid typhoid state.
	Dull red face: drugged, besotted appearance.
	High temperature: red: dusky: comatose.
	Drops asleep while answering.
	"Gastric 'flu": sudden attacks of violent diarrhœa and vomiting. Great prostration. (In such cases *Baptisia* will ensure as sudden a recovery.)
	'Flu-pneumonias with this besotted appearance.
	In the worst cases, mouth and throat are foul, and discharges very offensive. (*Merc.*)
	(Curious symptom) dissociation of parts: "scattered and can't get himself together". (*Petrol., Pyrogen.*)
Bryonia ..	White tongue: thirst for much cold fluid. (*Phos.*)
	From every movement, every noise, attacked with dry heat (rev. of *Nux, Gels.,* etc.).
	Wants to lie quite still, and be let alone.
	Especially with pleurisy, or pleuro-pneumonia.
	Headaches and pain all better for pressure, and worse for movement. (*Eup. per.*)
	The anxiety, dreams and delirium of *Bry.* are of business; in delirium he "wants to go home."
	Pains in head from coughing. Irritable.
Rhus tox. ..	Stiff, lame and bruised on first moving (opp. of *Pyrogen*), passes off with motion, till he becomes weak and must rest: then restlessness and uneasiness drive him to move again.
	The worst sufferings when at rest and kept without motion (opp. of *Bry.*).
	Illness from cold, damp weather: from cold damp when perspiring. (*Dulc.*)
	Anxiety, fear: worse at night. (*Acon.*)
	Restlessness: intense fever: thirst: great prostration. Weeps without knowing why. (*Puls.*)
	Typhoid forms of fever. (*Bapt.*)
	Severe aching in bones. (*Eup. per.*)
	A mental symptom of *Rhus* is fear of poison.
Mercurius sol.	Profuse, very *offensive* sweat.
	Very foul mouth. (*Bapt.*) Salivation. Offensive.
	Worse from sweating; or no relief from sweating.
	Colds extend to chest.

Camphor AND Nux IN INFLUENZA

Hahnemann discusses the effect of *Camphor* in the influenza epidemics "endemic in Siberia," which come among us occasionally. . . .
"*Camphor*," he says, "is of service, only as a palliative certainly — but an invaluable palliative, seeing that the disease is one of short duration."

"*On the other hand, Nux vomica, in a single dose, and that the smallest possible, will often remove the disease homœopathically in a few hours.*"

Read the pathogenesis of *Nux*, and see that this must be so. . . .

Nux   ..   "*After drinking, immediately shivering and chilliness.*
Chilliness on the slightest movement. On the slightest exposure to the open air, shivering and chilliness for an hour; dreads to go into open air.
By the slightest draught of air he gets chilled.
He cannot get warm.
Great coldness not removed by heat of stove, or by bed coverings.
Attack, as of fever: shivering and drawing in the limbs. . . ."

No wonder that Hahnemann says, "*Serious ailments from catching cold are often removed by it.*"

AFTER INFLUENZA BADLY RECOVERED FROM

Gelsemium   ..   Patients sometimes come to hospital, "cannot get well after 'flu a few weeks ago." They are found to have a temperature of somewhere about 99°. Not ill: *not well.*
If they are chilly, with heats and chills; if they feel a weakness and *heaviness* of limbs and eyelids, *Gels.* quickly puts them right.

China   ..   *Continued debility, with chilliness.*
Anæmic: pallid: weak.
Sensitive to touch: to motion: to cold air.
Worse alternate days.
Weariness of limbs, with desire to stretch, move, or change position.

Kali phos.   . .   General weakness and gloom.

Arsenicum   . .   *Chilliness: restlessness: anxiety: fear: fear of death (Acon.): prostration.*
Burnings, relieved by heat.
Oversensitive: fastidious.
Queer symptoms: — red-hot-needle pains.
Sensation of ice-water running through veins.
Or boiling water going through blood-vessels.
Thirst for sips of cold water.

Pulsatilla   . .   Flitting chilliness: chills in spots.
Cold creeps in back. Chilly in warm room.
Profuse morning sweat.
Heat as if hot water thrown over him.
One-sided chilliness — heat — sweat.
External warmth intolerable. Worse in a close room.
Palpitation with anxiety: must throw off clothes.
Better out of doors.
Better for slow motion (opp. *Bry., Eup. per.,* etc.).
Dry cough at night, goes on sitting up: returns on lying down again (*Hyos.*).
Thirstless: no hunger. Tearful; peevish.

Sulphur   . .   Partially recovers and then relapses.
Frequent flushes of heat. Uneasiness in blood.
Very sensitive to open air: to draughts (opp. to *Puls.*); worse for washing and bath. Takes cold.
Oppression, burning, stitches, congestion in chest.
Heat crown of head with cold feet.
Soles burn at night, must be put out of bed.
Hungry — starving at 11 a.m.
Drowsy by day: restless nights. Starts from frightful dreams.

Aconite ..	Throat *very red*: tingling.

Aconite ..
Throat *very red*: tingling.
Uvula feels long: comes in contact with tongue.
"Acute inflammation of all that can be seen and called throat." (Kent.)
Burning, smarting, dryness, great redness.
"Sudden onset in the night after exposure to cold, raw wind.
Plethoric person, wakes at night with violent, burning, tearing sore throat.
Cannot swallow. High fever, with great thirst for cold water.
Anxiety and fever."

Gelsemium ..
A *Gels.* develops several days after exposure: *Acon.* comes on in a few hours.
Gels. for colds and fevers of mild winters: *Acon.* for those violent winters and great cold winds (*Bell.*).
Gels. catarrhs excited by *warm, moist, relaxing weather.*
Sore throat, tonsils red: difficulty in swallowing, from weakness of muscles of deglutition. (*Bell.* from spasm, not weakness.)
Shuddering, as if ice rubbed up the back.
Hot skin: high temp. with cold extremities.
Weight and tiredness of whole body.
Sore throat, comes gradually: with muscular *weakness,* so that food and drink come back through nose. (*Bell.* from spasm.)
Great remedy of diphtheritic paralysis. (*Phyt.*)

Belladonna ..
Inflammation of throat. Tongue *bright red* or "strawberry": dry burning.
Fauces and tonsils inflamed and bright red. Esp. right side; extends to left (*Lyc.*).
Rapid progress. Constriction on attempting to swallow: ejection of food and drink through nose and mouth. (*Gels.* from paresis: *Bell.* from spasm.)
Dryness of fauces. Aversion to liquids.
Typical *Bell.* has congested, red, hot face and skin: big pupils, heat and dryness marked.

Phytolacca	Throat sore. Isthmus congested and dark red.
	Dark red inflammation of fauces: tonsils swollen.
	Feeling of a lump when swallowing saliva, or when turning head to left.
	Dryness, roughness, burning and smarting (fauces).
	"As if a ball of red-hot iron had lodged in throat."
	Throat so full, as if choked: or
	Pharynx dry, feels like a cavern.
	Every attempt to swallow sends shooting pains through ears (*Nit. a.*).
	Unable to swallow even water.
	Diphtheritic inflammation and ulceration of throat.
	Diphtheria, with above symptoms. Here *Phyto.* has made notable cures.
	Tongue fiery-red: feels burnt: or pain at root of tongue and into ear on swallowing.
	In less severe sore throats — ordinary ones! — one sees, not the smooth red swelling of *Bell.*, but a bluish-red inflammation (*Lach.*).
Nux	Sore throat.
	Colds settle in nose, throat, chest, ears.
	Sensitive to *least draught*: sneezing from itching in nose, and to throat and trachea.
	"Great heat: burning hot, but cannot move or uncover in the least without feeling chilly."
	Nux is hypersensitive (*Hep.*) irritable.
Apis	Burning, stinging pains in throat, better for cold, *worse for heat*.
	Œdematous condition: uvula and throat looks as if water would flow if pricked.
	Pains like bee-stings, with the thrust, and the burning following.
	Absence of thirst (*Gels.*).
	Must be cool: worse for heat: wants cool things.
	Especially worse from fire and radiated heat.
	Much throat trouble — even to diphtheria — with above symptoms.

Kali carb.   ..   Hoarseness and loss of voice (*Phos., Dros.*).
Catches cold with every exposure to fresh air.
"Lump in throat, must be swallowed."
Stinging pains when swallowing (*Apis*).
Uvula long, and neck stiff.
Always taking cold, and it settles in throat.
Chilliness: perspires much. Worse: cold air, water,
  draughts: better warmth.
"Fish-bone sensation in throat" so soon as he catches,
  or becomes, cold. (*Hep., Merc., Nit. a.,* etc.)
Hawks and hems.

Hepar   ..   "Seldom good in incipient colds and throats — more
  for ripened cold."
Fish-bone or crumb sensation (*Merc., Alum., Nit. a.,
  Arg. nit.*)
Worse any exposure: *worse cold dry wind.*
Intensely sensitive, mind and body.
Easily angry, abusive.
Throat extremely sensitive to touch (*Lach.*). Pain as
  if full of splinters: (*Nit. a.*) pain on swallowing.
The whole pharynx in a catarrhal state with copious
  discharge.
Larynx painful: painful as a bolus of food goes down
  behind the larynx.
Putting hand out of bed will increase the pain in
  larynx and cough. Croup after exposure to cold,
  dry wind (*Acon.*).

Dulcamara   ..   Sore throat from *damp, cold weather.*
Tendency to ulceration, which eats and spreads.
Catarrhal angina after catching cold.
Sore throat; fills with mucus: with yellow slime.
The tonsils inflamed, even quinsy (*Baryt. c.*).

Phosphorus   ..   Larynx raw, sore, furry. "Cotton" in throat.
Tonsils and uvula much swollen: uvula elongated:
  with dry, burning sensation.
Worse passing from warm to cold air.
Worse talking and coughing.
Hoarseness and aphonia, worse evening.

Arum triph. .. *Sore throats of speakers and singers.*
"Clergyman's sore throat" from straining voice, or a cold.
Arum triph. has a marked effect on larynx.
Hoarseness: lack of control over vocal cords.
If raises voice, it goes up with a squeak.
Graph. also for "uncertainty of voice: cannot control vocal cords: voice cracks."
And *Carbo veg.* has "deep voice, fails when he attempts to raise it."
But *Phyto.* also with real bad sore throats.
Corners of mouth and tongue cracked.
Excoriating saliva.
Tingling and pricking, lips, tongue, throat, nose: "in spite of soreness they pinch and scratch, and *pick and bore into sore parts.*"
Stinging pain in throat, which is ulcerated, raw and bleeding.

Alumina .. Like "Clergyman's sore throat" (*Arum triph.*).
Throat dry on waking, with husky weak voice.
It is dark red: uvula long.
Better hot drinks.
Splinter sensation, swallowing (*Hep., Nit. a.,* etc.).

Ignatia .. "A plug in throat," worse when not swallowing.
Tonsils studded with small, superficial ulcers.
Constriction about throat, with nervousness and insomnia. (Aphthous sore throat.)
Constriction also of larynx: "a feather there."
The more he coughs the worse the tickling.

Capsicum .. Throat feels "constricted, spasmodically closed."
Worse when not swallowing (*Ign.*).
The pain is smarting, *as from cayenne pepper.*
Chill or shuddering after every drink.
Odour from mouth like carrion.
"*Caps.* is loose, flabby, red, fat and cold."
"Throat looks as if it would bleed, so red. It is puffed, discolored, purple, mottled."
Throat remains sore a long time after a cold, or sore throat. (*Sulph.*) Does not get very bad, but gets no better.
Nose and cheeks red, and cold.

Aesculus   .. Useful in coryza and sore throat.
Coryza, thin, watery, burning: with *rawness*.
Sensitive to inhaled cold air. (*Phos., Rumex.*)
Violent burning in throat, with raw feeling.
Fauces dark, congested.
"After the sore throat, engorged veins left."
HOT, DRY, STIFF, ROUGH. Full feeling internally, throat
and anus.
Chronic sore throat with hæmorrhoids.

Pulsatilla   .. Catarrh of throat. Veins distended: throat bluish-
red.
Redness and varicose condition of tonsils.
Stinging pains (*Apis*) worse swallowing saliva.
Better cold, fresh, open air (opp. to *Phos.*).
Worse warm air, room; worse getting feet wet.
(A *Puls.* patient: weepy: wants fuss and help.)

Sulphur   .. Sore throat with great burning and dryness.
Chronic sore throat. Tonsils enlarged, with purplish
aspect lasting for weeks and months; a sore and
painfully sensitive throat.
Inflammation purplish, venous. . . .
In a sulphur patient: "the ragged philosopher":
argumentative and speculative. Intolerant of heat.
Loves fat. Intolerant of clothing: kicks covers off,
and thrusts feet out.

Baryta mur.   .. "Less greasy than *Merc.*" Warm, damp skin.
Saliva sticking round tonsils.
Tonsils very large, look like big plums.
"A lump in throat" pain.
Pains shoot to neck (*Phyt.* to ears).

Baryta carb.   .. Every little exposure to *damp or cold* awakens anew
inflammation of tonsils — throat — fauces (*Dulc.*).
Granulations, throat: worse every cold spell.
A very sore throat that comes slowly after days of
exposure.
Children with big tonsils; intellectually and physically
dwarfish: slow to develop.
Even the sore throat is of very slow development.

Sepia   .. Left side inflamed: much swelling but little redness.
                 Sensation of lump in throat (*Ign.*).
                 Waking with sensation as if had swallowed some-
                     thing which has stuck in throat.
                 Contraction of throat when swallowing.
                 Sepia is chilly: indifferent; intolerant alike of cold
                     and of close places.

Cinnabaris.   .. Throat swollen: tonsils enlarged and red.
                 "Sensation of something pressing on nose, like a heavy
                     pair of spectacles."
                 Throat very dry, awakening from sleep.

Natrum ars.   .. Throat dark-red, swollen, covered with yellow, gela-
                     tinous mucus which gags the patient when he at-
                     tempts to hawk it out.
                 Sneezing from draught, or breathing cold air.

Mercurius   .. Smarting, raw, sore throat.
                 Sore throat with every cold.
                 Tongue: thick, yellow, moist covering.
                 Profuse sweating without relief.
                 Thirst with salivation.
                 Bad smell from mouth.
                 Discharge (nose) yellow-green, thick, mucopurulent.
                 Worse at night; worse in bed.
                 ("Rarely give *Merc.* if tongue is dry.")

Nitric acid   .. One of the "fish-bone in throat" remedies.
                 Ulcers in throat, irregular in outline.
                 "A morsel stuck in pharynx," "as if pharynx con-
                     stricted."
                 Swallowing difficult: distorts face and draws head
                     down.
                 Swallowing even a teaspoonful of fluid causes violent
                     pain extending to ear (*Phyto.*).
                 Suddenly appearing, or slowly creeping ulcers on
                     fauces and soft palate.
                 Large deep ulcers, with bluish margins.
                 Nit. a. is chilly: loves salt and fat: is depressed and
                     anxious. Its pains are splinter-like, as if sticking in
                     the part, worse for touch.

Aurum   .. Tonsils red and swollen; parotid gland on affected
                side feels sore (*Phyto.*).

                Ulceration of palate and throat (*Nit. a.*) and espec-
                ially after *Mercury* and Syphilis.

                Aurum especially where the patient is depressed to
                the verge of suicide. Loathing of life.

Kali bich.   .. Ulcers, throat, which tend to perforate.

                Tonsils swollen and inflamed: ulcerated; deep ulcers;
                dropsical, shiny, red, puffy.

                Discharges ropy and stringy.

                Nose, throat, bronchi, bladder, all partake of this
                catarrhal condition, with discharges thick, yellow,
                ropy and stick like glue; tough, jelly-like: form
                hard masses.

                Exudate in throat looks like fine ashes sprinkled on
                the part.

Cantharis   .. Inflammation of throat with severe *burning* and raw-
                ness. Vesication.

                Great constriction of throat and larynx, with suffo-
                cation on any attempt to swallow water. (*Bell.*,
                Merc. cor., *Ars.*, *Arum triph.*, *Caps.*)

Mercurius cor. Symptoms "almost identical with *Canth.* But *Merc.
                cor.* has more swelling, throat and tongue, and deep
                ulcers, rather than the extensive vesication of
                Canth."

                Intense burning in throat (*Ars.*, *Ars. i.*, *Caps.*).

                Uvula swollen, elongated, dark-red.

                Throat symptoms very violent.

                "Any attempt to swallow = violent spasms of throat
                (*Bell.*) with ejection of the solid or liquid; but dis-
                tinguished from *Bell.* by its intense *destructive* in-
                flammation of throat."

Mercurius cy. Throat feels raw and sore.

                Looks raw in spots, as if denuded.

                Broken-down appearance of mucous membrane, bor-
                dering on suppuration.

                One of our most frequently-useful remedies in folli-
                cular tonsillitis: in diphtheria also, for which it
                has a great reputation.

                In poisonings *Merc. cy.* has produced membrane in
                throat, mistaken for diphtheria.

Lycopodium .. Has peculiar hours of aggravation: 4-8 p.m. Affects right side (in throats, quinsy, diphtheria): but may extend across to left side.

Also extends from above downwards, as when diphtheria begins in upper part of pharynx, or in nose, and spreads downwards.

Generally better from swallowing warm fluids: or better from holding cold water in mouth.

(*Lach.* is better for cold, and has spasms of throat from attempting to drink warm drinks.)

"The throat is extremely painful, it has all the violence of the worst cases of diphtheria."

Lachesis .. Left throat especially affected: left tonsil: tends to pass from left to right (opp. to *Lyc.* which goes from right to left). *Lac. can.* (in throats also, and in diphtheria) goes *from side to side and then back again*.

Throat bluish-red (*Phyt., Nat. ars., Lach.*).

Sense of constriction: "Throat suddenly closing up" or "lump in throat that he must constantly swallow."

Rawness and burning.

External throat is *excessively sensitive to touch* (*Hep.*).

Can swallow solids better than liquids: worse empty-swallowing. Even relief from swallowing solids. *Nothing must touch larynx or throat.*

All worse after sleep: sleeps into an aggravation: or wakes smothering.

One of our great diphtheria remedies — left side, or left to right; with above symptoms; but without the filthy mouth and tongue of the *Mercs.*

Merc. iod. flav. Throat right side, then left (*Lyc.*). Left to right (*Lach., Merc., iod. rub.*).

Tongue yellow at base. Better cold drinks.

Lac caninum .. "Throat closing: will choke!"

Very sensitive to external touch (*Lach.*).

Swallowing almost impossible.

Pain in throat pushes toward left ear. (*Phyto.*, shoots to ears.)

Pain, membrane, goes from side to side and back.

Throat dry, husky, as if scalded.

Sore throat before menses since diphtheria, with patches of exudation on tonsil. Glazed, shiny red throat. A grey, fuzzy coating. Better cold, or warm drink: Worse empty swallowing.

Has cured tonsillitis, diphtheria: has been used as prophylactic against diphtheria.

Lac can. is intensely sensitive and obsessed: sees faces: — sees spiders, snakes, vermin.

Cannot bear to be alone.

Thinks she has a loathsome disease: that everything she says is a lie.

Baptisia .. Pain and soreness of fauces.

Fauces dark-red; dark putrid ulcers: tonsils and parotids swollen.

Unusual absence of pain, in an extremely bad throat, is a characteristic of *Baptisia*.

Œsophagus feels constricted: can only swallow water.

But all this with the *Baptisia* "typhoid condition": — drowsy, dull red: as if drugged; lapses into a comatose condition. *Rapid onset of very severe symptoms, and rapidly curative in the Baptisia case.*

Pyrogen .. Septic throats, with extreme fetor.

Taste as if mouth full of pus. Carrion-like odour. Offensive sweats.

Tongue, red glazed; then dark red, intensely dry, or flabby: yellow-brown streak down centre.

Pulse very high: or out of proportion to temp.

Diphtheria with extreme fetor.

Quinsy with rapid suppuration.

A symptom of *Pyrog.* extreme restlessness.

SOME COUGH MEDICINES

Aconite   ..   Constant short *dry* cough, with feeling of suffocation, which increases with every respiration.

Cough hoarse, dry, loud; spasmodic: dry, hard ringing.

Cough wakes him from sleep, dry, croupy, suffocating.

Anxiety and fear. Restlessness. Worse at night.

Comes down suddenly *after exposure to cold, dry winds.*

Dry cough. Sensation of dryness whole chest. "No expectoration except a little watery mucus and blood. Otherwise dry."

Belladonna   ..   *Dry* cough, from *dryness* larynx.

Cough with red injected throat.

Violent scraping in larynx exciting dry cough.

Tickling and burning in larynx with violent paroxysms of cough. As if head will burst. (*Phos., Nux., Bry.,* etc.)

Child begins to cry immediately before cough comes on.

Attacks of cough end with sneezing.

The typical *Belladonna* patient is red, and burning hot, with dilated pupils.

Cough begins with peculiar clutching in larynx as if a speck of something had got into larynx.

Dry cough: spasmodic barking, short.

Kent. The *Bell.* cough is peculiar. As soon as its great violence and effort have raised a little mucus, he gets peace, and stops coughing. *Then air passages grow drier, and drier, and begin to tickle, then comes the spasm,* as if all air passages were taking part in it, and the whoop, the gagging and (?) vomiting. (A great whooping-cough medicine with spasms larynx, causing whoop and difficulty of breathing.)

Bryonia   ..   Hard, *dry* cough, with soreness in chest.

Dry spasmodic cough: worse night, after eating and drinking, when entering a warm room, after taking a deep breath.

Cough with stitches in chest: with headache, as if head would fly to pieces. (*Bell., Phos.,* etc.)

When coughing must press hand to sternum.

Cough compels to spring up in bed.

Cough shakes whole body.

Wants to sigh: to breathe deeply, which hurts.

Bry. is one of the worse cold, dry medicines: worse East wind (*Hep., Nux., Spong.,* etc.).

Bry. is always worse from movement: better for pressure.

Irritable: wants to be let alone: thirsty.

Nux   ..   Dry, teasing cough with great soreness of chest.

Coryza travels down to chest.

Feverishness, when patient *cannot move or uncover without feeling chilly.*

Spasmodic cough with retching (*Dros., Rumex*).

Worse cold, dry, windy weather.

Cough causes headache as if skull would burst: *Bell., Phos.,* etc. — or bruised pain about umbilicus, as if shattered and torn.

Tickling and pain in larynx with cough.

Acute catarrhal laryngitis: asthma — whooping cough.

"Something torn loose in chest."

Nux is hypersensitive, mentally and physically. Angry, easily offended.

Hepar   ..   *Worse for cold, dry weather.*

Better in warm, moist weather.

Cough when any part of the body becomes uncovered (*Rhus, Rumex*).

Worse breathing cold air (*Rumex*): worse putting a hand out of bed.

Suffocative coughing spells.

Croup from cold, dry wind, or cold air.

In croup, after *Acon.* and *Spongia.*

Phosphorus ..	Dry, tickling cough: irritation in larynx and below sternum.

Hard, dry, tight cough, which racks the patient and is very exhausting.

Racking cough. Violent cough.

Dry cough, with pain in head as if it would burst. (*Bell., Nux,* etc.)

Violent pain in chest with coughing, obliged to hold chest with hand. (*Bry.*)

Cough with pain chest and abdomen, obliged to hold abdomen with hand. (*Dros.*)

There may be involuntary stool when coughing.

Oppression and constriction, as if a great weight lying on chest.

Tightness across chest, better external pressure.

Violent, shaking cough. Trembles with cough.

Cough worse laughing, talking, reading aloud, eating, lying on left side.

Sputum saltish, yellow, sour, purulent, bloody, rusty.

Cold sputum, tasting sour, salt or sweet.

Worse open air. Going from warm to cold room (*Rumex*) *or vice versa.*

The typical *Phos.* patient is chilly, with thirst for cold drinks. Thirst for ice-cold water

Craves salt.

Sensitive to thunder.

Nervous alone — in the dark.

Suspicious. Anxious. Indifferent.

Causticum ..	Dryness: rawness: hoarseness: aphonia.

Cough hard, and racks the whole chest.

Chest seems full of mucus, "Feels if he could only cough a little deeper he could get it up.

"Struggles and coughs till exhausted or till he finds that a drink of cold water will relieve: ice-cold."

With each cough escape of urine.

Obliged to swallow the sputum raised.

Inability to expectorate.

Part of the *Causticum* local paralyses.

Greasy (*Puls.*) tasting expectoration.

Spongia   .. Chest dry. No wheezing or rattling, with respiration or cough.

Croupy cough: sounds like a saw driven through a board.

Wakes out of sleep with suffocation, with loud violent cough, great alarm, anxiety and difficult breathing. (*Acon.*)

Cough worse talking, reading, singing, swallowing, lying with head low.

Later tough mucus, difficult to expectorate: has to be swallowed. (*Caust.*)

Rhus tox.   .. Dry, teasing cough, from tickling in bronchia; from uncovering even a hand.

Nocturnal dry cough.

Cough with taste of blood, though no blood to be seen.

Cough during sleep.

Worse cold, wet weather. Worse uncovering.

Restlessness: must move.

Sepia   .. Violent cough with retching and gagging.

Thick, tenacious, yellow expectoration.

Severe cough on rising in a.m., with much expectoration.

No expectoration in the evening.

Or expectoration at night, none by day.

The *Sepia* patient is tired, indifferent, wants to get away.

Offensive axillary sweat.

Scilla   .. Gush of tears with coughing.

Cough causes sneezing, flow of tears, spurting of urine (*Caust., Phos., Rumex,* etc.), even involuntary stools. (*Phos.*)

Cough with expectoration in a.m. and none in evening.

Stannum   .. Loose cough, with heavy, green, sweet sputum (or salty).

Sensation of great weakness in chest.

Chest feels empty.

| *Drosera* | .. | Crawling in larynx which provokes coughing. |

Violent tickling in larynx brings on cough, and wakes him.

Spasmodic cough till he retches and vomits.

Cough coming from deep down in chest.

Provokes pain in hypochondrium: must hold it in coughing.

Oppression of chest so that breath could not be expelled.

Cough, the impulses follow on another so violently that he can hardly get his breath.

Hoarseness. Clutching, cramping, constricting and burning in larynx.

Cough worse at night.

Coughs of phthisis: asthma. Whooping-cough.

(Here Hahnemann urges a single dose of *Dros.* 30, not to be lightly repeated.)

N.B. — *Dros.* is especially indicated when there is a history of weak resistance to T.B.

| *Rumex* | .. | Cough on changing rooms, *from breathing cold air.* (*Phos.*) |

Cough provoked by changing from warm to cold.

Covers mouth up.

Every fit of coughing produces the passage of a few drops of urine. (*Caust.*, etc.)

Tough, stringy, tenacious mucus.

(Symptoms very like *Dros.*).

Much tough mucus in larynx with constant desire to hawk it but without relief. Hoarseness.

Dry spasmodic cough like early stage of whooping-cough (*Dros.*).

Dry at first. In paroxysms, preceded by tickling in throat pit with congestion and slight pain in head and wrenching pains right chest. The most violent paroxysms were a few minutes after lying down at night (11 p.m.), after which slept all night. Paroxysms also on walking, and through day. Later, expectoration of adhesive mucus in small quantities, detached with difficulty.

Breathlessness, as when passing rapidly through the air. Sensitive to open air.

Ipecacuanha   ..   Spasmodic or asthmatic cough. Suffocative cough.

Child becomes blue and stiff.

Respiration wheezing. Rattling.

Violent dyspnœa with wheezing and great weight and anxiety in chest.

Loss of breath with cough: with inclination to vomit without nausea.

Or, more often, *Ipecac.* has intense nausea — nausea unrelieved by vomiting; with clean tongue.

Arsenicum   ..   Wheezing respiration with cough and frothy expectoration.

Air passages seem constricted, cannot breathe fully.

Asthma type of cough.

Great prostration and debility.

Very sensitive to cold.

"Catarrh keeps traveling down. From nose to larynx, with hoarseness; down trachea with burning and smarting worse from coughing. Then constriction of chest, asthmatic dyspnœa, with dry hacking cough and no expectoration. With the *Ars.* anxiety, prostration, restlessness, exhaustion, sweat.

"Then constriction, wheezing, suffocation. Expectorates great quantities of thin, watery discharge. Expectoration is excoriating. Burning in chest."

Patient is worse after midnight. 1 a.m.

Kali carb.   ..   Cough at 3 a.m. or worse at 3 a.m.

Cough asthmatic: must lean forward, head on knees.

Cough with cutting or stitching (*Bry.*) in chest, with respiration, or between breaths. (*Bry. with* only.)

Sputum, of small round lumps: of blood-streaked mucus: of pus.

Kali bichr.   ..   Cough with white mucus, "tough as pitch, can be drawn out into strings."

Membranous shreds with cough.

Pulsatilla   ..   Cough caused by inspiration.
Worse warm room: coming into warm room.
Cough in the evening: when lying; prevents sleep.
Dry in the evening, loose in the morning.
Cough from tickling or scraping in larynx.
Paroxysmal. Gagging and choking.
Dry, teasing cough, wants windows and doors thrown
open. (*Sulph.*)
Discharges thick, bland, yellowish-green.
The typical *Pulsatilla* is tearful: is tolerant of heat
and of close places: better in cool, fresh air. Not
hungry, or thirsty.

Sulphur   ..   Suffocated. Wants doors and windows open (*Puls.*)
at night. Cough at night.
Congestion of blood to chest: to head.
Burning chest: head: face. In soles at night.
For coughs, and to clear up coughs in a *Sulph.* pa-
tient: — starving about 11 a.m.
Red lips, red lids: red orifices. Worse for bath.

Calcarea c.   ..   Tickling cough.
Sputum mucous, purulent, yellow, sour, offensive.
Worse cold: worse wet: worse wind.
Head and neck apt to sweat at night.
Cold damp feet (*Sepia*).

Tuberculinum   Hard, dry cough. Craves air (*Puls.*).
Better in cold wind. Suffocation in warm room.
To clear up coughs or pneumonias that hang fire,
where there is a T.B. history.
Night sweats.

SPASMODIC CROUP

There is a celebrated group of homœopathic remedies for Spasmodic
Croup, sold for years as "Boeninghausen's Croup Powders." They are
five in number.

Aconite, Hepar, Spongia, Hepar, Spongia: in that order, and should
so many be required.

Give at two- to four-hourly intervals, according to the urgency of the
case.

THE COMMON REMEDIES OF ACUTE CHESTS:—

EARLY CASES

Aconite .. Sudden onset: from chill: in cold dry weather.
First stage of pneumonia, bronchitis, pleurisy.
Cough hard, dry, painful. Chest tight.
Dry, hot skin.
Full, hard pulse. Rapid, difficult breathing.
Worse at night.
Lungs engorged. Sits erect. (*Chel., Lach.*)
May grasp larynx (*Ant. t., Phos.*). . . .
Always, with *Acon. restlessness, anxiety,* FEAR.

Ferrum phos. .. Early inflammatory diseases: pneumonia, etc., with
very few indications.
Lacks the restless anxiety of *Aconite*, the burning,
and brain symptoms of *Belladonna*, and the in-
tense thirst of *Phos.*
Breathing oppressed, short, panting.
Expectoration of clear blood.
Pains and hæmorrhages caused by hyperæmia.

Veratrum viride Sudden, violent congestion of lungs.
Bloated, livid face: faint, attempting to sit up.
Slow, heavy breathing. Must sit up (*Ant. t.*).
Dry, red streak along center of tongue.
Rapidly oscillating temperature.
Hyperpyrexia, with sweat.
Rapid, full pulse. Engorgement severe, with violent
excitement of heart.

Belladonna .. Pneumonia, etc., with cerebral complications.
Great nervousness: delirium.
Sleepy, yet cannot sleep.
Dilated pupils.
Flushed face, congested eyes: skin dry, hot.
Bronchitis with paroxysms of dry, hard spasmodic
cough.
Pleurisy, esp. right side: great pain, extreme soreness.
Worse if bed jarred.
Cannot lie on sore side (opp. to *Bry.*).

Ipecacuanha .. "Especially the infant's friend, commonly indicated in the bronchitis of infancy."

Bronchitis, broncho-pneumonia, pneumonia.

"Child coughs, gags, suffocates: coarse rattling often heard through the room."

Spasmodic cough, with nausea, and vomiting.

Rapid onset (Acon., Verat. v., Bapt.).

(Compare *Ant. tart.*; both have rattling cough and breathing, and vomiting. *Ipecac.* for stage of irritation, *Ant. tart.* for stage of relaxation.

Ipecac. comes on hurriedly: *Ant. tart.* at the close of a bronchitis, or broncho-pneumonia, with threatened paralysis of lungs: while chest is full of mucus, nothing can be raised.)

Chelidonium majus.

Pneumonia, generally right-sided.

Pleura generally involved, and (?) diaphragm.

If stirs, pain shoots through him like a knife.

Sits up with pain that transfixes chest. Worse movement (*Bry.*; but *Bry.* must lie still).

Tight girdle sensation. Apt to get jaundiced.

Tongue coated; tooth-notched (*Merc.*, etc.).

Deep-seated pain in whole of right chest.

Pain lower angle right shoulder-blade: from chest to shoulder-angle. (Characteristic.)

Cough loose and rattling, but expectoration difficult (*Ant. t., Ammon. carb., Kali carb.*).

"*In catarrhal pneumonia of young children* very like *Ant. tart.*; chest seems full of mucus, not easily expectorated."

Gelsemium .. Influenzal pneumonia. Chills up and down back.

Paralytic weakness. Limbs heavy: eyelids heavy.

Dusky-red face (*Bapt.*). Confused, dull, dazed, thirstless, severe congestive headache.

Baptisia .. Sudden onset: rapidly goes into a typhoid state.

Influenzal pneumonias, typhoid pneumonias.

Face besotted: dusky: purple (*Lach.*): bloated.

Tongue dry, brown down centre.

Besotted: mind confused: tries to answer or speak, but it flits away into stupor.

Baptisia (cont.)   In delirium, dual personality: tries to get the pieces together.

Discharges pungent: fœtid.

Pyrogen   ..   "*Baptisia,* only more so."

General aching and soreness.

"Bed too hard." (*Arnica.*)

Intense restlessness. ("*Rhus,* only more so.")

Offensiveness. (*Bapt., Kreos.*)

Fiery-red, smooth tongue.

Quickly oscillating temperature.

Pulse quick, or reverse: out of proportion to temperature. Delirium with dual personality.

Opium   ..   Insensitive. Comatose.

Stertor: blows out cheeks in expiration.

Hot sweat.

Nitric acid   ..   Inhalation of *Nitric acid* fumes causes rapid congestion and inflammation of lungs.

Chest feels crowded: oppression, worse bending backwards. Sensation of a spring released: — of a big hole in *right* temple.

Shattering cough.

Sputum sticks like glue: yellow, acrid, bitter, salt: flaps during respiration.

Expectoration of black, coagulated blood.

Stitches in right chest.

Fear of death, anxious about his illness (*Acon.*).

The typical *Nit. a.* patient is brown-eyed, chilly, intolerant of fuss; loves fat and salt.

Mercurius   ..   Bronchitis: cough worse evening and night.

Tickling in chest: feels dry.

"As if chest would burst."

Copious sweating without relief; "The more he sweats the worse he is."

"Rarely give *Merc.* if the tongue is dry."

"Pneumonia with excessive, offensive sweat, offensive mouth and breath, offensive expectoration." (The action of *Merc.* is pretty in such cases!)

Broncho-pneumonia, infantile broncho-pneumonia, bilious pneumonia (*Chel.*).

Tongue foul: tooth-notched (*Chel.*).

Mercurius (cont.)   Stabbing pains from base right lung to back.

Bloody, thick-green expectoration.

Suppuration of lungs: large quantities of pus.

MORE ADVANCED CASES

Bryonia   ..   Takes the place of *Acon.* when hepatization has begun.

Cough hard, painful. Expectoration thicker.

Anguish from oppressed breathing (*Acon.* from fever).

Lies perfectly still. (Opp. to *Rhus.*)

Every breath causes intense pain, in pneumonia or pleuro-pneumonia (*Kali carb.*).

Breath short, rapid, as deep breathing means great pain.

Lies on painful side, to keep it still. (Opp. of *Bell.*)

Stitching pains, better pressure: (*Bell.,* has throbbing pains, worse pressure.)

Lips dry. Tongue coated: dry.

Thirst for large quantities.

Constipation; dry, dark, hard stools.

Probably our most frequently-useful medicine in pneumonia.

Kali carb.   ..   Pneumonia, or pleuro-pneumonia with stabbing pains (chest) worse motion, worse respiration (*Bry.*) but (unlike *Bry.*) *also independently of respiration.*

Hepatization of lungs, with much rattling of mucus during cough.

Affects especially *lower, right chest* (*Phos., Merc.*)

Hepatization right lung, cannot lie right side: (*Bry.* lies on affected side — or back).

Infantile pneumonia, or broncho-pneumonia, with intense dyspnœa, much mucus, raised with difficulty, though constantly coughing.

Child oppressed, can neither sleep nor drink.

Wheezing, whistling, choking cough (*Ant. t.*).

Worse 2, 3 or 5 a.m.

Natrum sul.   ..   Pneumonia of *left lung,* and *left lower lobe.*

Pneumonia with asthma.

"Humid asthma of children."

Natrum sul. (cont.) Important *time aggravation,* 4 or 5 a.m.

Nat. sul. is *worse in damp weather; from damp dwellings.*

Phosphorus .. "Great weight on chest." Constriction.

Pneumonia with anxiety, oppression.

Expectoration of bright-red blood: or sputum rust-colored; purulent; saltish, sweet, cold.

Especially right lower lobe (*Kali carb., Merc.*) but *Phos.* lies on right side, *Merc.* on left.

Stitching pains in chest: in left chest, better lying on right side. (*Bry.* better lying on and steadying sore side, opp. to *Kali c.*)

Pleurisy, pleuro- or broncho-pneumonia, typhoid pneumonia — *with Phos. symptoms.*

To clear up hepatization (*Tub. bov., Sulph.,* etc.).

Dryness of air passages.

Hard, dry, tight cough; racks him. Trembles with cough. Suppresses cough, it hurts so.

Bronchitis with yellow, blood-streaked sputum.

Thirsty for cold water (*Bry.*).

Better for sleep (opp. to *Lach.*).

Wants company: fear alone.

Typical *Phos.* is tall, slender, "artistic" type.

Ranunculus .. Acute, stabbing pains chest, with effusion.
bulbosus

Anxiety, dyspnœa and distress.

Sore spots left in chest after pneumonia.

Sensation of sub-cutaneous ulceration.

Everything sore, bruised, *very sensitive to touch.*

Bright red cheeks with clean tongue. (*Ipecac.*)

Short, very oppressed breathing.

Dry heat: prostration from the start.

Small, very rapid pulse.

Cardiac and vascular excitement: nausea, even faintness, on motion (*Bry.*).

Rhus tox. .. Pneumonia has taken a typhoid form. (*Bapt.*)

Pleuro-pneumonia, with stitching pain. (*Bry., Kali carb.,* etc.).

Much fever: aching bones: market prostration. Dry hot skin.

Restlessness; relieved by motion.

Pain and dyspnœa worse at rest. (opp. *Bry.*)

Rhus tox. (cont.)   Bloody expectoration: or cold, green putrid-smelling sputum.

Tongue, red tip: dry. (Red line, center, *Verat. v.*)

? Incontinence of stool and urine.

Lachesis   ..   Worse after sleep. *Sleeps into an aggravation.*

Throat sensitive to touch.

Cyanosis.

Fits of suffocation: must sit up: or worse sitting erect, must bend forward (*Kali carb.*).

Least thing near mouth produces suffocative dyspnœa.

Oppression of chest: constriction (*Phos.*) worse afternoon: worse after sleep. Worse lying on left side (*Phos.*). Worse covering mouth or nose.

Asthma *during* sleep. (*Sulph.*).

Dry, hacking cough: worse touching throat: after sleep.

Tickling cough.

Cough "as if some food had got into wrong passage."

Hepatization, esp. of left lung.

Threatened paralysis of lungs with much dyspnœa, and long-lasting, suffocating paroxysms.

($<$ Pressure, *Lach*: $>$ pressure *Bry*.)

Left side, may go over to right.

Face puffy, purple, mottled. (*Bapt., Ant. t.*)

Lycopodium   ..   Unresolved pneumonia.

Fever worse 4-8 p.m.

Frowning forehead, in chest troubles.

Fan-like motions of alæ nasi.

Short, rattling breathing.

Wakes angry or cross.

A little food fills up.

Fulness and noisy flatulence.

Worse eating and drinking cold things.

Bronchitis, capillary bronchitis, broncho-pneumonia, pneumonia, *with above symptoms.*

Kali bich.   ..   Yellow, thick, lumpy, tough, stringy or sticky secretions. (*Sang.*) Sputum sticks to teeth, tongue, lips, draws out in strings — coughs up casts.

Worse 2-3 a.m.   Worse from cold.

Capsicum .. Chest too full: not enough room in it.

Cannot get air deep enough into lungs.

With every explosive cough, there escapes a volume of pungent, fœtid air. (*Sang.*)

Cough *causes distant pains,* or *raises foul air.*

Sputum dirty-brown, not rusty.

"Children of beer-drinkers: of over-stimulated men."

Fat; flabby; red, cold face. (Red, hot, *Bell.*)

Sanguinaria .. Cough ceases as soon as patient passes flatus.

Circumscribed redness of cheeks.

Distressing dyspnœa. Rusty sputum.

Hands and feet burning, or cold. Tongue red and burning.

Coughs, raises foul air (*Caps.*) tough bloody plugs or purulent sputum: ends with belching.

Feels very faint, with sweat and nausea.

"Sudden chill: burning in chest: Symptoms of pneumonia: Rusty sputum; violent cough, felt as a concussion at bifurcation of trachea; as if a knife were in the parts; as if torn asunder; and after cough copious, loud, empty eructations, no other remedy has this." (Kent.)

DESPERATE CASES

Cantharis .. Inflammation of lungs, gangrenous type, prostration, and the *lung affected burns like fire* (*Tereb., Kreos., Carbo v.*), or as if full of boiling water.

Esp. with frequent micturition with burning, cutting pain.

Antimonium .. Sudden and alarming symptoms of suffocation;
tartaricum

Oppression and short breathing: must sit up.

Accumulation of mucus in chest with coarse rattling: expectoration of thick white mucus after great efforts to raise it. Chest filling up; threatened paralysis of lungs.

Capillary bronchitis: Broncho-pneumonia.

Especially infants and old people.

Drowsiness. Weakness. Lacking in reaction.

Must sit up.

Sickly, sunken, pale, bluish face: twitching: covered with cool sweat.

Ammonium carb. Somnolence: drowsiness (*Ant. t.*). Great debility.

Rattling of large bubbles in lungs.

Bluish or purplish lips (*Ant. t., Lach.*).

Coughs continually, but raises nothing, or with great difficulty (*Kali carb.*).

VERY LIKE ANT. TART. — but *Ammon. carb. is worse for cold, Ant. tart. is worse for heat.*

Chests of old people; typical winter coughs.

Kreosotum .. Dreadful burning in chest. (*Tereb., Canth.,* etc.) Constriction.

Bronchitis: bronchiectasis, with *fearfully offensive sputum.* Gangrene of lung.

Bloody, greenish-yellow, pus-like sputum.

(One remembers an elderly woman, dying of bronchitis, where the stench of breath and sputum was so terrible that she was screened. *Kreos.* 200, promptly cleared whole condition up, beginning with the intolerable odour; she made a good recovery.)

Arnica .. Says he is well, when desperately ill.

Carbo an. .. Pneumonia, suppuration of right lung.

Burning in chest, or coldness in chest.

Suffocative cough, shakes brain, which feels loose. Sputum greenish, brown, syrup-like.

Destruction of lung tissue, and decomposition of fluids expectorated.

On closing eyes, feels smothering.

Terebinth .. Capillary bronchitis, drowsy, lungs clogged up; urine scanty, dark with blood.

Typhoid pneumonia: *unbearable burning* (*Canth., Carbo v.*) and rightness across chest: great dryness: or profuse expectoration.

Hepatization of lungs.

Carbo veg. .. The homœopathic CORPSE-REVIVER.

Burning in chest, as from glowing coals.

Capillary bronchitis.

Pneumonia, third stage. Patient moribund.

Fœtid sputum.

Cold breath and sweat: wants to be fanned.

Air-hunger. Threatened paralysis of lungs.

Cold throat, mouth; tongue cold.

Face yellow-grey: greenish: hippocratic.

Patient collapsed — "almost gone."

BUT A PNEUMONIA MAY NEED

Calcarea   . .   Bronchial catarrh of teething children.

To clear up pneumonia, or broncho-pneumonia in fair fat children of "plus tissue minus quality." Head sweats profusely in sleep. Cold, damp feet. Rickety children: big head and big abdomen.

Apis   . . . .   Constant sensation (chest) as if he couldn't live.

Anguish of mind. Impossible to get another breath, so great the suffocative feeling.

"Pleurisy with exudation: one of the best remedies to bring about absorption. *Apis* and *Sulph.* will cure most cases."

Apis cannot stand heat. (*Puls., Sulph.*)

Sulphur   . .   Torpid condition: *Bry.* helped but he does not rally.

Load on chest. Flushes without much fever.

Deficiency of reaction; to help absorption.

Especially in the typical *Sul.* patient — shock-headed: argumentative: not too tidy or clean: feels the heat: throws off the clothes and won't be covered: very red lips.

Psorinum   . .   Patients convalesce very slowly; are chilly, offensive; with despair of recovery.

Psor. is a chilly *Sulphur.*

Tuberculinum bovinum   . .   has promptly cleared up many a pneumonia, where it hangs fire, in persons of *tuberculous family history.* (In rare cases one of the other nosodes may be needed on such indication.)

N.B. — An imporant point in treating pneumonia, is not to imagine that you have cured because the temperature has dropped to almost normal, and so stop the medicine. Don't be happy till the patient has been normal or sub-normal for 48 hours.

*   *   *

It is only in the earlier stages of pneumonia in patients previously healthy, that the first prescription may be expected to finish the case. You may need to retake the symptoms and prescribe again.

*   *   *

Again. — At the end of pneumonias and broncho-pneumonias, treat afterwards, so as not to get further attacks.

SOME ASTHMATIC CONDITIONS WITH THEIR REMEDIES

(N.B. — The big-type remedies for Asthma in Children are
CHAM., IPEC., NAT. S., PULS., SAMB.)

And N.B. — *Periodicity* and *Special hours* are sometimes very important in selecting the remedy for asthma: but allow for summer-time: remedies take no account of this!

Arsenicum	..	Worse at night: after midnight.

Arsenicum ..
Worse at night: after midnight.
Worst hour 2 a.m. (1 to 2 a.m.).
Periodic attacks: spasmodic.
Worse cold air (rev. of *Puls.*).
Better bending forward (*Kali carb., Kali bi., Lach., Spong.*); > rocking (*Kali carb.*).
Leaps from bed; < lying; lying impossible (*Kali carb.*).
Worse motion.
Great debility and burning in chest.
Ars. is typically RESTLESS; ANXIOUS; IN FEAR.
ANGUISH. *Agonizing fear of death* (ACON.).
Worse for ices.
Better for heat applied and hot drinks.
Hippocratic face.

Kali carb. ..
Worst hours 2 to 3, and 3 a.m. (*Samb.*), or 2 to 4 a.m.
Better sitting upright, sitting *forward,* head on table or knees; > rocking (*Ars.*).
Worse lying; lying impossible (*Ars.*).
Worse drinking; worse motion.
Sensation of no air in chest.
< draughts (*Hep., Nux*).

Kali ars. ..
Worst hour 2 to 3 a.m. (*Kali carb.*).
Worse touch: noise.
Can't get too warm, even in summer.
Worse every other day, or every third day.

Aralia rac. ...
Asthma; loud wheezing with cough.
Worse evening and night; *after first sleep*; after short sleep; after a nap.
Would suffocate if did not sit up.
Expectoration warm and salty.

Sambucus .. *Attacks* 3 *a.m. (Kali carb.)*. Must spring out of bed (*Ars.*).

Sudden attacks in the night. Child wakes; sits up; *turns blue*; *grasps for breath*; seems almost dying. Then it goes to sleep, to wake up with another attack, again and again.

Asthma with suffocative attacks; may be well when awake, but sleeps into the trouble (*Lach., Aral.*).

Samb. has dry heat when asleep, profuse sweat when awake. (Profuse sweat when asleep *Con.*)

Cuprum .. Spasmodic asthma. Violent sudden attacks, last one to three hours, suddenly cease (*Samb.*).

Dreadful spasmodic breathing. Great rattling.

The more the dyspnœa the more the thumbs will be clenched and fingers cramped.

Spasmodic asthma, and violent dry spasmodic cough: "will be suffocated."

A characteristic: *strong metallic taste* (*Rhus*).

Natrum sulph. *Worst hour,* 4 *to* 5 *a.m.*

Worse wet weather: warm wet (*worse cold dry Acon., Hep., Nux*).

Great dyspnœa; violent attacks.

Profuse greenish purulent expectoration.

Dyspnœa with cough and copious expectoration. Humid asthma.

"If in a child, give it as first remedy."

Worse lying on left side.

In pneumonia of left lower chest.

Loose cough with soreness and pain through left chest (*Bry.*, with *dry* cough).

Springs up in bed (*Ars.*) and holds chest.

Pain lower left chest (lower right chest, *Ars.*).

Dulcamara .. "Asthma humidum:" loose cough and rattling of mucus. *Worse cold, wet weather* (*Nat. sul.*).

From suppressed sweat. From going from heat into icy cold. (Its "chronic" is *Sulph.*)

Ipecacuanha .. "Violent degree of dyspnœa, with wheezing and great precordial weight and anxiety."

Asthmatic bronchitis. Suffocates and gags with cough; spits up a little blood (*Ferr.*).

Has to sit up at night to breathe.

Gasps for air at the open window.

Worse warmth; better open air (*Puls.*).

"Suffocative cough; stiffens out, turns red or blue, gags or vomits."—KENT.

"Hands and feet drip cold sweat."

Antimonium Dyspnœa: must be supported in sitting position.
tart. ..

Great accumulation of mucus with coarse rattling (Ipec., but *Ipec.* has great expulsive power), *filling up with it, with inability to raise it.* Especially in children and old people.

Suffocative shortness of breath. Chest seems full, but less and less is raised (*Zinc.*).

Increasingly weak, drowsy, sweaty and relaxed.

Great drowsiness — almost to coma.

Face pale, or cyanotic.

Nausea and loathing of food. Thirstless.

Irritable: won't be touched or disturbed.

Aconite .. *Aconite* is sudden, violent, acute.

"AGONY: sits straight up: can hardly breathe. Pulse a thread. Sweats with anxiety."

Asthma from active hyperæmia of lungs and brain.

Face red: eyes staring; after emotions.

"A great storm, sweeps over and passes away."

From exposure to cold, dry wind (*Hep., Spong.*).

Fear: anxiety. "Going to die." Restlessness.

Anxious, short, difficult breathing (? with open mouth). (With protruding tongue, *Psor.*)

"Never give *Acon.* where the sickness is borne with calmness and patience."

Ailments from fright, shock, vexation, COLD, DRY WINDS.

Spongia   ..   Cardiac dyspnœa, and the most violent forms of asthma.

Dryness of air passages; whistling, wheezing, seldom rattling.

Must sit up and bend forward (*Ars., Kali carb.*).

At times, after dyspnœa, white, tough mucus, difficult to expectorate (? has to be swallowed).

Feels *as if breathing through a sponge.*

Worse cold, dry wind (*Acon., Hep.*).

Anxiety and fear (*Acon.*).

Kali nit.   ..   Asthma with violent dyspnœa: rapid gasping breathing; faintness; nausea.

Thirsty, but can only drink in sips between breaths.

Dull stitches or burning pain in chest.

External coldness; internal burning.

Stramonium   ..   *Violence. Face flushed. Staring look.*

Desire for light and company. Cannot bear to be alone.

Worse in dark and solitude.

Yet worse bright light. Looking into light.

Chamomilla   ..   Asthma *after a fit of anger* (*Ars., Rhus., Ign.*).

Suffocative dyspnœa. "Chest not wide enough."

Windpipe as if tied together with a string (? with or from accumulation of flatus).

Better bending head backwards; in cold air; from drinking cold water.

Hard, dry cough; coughs in sleep (*Arn., Lach.,* etc.).

Coughs when angry. Impatience of suffering.

Irritable and capricious.

One cheek flushed.

Ferrum   ..   Asthma after midnight: must sit up.

Better walking slowly about and talking.

Suffocative fits, with warmth of neck and trunk, and limbs cold.

Oppression from organism of blood, expectoration of blood (*Ipec.*).

Apis ..	"Cough impossible, lest something burst," or tear loose. All tense and stretched.
	Throat feels strangled. Suffocation: *can't bear anything about throat* (*Lach.*).
	Warm room unbearable. Worse warm drinks; heat of fire. *Better cold.*
	"As if every breath would be his last."
	Worse bending forwards or backwards (reverse of *Kali carb.*, etc.; reverse of *Cham.*).
	Attacks with violence and rapidity.
Cactus ..	Especially useful in acute attacks.
	Chest constricted, squeezed, caged; as if normal movement prevented by an iron band.
	Congestion of blood in chest — cannot lie down.
	Cardiac asthma (*Aur., Naja., Lach.*).
Lachesis ..	May occur in sleep (*Sulph.*) and not wake.
	Attacks of suffocation in sleep; when falling asleep; on waking; after sleep (*Samb.*).
	Better bending forward (*Ars., Kali carb.*).
	Worse covering mouth, nose; touching throat.
	Worse motion of arms; after talking.
	Wants doors and windows open (*Apis, Puls.*)
	Useful in cardiac asthma (*Cact., Aur., Naja*).
	Typical *Lach.* is purple, suspicious, loquacious.
Naja ..	"*A great remedy for asthma, especially cardiac asthma*" (*Caclt., Aur., Lach.*). "The breathing is so bad that he cannot lie down."
	Nervous palpitation; can't speak for choking.
	Wakes suffocating, gasping, choking (*Lach.*).
	Inability to lie on left side.
	"Our most useful remedy in a cardiac state with very few symptoms."
Aurum ..	Suffocative fits with spasmodic constriction of chest.
	Asthma from congestion of chest.
	Face bluish red, cyanotic.
	Palpitation: falls down unconscious.
	Cardiac dyspnœa.
	Deepest depression; hopeless; suicidal.
	Worse warm wet (*Nat. sul., Lach., Carbo veg.*).

Lobelia .. Extremely difficult breathing from constriction of
chest (*Cact.*). Want of breath, *hysterical.*
Asthma with sensation of lump above sternum.
Worse shortest exposure to cold during paroxysm.
Deep breath relieves pressure in epigastrium.
Attack often preceded by prickling all over, even to
fingers and toes.
Urine; deep red, with much red sediment.

Ambra .. Difficult breathing with cardiac symptoms.
Asthmatic dyspnœa; from any little *exertion; from
music; from excitement.*
"Asthma of old people and children."
Violent spasmodic cough with eructations.
Distension with much flatulence; < after eating.
Worse presence of others. Can only pass stool, or
urinate (*Nat. m.*) when alone.
"Hysteria of old age."

Nux .. "Asthma from every disordered stomach."
"Connected with imperfect and slow digestion."
"Something disagrees, and he sits up all night with
asthma.'
Nux is oversensitive; to noise, light, least draught.
Is *touchy.*
Craves stimulants; something to brace him up.
"Selects his food, and digests almost none."
Worse morning: after eating; *from cold air.*

Lycopodium .. *Asthma with great distension.*
Feels will burst: must loosen clothes.
Asthma and dyspnœa in catarrh of chest.
Forehead frowning; alae nasi flap; inability to ex-
pectorate (*Zinc.*).
Hours of aggravation (especially of fever), 4 to 8
p.m.

Carbo veg. .. Asthma with great flatulent distension.
Desperate cases of asthma; patient appears to be
dying.
Air hunger: "Fan me! fan me!"
Coldness and collapse: cold face, breath.
Asthma *ever since* whooping-cough, etc.

Bromium .. *Asthma of sailors as soon as they go ashore.*

Asthma of fair and fat children, "like *Puls.* but where *Puls.* fails."

Gasping, wheezing, rattling; spasmodic closure of glottis.

"Can't breathe deeply enough."

Must sit up in bed. Constriction.

"Air passages full of smoke."

Peculiar symptom: Coldness in larynx.

Worse from dust.

AMONG HAHNEMANN'S CHRONIC REMEDIES OF CONSTITUTIONS

(His "Anti-Psorics, Anti-Syphilitics and Anti-Sycotics") that may be needed for Asthma, are

Sulphur .. The more chronic cases with dyspnœa and oppression of chest.

Chest, rattling and heat: *especially* 11 *a.m.*

Sensation of a band, or load.

"Every cold ends in asthma" ("*Dulc.* but the deep acting remedy to follow may be *Sulph.*").

Sulph. is warm; hungry; often craves fat; kicks off the bedclothes or puts feet out.

The "ragged philosopher" type.

Psorinum .. Asthma; anxious dyspnœa and palpitation.

Worse sitting up; *better lying; the wider apart he can keep his arms, the better he breathes.*

Worse in open air.

Thinks he will die; will fail in business.

"A chilly edition of *Sulphur.*"

From suppressed eruptions (*Ars., Sulph.*).

Pulsatilla .. After suppression of rash (*Ars.*), of menses; in hysteria.

Worse evenings; after eating. As if throat and chest constricted; or as if fumes of sulphur had been inhaled. (Full of smoke, *Brom.*)

In the *Puls.* type; mild, weepy, craves sympathy; *intolerant of heat; craves air.* Not hungry; not thirsty; not constipated.

Changeable, symptoms, mental and physical.

Silica   ..   "Humid asthma. Coarse rattling. Chest seems filled with mucus; seems as if he would suffocate.

Asthma of old 'sycotics', or children of such. Pale, waxy, anæmic, with prostration and thirst."— KENT.

Asthma from suppressed gonorrhœa (*Thuja*).

Worse cold; draught; thunderstorms.

From checked perspiration or foot-sweat.

Often fetid, or suppressed fetid foot-sweats.

Head sweats profusely at night.

Zincum   ..   Can't expectorate: if he can is relieved.

Kali bichrom ..   With *ropy mucus;* stringy, tough, lumpy.

Worse cold, damp.

Tuberculinum ..   *In persons with a T.B. history or family history.* Even tentative panel doctors are finding this.

"Takes cold every time he gets a breath of fresh air." Yet craves fresh air.

Drosera   ..   *Asthma with T.B. History* — or family history; or after whooping cough.

Asthma, where the cough is violent, especially with spasmodic and constricting pains in abdomen, throat, chest, etc.

Worse at night.

Thuja   ..   Short breath from mucus in trachea (*Ars.*). from fullness and constriction upper abdomen.

Sensation of adhesion of lungs.

Drops in sleep.

Worse from onions.

Cases that follow vaccination; or many vaccinations; or bad vaccination.

After gonorrhœa, or offensive green discharges.

Greenish expectoration (*Nat sul.*) — in a.m.

Copious sweat; offensive; pungent; sweetish.

Peculiar symptom, sweat only on uncovered parts.

Worse cold damp (*Nat. sul.*) 3 a.m. (*Kali carb.*).

A left side remedy. "Often the chronic of *Ars.*"

Medorrhinum .. "Asthma: choking from weakness or spasm of epi-
glottis.

Larynx stopped so that no air can enter.

Only > by lying on face and protruding tongue."

Better seaside (Brom.).

Where asthma is connected, even remotely, with
gonorrhœa (*Thuja*).

Lueticum .. *Worse at night; night a dreadful time.*

"In syphilitic-looking kids."

"Attacks only at night, after lying down, or during a
thunderstorm."

Aggravation from sunset to sunrise.

Queer sensation, "as if sternum were being drawn to
dorsal vertebrae" (as if navel drawn to spine, *Plat
Plumb.*).

COMMON STOMACH AND DIGESTIVE REMEDIES
WITH INDICATIONS FOR THEIR USE

Nux   ..   Putrid or bitter taste in mouth, but food and drink taste right.

Repugnance to food.

Want of appetite, and constant nausea.

Dislike to accustomed tobacco smoking and coffee.

Eructation of bitter and sour fluid.

Nausea in morning (*Sep.*) — after dinner:

Qualmish nausea after eating:—

Inclination to vomit.

Contractive, squeezing stomachache.

Contractive pain in abdomen.

Distension and tenderness over stomach.

Flatulent colic upper part of abdomen, in the evening, lying.

Flatulence rises and presses under short ribs.

After a meal, flatulent distension (*Lyc.*): — immediately after drinking.

Cutting bellyache with inclination to vomit: — as if diarrhœa would occur.

Vomiting of sour smelling and tasting mucus.

Constipation from irregular peristalsis: frequent, ineffectual desire for stool: or passes small quantities with each attempt.

The typical *Nux* patient is: —

Very chilly and worse cold.

Very particular (*Ars.*), careful, zealous.

Gets excited, angry, even spiteful and malicious.

Easily offended.

Anxiety: sadness: scolding crossness.

Oversensitive to noise, slightest noise, strong odours, bright light, music.

Feels everything too strongly — music, singing.

May be suicidal, but afraid to die.

Sensitiveness; nervousness; *chilliness.*

Worse dry winds, east wind. Better warm wet weather. (*Acon., Asar., Bry., Caust., Hep., K.c.,* etc.)

Spasms from disorderly peristalsis. Reversed peristalsis.

Pulsatilla   ..   In mouth, taste, as from putrid flesh, with inclination to vomit.   Dislike to butter — to all fats.

Bilious eructation in the evening.

Diminished taste to all food. Adipsia.

Frequent eructation; taste of what was previously
eaten.

Sensation of sickness in epigastric region, especially
after eating and drinking.

Inclination to vomit, with rumbling and grumbling
in subcostal region.

Aching and drawing pain, stomach, in the morning.

Immediately after supper flatulent colic: flatulence
rumbles about painfully, especially in upper part
of abdomen.

Flatus discharged with cutting abdominal pain in
the morning.

Bellyache as if diarrhoea must ensue, yet only a natural stool occurs. Bellyache after stool.

Urgings to stool — to soft stool with mucus.

Frequent mucus stools with a little blood.

Bad taste: dryness in mouth with no thirst.

Worse for pastry, cakes, rich, fat foods.

Not hungry: not thirsty: not constipated.

The typical *Pulsatilla* patient is: —

Mild, gentle, yielding: cries easily: — can hardly give
her symptoms for weeping.

Sandy hair, blue eyes: inclined to silent grief with
submissiveness.

Conscientious about business. Loves steady work,
hates hustle.

Changeableness in everything: — in disposition: in
the pains that wander from joint to joint: in character of stools — menses, etc.

Pulsatilla feels the heat.

Worse warm room, warm applications.

Better in cool, open air: by walking slowly: but the
pains of *Puls.* are accompanied by chilliness.

Loves sympathy and fuss.

"Little suited to persons who form resolutions with
rapidity, and are quick in their movements." (The
antithesis of *Nux*.)

Sepia   ..   Nausea. Morning nausea (*Nux*).

Nausea after eating, or, often relieved by eating.

Vomiting of food and bile in the morning.

Nausea and morning sickness of pregnancy. (*Ipec.*)

Peculiar faint, sinking emptiness and goneness at pit of stomach. (*Sulph.*)

Sagging of all viscera. Bearing-down in pelvic organs. (*Lil. tigr.*)

Aversion to food — meat — fat — bread (during pregnancy) to milk, which causes diarrhœa.

Nausea from the smell of food and cooking (*Colch., Ars.,* etc.).

Characteristic symptoms:—

Indifference: indifference to loved ones. (*Phos.*)

Wants to get away: to be alone. (*Nat. mur.*)

Hates fuss and sympathy (*Nat. mur.*): — talking; talking of others. Hates noise.

Flashes of heat with perspiration, and faintness.

General relaxation, mental and physical. Faintness — kneeling and standing.

Often, yellow saddle across nose and cheeks.

Ipecacuanha   ..   Nausea with empty eructations and great flow of saliva. VOMITING.

Vomiting with a clean tongue.

Persistent nausea: not relieved by vomiting.

Distress as if stomach hung down, relaxed.

Griping, as from a hand in abdomen: esp. about umbilicus.

Diarrhœic, as if were fermented, stools.

Sulky: despises everything: desires that others should not esteem or care for anything.

Phosphorus   ..   Excessive thirst. Thirst for cold drinks.

Regurgitation of food. Empty eructations.

Nausea. Vomiting. *Burning in stomach.* (*Ars.*)

Thirst for cold water. (Or unable to drink water, even the sight of it causes nausea and vomiting. Must close eyes when bathing.)

Water vomited as soon as warm in stomach.

Goneness, as if stomach had been removed.

Weak, empty, gone sensation whole abdomen.

Stomach pains better for cold food, ice cream.

Phos. (cont.)   Profuse diarrhœa. Blood in stools.

Sphincter relaxed: involuntary stool. Oozing of stool from unclosed sphincter. (Comp. *Apis.*)

The typical Phos. patient is: —

Tall, thin, the artistic type. Fine, dark hair.

Easy bleedings of bright blood. Small wounds bleed much. Bruises easily.

Desire for salt — for cold drinks — for ices.

Fear alone — dark — thunder; "someone-behind."

Relief from rubbing: from a short sleep. (*Sep.*)

Burnings; stomach, intestines, up spine, between scapulae (*Lyc.*)

(N.B. — *Ars.* burnings everywhere are better for heat; distinguishes from *Phos.*)

Answers slowly. Indifferent: to loved ones (*Sep.*).

Arsenicum   ..   *Burning* pain stomach, relieved by heat. (Rev. of *Phos.*).

Burning, violent pain, like red-hot coals.

Epigastrium sensitive to slightest touch.

Great anxiety about epigastric region.

Acute gastritis; painful vomiting of grass-green solids; or fluids; or after drinking.

Hæmatemesis, often with black stools.

Violent pains in abdomen with great anguish: rolls about on the floor and despairs of life.

Periodic colic.

Burning in intestines. Abdomen distended.

The great remedy of PTOMAINE POISONING.

The burning pains of *Ars.* are everywhere relieved by *heat*.

Diarrhœa, worse after midnight and after eating, with great prostration.

Vomiting and stool may be simultaneous.

Intense thirst: —for small quantities: — for cold drinks, which disagree.

Characteristic symptoms: —

Great anguish. Anxious impatience. GREAT ANXIETY. GREAT RESTLESSNESS.   GREAT PROSTRATION.

Worse at night: after midnight: 1 to 3 a.m.

Worse cold air: cold drinks: cold applications.

Chamomilla .. Putrid breath after dinner. Ptyalism.

The pains are aggravated by eructation.

After a meal distension, with heat of face.

Obstructed flatus. Vomiting of bile.

Typical characteristic symptoms: —

A spiteful, sudden, irritable incivility.

Moans, weeps and howls in sleep.

Shivers at cold air. Redness in one cheek.

Evenings, burning cheeks with transient rigor.

Extreme restlessness, anxious tossing, with tearing pain in abdomen.

Howling on account of a slight, even imaginary insult — perhaps of long ago. (*Staph.*)

Wants this or that; then refuses it, or knocks it away. (*Staph.*)

Oversensitive to pain. *"Unsuited for persons who bear pain calmly and patiently."*

Sulphur .. Burning in stomach. (*Phos., Ars.: Phos.* desires cold drinks, ices; *Ars.* hot drinks.)

Empty, weak sense (stomach) about 11 a.m.

Big appetite: craves food at 11 a.m.

Or, drinks little, but eats much. Worse for milk.

Desires sweets, fat, alcohol, beer and ale.

Liable to early morning diarrhoea.

In the typical *Sulph.* patient, worse for heat: intolerant of clothing and its weight.

Natrum carb. .. "Greedy persons: love sweets and nibbling."

Excessive flatulence: always belching with sour stomachs and rheumatism.

Better eating. When chilly eats, and is warm.

All-gone feelinng and pain in stomach, which drives him to eat. (At about 11 a.m. *Sulph.*)

At 5 a.m. so hungry; is forced out of bed to eat something, which also ameliorates the pain

At 11 p.m. hungry. (11 a.m. *Sulph.*)

Fatigue and weakness; mind and body. Nervous exhaustion. Confusion. Bad tempered.

Cannot digest milk: diarrhœa from milk.

Flatulence and looseness of bowels from starchy foods.

(Patients who take much carbonate of soda to neu-

Nat. carb. (cont.)	tralize acidity, with temporary relief. Where indicated acts curatively in potencies.)
Bryonia ..	After eating, pressure in the stomach; it was as if a stone lay there and made him cross.
	Stomach extremely sensitive to touch and pressure.
	Vomiting: of bile: of what has been eaten.
	Mouth dry: tongue white: thirst for large quantities at long intervals. (Comp. *Phos.*)
	Patient cannot bear a disturbance of any kind, either mental or physical.
	Cannot sit up in bed, as it makes him so sick and faint.
	Better lying quite still, and left alone.
	Stools dry, hard, as if burnt; dark.
	Nausea on waking: from slightest motion.
	Unnatural hunger: of loss of appetite.
	Desires acids, sweets, oysters, etc.

Characteristic symptoms: —

Worse for motion. Dryness of mucous membranes. Pains stitching in character, provoked by motion.

Anxious; irritable.

Dreams of quarreling, and of business.

Antimonium crud. ..	A characteristic symptom is *Thick, milky white coating on tongue.* (*Bry.*)
	Deranged stomach from eating what does not agree. Easily disturbed digestion.
	Gastric catarrh: nausea and vomiting.
	Loathing; for food and drink.
	Desire for acids, pickles. Worse for vinegar.

The typical Ant. crud. patient is: Sentimental: peevish: dislikes to be touched or looked at.

Colocynth ..	Frequent vomiting. Vomiting caused by PAIN. Annoyance or distress may result in extreme pain in any part of body, causing vomiting.
	Agonizing pain in abdomen, *only relieved by bending double and pressing hard into abdomen.*
	Colics, better heat and pressure. (*Mag. phos.*)
Robinia ..	A great remedy for HEARTBURN and acidity. Everything turns to acid.
	"The chief keynote of *Robinia* is acidity, especially if the time of aggravation is night."

Lycopodium .. Fullness, flatulence, distension and bloating of stomach and abdomen (*Arg. nit., Chin.*).

Discomfort, pressure, tenderness, heaviness in stomach after eating a little. *Must loosen clothing.* Very sensitive to pressure there.

Sudden, easy repletion. Loses appetite after first mouthful: — *or,* eating increases appetite.

Acidity — waterbrash — heartburn.

Typical nervous dyspepsia of the brain-worker coming on in afternoon and better in evening after gettting home and being at peace — often felt only on leaving office in evening. Hunger headache.

The typical Lycopodium patient: —

Craves sweets (*Arg. nit.*), hot drinks.

Is worse for cold food, flatulent food, cabbage, onions, oysters.

Is generally better in the morning.

Worse 4-8 *p.m.* is very typical of *Lyc.* In fevers, and pneumonias, also.

Worse afternoons and evenings, better later.

Likes, and fears to be alone. "Wants to be alone with someone in the next room."

One of the "anticipation drugs." Dreads ordeals — speaking in public — singing.

In *Lycopodium* the intellectual predominates over the physical; and it is the intellectual that is apt to suffer — memory, etc.

Argentum   Flatulent dyspepsia. (*Lyc., Carbo veg.,* etc.)
nitricum .. Gastric derangements accompanied by belching.

"Belching after every meal, as if stomach would burst; belching difficult, finally air rushes out with great noise and violence."

Irresistible craving for sugar, and sweets.

Fluids "go right through him."

Red painful tip to tongue, papillae prominent.

Characteristic symptoms: —

Apprehension: Anticipation, even to diarrhœa (*Gels.*). Examination funk (*Aeth.*).

Queer fears: of high places: or corners: of walls closing. Worse shut in anywhere.

Hurried feeling. Must walk fast (*Lil. tigr.*)

Carbo veg.   ..   Great distension of the abdomen with gas.

Constricting and cramping pains from distension.

Belching, and sour disordered stomach.

Burning in stomach: anxiety: distension.

Constant eructations, flatulence, heartburn, water-brash.

If he eats or drinks, abdomen feels as if it would burst. (*China,* etc.)

Worse lying down.

Aversion to fats and to milk.

Longs for coffee (*Bry.*), acids, sweets and salt things (*Arg. nit.*).

"Aversion to the most digestible things and the best kinds of food." "Mince pie fiends."

RELIEF FROM BELCHING: headaches better from belching; rheumatism and other sufferings better from balding. Always belching.

In *Carbo veg.* the face flushes to the roots of the hair after a little wine.

A chilly patient — with air-hunger. COLDNESS.

Burnings. Internal burnings with external coldness.

"Sluggish, lazy, turgid, full, distended, swollen, puffed." "Veins large, relaxed, paralysed."

Carbo animalis   The rapid and magical relief of abdominal distension after abdominal operations that follows a dose of *Carbo an.* 200 must be seen to be believed.

Colchicum   ..   *Colchicum* has great meteoric distension of the abdomen. (*Lyc., Carbo veg., Carbo animalis, China.*)

Aversion to food: loathing the sight, and still more the smell of it (*Sep., Ars.*).

The smell of fish, eggs, fat, meats and broth causes nausea even to faintness. Smell of cooking gives extreme nausea.

Great distension of abdomen with gas.

Violent burning in epigastrium.

His suffering seems intolerable to him: external impressions, light, noise, strong smells, contact disturb his temper (*Nux*).

Gouty patients. Worse extremes of heat or cold.

Asafoetida   . .   In dyspepsia, "If you have seen a typical case of *Asaf.* you will wonder where all the air comes from: it comes up in volumes.

"Expulsion of wind like the sound of a small pop-gun going off almost every second."

Loud belching: flatus is not passed down, but all upwards.

Offensive: *Asaf.* is offensive everywhere: "horribly offensive" liquid stools of most disgusting smell.

Puffed, venous, purple faces. *Asaf.* is "fat, flabby and purple."

Hysterical spasm of œsophagus and trachea.

Graphites   . .   Aversion to animal food and sweet food.

Constrictive or *gnawing* pain in stomach: in empty stomach: with relief from eating.

Pain in upper abdomen. Great distension in abdomen.

The three characteristic symptoms of *Graphites* in stomache complaints are: —

Relief from eating.

Relief from hot food, and drink. (*Chel.*)

Relief from lying down.

Ornithogalum . .   Dr. Robert Cooper's little proved, but valuable remedy in gastric ulcer, even malignant.

Distension of stomach and abdomen.

Belchings of mouthfuls of offensive flatus.

Must loosen clothes.

Writhing in agony. Pains worse at night, spread to heart and shoulders.

As if an iron brick were being forced through stomach and chest.

Cooper says, "*Ornithogalum,* in those sensitive to it, goes at once to the pylorus, causes painful spasmodic contraction of it, and distends the duodenum with flatus, its pains being invariably increased when food attempts to pass the pyloric outlet of the stomach." Cooper gave a single drop of the φ (allowed to act for several weeks.)

SOME REMEDIES OF CONSTIPATION*

Nux   ..   Constant urging for a stool which never comes or a small stool is passed with urging, leaving sensation of more remaining behind.

Always as if evacuation were incomplete.

Ineffectual desire for stool.

Tearing and sticking and contracting pain, as from piles in rectum and anus after a meal; and especially *on exerting the mind, and studying.* (Comp. *Caust.*)

Bright blood with fæces, with constriction and contraction during stool.

Nux is the medicine of the sedentary, the studious, the hypersensitive and the *irritable.*

The key to the *Nux* constipation (and colic) is *irregular peristalsis.* Spasmodic constrictions (*Strych.*) which drive the intestinal contents at once backwards and forwards.

Strychnine   ..   Obstinate constipation, with griping pains (*Nux*).

Bryonia   ..   Chronic constipation, with severe headache.

No desire; or urging with several attempts before result.

Stool unsatisfactory, after much straining with rush of blood to head. (Nose bleed. *Coff.*)

Stools hard, dark, dry; as if burnt (*Sulph.*).

Stools too thick; too large (*Sulph.*).

Obstruction from induration of fæces.

Distended abdomen; rumbling and cutting, yet obstinate constipation. After stool long-continued burning in rectum (*Thuja*).

Bryonia is irritable (*Nux*): everywhere DRY: < motion; white tongue; great thirst.

Natrum mur. ..   Constipation: obstinate retention of stool.

Irregular; hard, dry; on alternate days.

During M.P. Anus contracted, or torn.

Knows not whether flatus or stool escapes; dryness of mucous linings, with watery secretion in other parts.

Nat. mur. is irritable; weepy; hates fuss.

Craves salt. Aversion to fats; to bread.

---

* N.B. — "To every action there is an equal and contrary reaction," and most of the great remedies of constipation are also great remedies for diarrhœa.

Sulphur .. Stool with "something left behind" (*Nux*).
Hard, as if burnt (*Bry.*). Extreme constipation.
Stool every 2, 3 or 4 days, hard and difficult.
Stools large, painful: held back from pain.
Sulphur is a warm patient; hungry about 11 a.m.;
kicks off the clothes at night; puts feet out; hungry
for fat, for everything.
Red orifices; acrid excoriating discharges.

Lac deflor. .. Large painful stools (*Sulph.*). Dry (*Bry.*).
Invincible constipation with chronic headache.
Constipation *with coldness;* cannot get warm.
Lac deflor. is supersensitive to cold: to least draught.
Complaints from putting hands into cold water.
Worse milk: aversion to milk.

Graphites .. Stool large, hard, knotty, in agglomerated masses,
mixed with *tough slimy mucus.*
"Sometimes great quantities of mucus with hard stool,
as much as a cupful of thick, tough, stinking mucus."
Hæmorrhoids with burning rhagades.
Itching; smarting, sore pain at anus.
(Characteristics of *Graph.*) Obesity; relief from eat-
ing; from hot foods and drinks.
Skin troubles, with sticky oozing.

Collinsonia .. Obstinate constipation with hæmorrhoids.
Piles with constipation, (even diarrhœa) bleeding, or
blind and protruding; feeling of sticks (*Æsc.*),
gravel, or sand in rectum.
Chronic, bleeding, painful hæmorrhoids.
Very constipated, with colic.

Æsculus .. Hard, dry, difficult stools.
Rectum dry, hot: "full of small sticks."
Knife-like pains shoot up.
Severe lumbo-sacral backache.
Stool followed by fullness in rectum, and intense pain
for hours (*Nit. ac., Aloe, Ign., Sul.,* etc.).
Painful, purple external piles, with burning (*Collin-
sonia's* bleed more).
(A queer sensation, a bug crawling from anus.)

Nitric acid .. Pain with stool as if something would be torn. *Sticking* pain (rectum), during stool, and lasting many hours after (*Æsc.*).

Fissures and hæmorrhoids. Great pain after stool (even soft stool) *lasts for hours.*

Burning in anus. Itching in rectum.

Nitric acid affects especially parts where skin and mucous membrane join.

Its pains are *splinter pains,* worse for contact.

Nitric acid patient is very like the *Sepia* patient, but loves fat and salt (unlike *Sepia*).

Arsenicum .. Constipation with tenesmus: with pain in bowels. (More characteristic, diarrhœa and purging.)

Hæmorrhoids: with stitching pain walking and sitting, *but not at stool:* pain like slow pricks of a hot needle: protrude like coals of fire.

Burning pains anus, *relieved by heat.*

Diarrhœa alt. constipation — in an *Ars.* patient, with restlessness, anxiety and prostration.

Opium .. Almost unconquerable chronic constipation.

Constipation from inaction, or paresis — for 6 or 8 weeks, with loss of appetite.

Peristaltic action entirely suspended: even reversed peristalsis with fæcal vomiting.

Fæces protrude and recede (*Sanic., Sil., Thuja*).

Or. stool invol. after a fright — from paresis.

Stools hard, round, black balls; obstruction from indurated fæces.

Opium has the most startling opposite conditions. Inveterate constipation—persistent diarrhœa. Coma, to complete insensibility — exalted sensibility, "Can hear the flies walk on the walls, and distant clocks chiming;" sleepy but cannot sleep; hears noises not generally noticed.

Stramonium .. Stool and urine suppressed.

Obstinate constipation.

Cannot bear solitude, or *darkness.*

Face red and bloated.

Painlessness with most complaints.

Plumbum .. Obstinate habitual constipation.

Paresis of intestines. Cannot strain at stool: cannot expel the fæces.

Obstruction from induration, from impaction.

Urging and terrible pain from constriction and spasm of anus ("Where *Platina* fails")

Violent colic. Abdominal wall "drawn to spine by a string" (*Plat.*).

As if abdomen retracted and drawn towards spine: retraction both objective and subjective.

Boat-shaped abdomen.

Stools like sheep's dung: balls in conglomerate masses.

Typical *Plumbum* has slowness; torpor; emaciation: must stretch for hours.

A keynote, "Paralysis with hyperæsthesia."

Alumen (*Alum*) Ineffectual urging: or several days without desire for stool. No ability to pass stool.

Long useless straining, then after many days stool is passed — an agglomeration of little hard balls.

After stool, sensation as if rectum still full (*Nux*).

Cramps and colic: sensation of abdomen drawn to navel (*Plumb., Plat.*).

Hæmorrhoids ulcerate: prolonged suffering after stool (*Nit. ac., AEsc.,* etc.).

Antidote to lead poisoning: and for lead constipation. Symptoms very similar to lead.

Platina .. Difficult stools: sticks to anus and rectum like putty.

Frequent urging with inability to strain at stool (*Alum.*).

Inveterate constipation and unsuccessful urging (*Nux*).

Stool, hard, scanty, or sticky. Undigested.

Peculiar symptom of *Platina*. Feels tall: everything looks small to her.

Mentally also, pride, and looks down on others.

Another curious symptom, navel feels retracted by a string (*Plumb.*).

Alumina   .. Inactivity rectum and bladder.

Great straining to pass even a soft stool.

Must strain at stool to urinate.

No desire for and no ability to pass stool with large accumulation. Great straining.

Rectum seems paralysed: has not strength to press the contents out.

Stool hard, knotty, covered with mucous, or soft, clayey, adhering to parts (*Plat.*).

Patients are asking for help in regard to a curious and very obstinate form of constipation, evidently from the use of aluminum cooking pots, because it promptly disappears when these are discarded, the bowels resuming their normal functioning. This is how these aluminum sensitives describe their constipation:

No desire whatever for stool.

No physical inconvenience from "No stool for days, even a fortnight!"

"Nothing seems to go down lower than the upper left abdomen" (*the splenic flexure*).

"Rectum seems not only inactive, but empty."

Veratrum alb. .. Digestion good; but defæcation almost impossible from inertia of rectum.

No desire for stool: which is large, hard, in round black balls. No expulsive action.

Verat. is cold: sweats much. Cold sweat on forehead.

Causticum   .. Frequent ineffectual efforts to stool, with pain, anxiety and redness of face (with nosebleed, *Coff.*).

Rectum active: fills with hard fæces, which pass involuntarily and unnoticed (*Aloe*).

Passes little balls unnoticed.

Stool tough and shiny: shines like grease.

Passes better standing.

Hæmorrhoids: impeding stool: swell; itch; stitch; worse walking; thinking of them; preaching or straining voice. (Comp. *Nux.*)

Causticum is intensely sympathetic with suffering.

A remedy of local paralysis. Urine involuntary when sneezing or coughing. Enuresis in children.

Phosphorus .. Inveterate constipation.

Fæces slender, long, dry, tough and hard, voided with difficulty. "May be compared to a dog's stool in appearance and manner of evacuation."

Paralysis of bowel, so that it is impossible to strain at stool (*Alum.*).

(*Phos.* has also a paralytic condition in which anus stands open (*Apis*) and stool oozes out.)

Hæmorrhage from bowel.

Typical *Phos.* is the slender, artistic type: fears dark — alone — thunder; craves salt, ices, cold drinks: Chilly (*Apis,* warm).

Apis .. Constipation: sensation (abdomen), "something tight, will break if effort used." (See *Plumb., Plat.*)

Bowels seem to be paralysed.

No stool for days — for a week.

Or stools occur with every motion of the body as if anus were constantly open (*Phos.*).

Anus swelled: oozing blood.

Apis feels the heat; cannot stand heat.

Is *thirstless.* (Reverse of *Phos.*)

Its pains everywhere are STINGING and burning.

It is one of the remedies for dropsical conditions.

Conium .. Ineffectual urging; hard stool.

Inability to strain at stool; inability to expel contents because of the paralytic weakness of all the muscles that take part in expulsion.

Strains so much at stool that uterus protrudes.

At every stool tremulous weakness and palpitation.

Conium has dizziness; numbness; paralytic weakness, mental and physical.

A queer symptom: sweats copiously during sleep — on merely closing eyes.

Ruta .. Large stool evacuated with difficulty, as from loss of peristaltic action of rectum. (*Alum., Phos. ac.*).

Frequent urging to stool, but only rectum prolapses *Ign.*). The slightest stooping, or crouching down, caused rectum to protrude.

Sepia	..	Ineffectual urging: or days with no urging, then the effort as if in labor.

Sepia .. Ineffectual urging: or days with no urging, then the effort as if in labor.

Stool not hard, but much straining.

Constipation of pregnancy.

"A ball in rectum;" fullness, prolapse.

Straining and sweating with stool.

Sepia is dull and indifferent, has heaviness and sagging of all viscera; tendency to prolapse.

Mezereum .. Stool hard as stone: threatens to split anus: dark hard balls; much painless straining.

During stool prolapsus ani with constriction: it is difficult to replace.

Before stool copious discharge of fetid flatus.

"Frightened in the stomach" (*Calc., Kali c., Phos.*).

Cocculus .. Paralytic condition rectum. Inability to press at stool, or to evacuate stool.

Disposition to stool; but peristalis wanting in upper intestines.

Inability to use muscles of evacuation.

After stool violent tenesmus, even to fainting.

Nausea at thought or smell of food (*Colch., Ars., Sep.*).

Lachesis .. Stool lies in rectum without urging.

Drawing and constriction of anus (*Lyc.*).

Pain extends from anus to navel.

Lach. cannot bear touch (abdomen or throat).

Foul stools. Piles, worse coughing.

Lach. sleeps into aggravation of symptoms.

Lach. is purplish and loquacious.

Calcarea .. Old, lingering, stubborn constipation.

Constipated stool white, like chalk.

Patient generally better when constipated. (Diarrhœa, and no worse, or better, *Phos. ac.*)

Hard, difficult, light-colored stool. Undigested stool (*Chin.*). Smells like bad eggs.

Sour eructations, vomit, stool, sweat.

Head and neck sweat at night (*Sil., Sanic.*).

Coldness of single parts: sensation of cold damp stockings (*Sepia*).

Staphisagria .. Frequent desire for stool with scanty evacuations, hard or soft. Difficult evacuations.

Staph. is sensitive, angry, petulant. Dwells on old injuries, insults: on things done by himself or others.

Thuja .. Difficult evacuation after 2, 3, or 8 days; subsequent burning in anus (*Bry.*).

Moisture at anus. Anus fissured; painful; surrounded with flat warts.

Violent pains compel cessation of effort (*Sul.*).

Stool recedes (*Sil., Sanic.*).

Sensation of something alive in abdomen (*Croc.*).

Great remedy for the much vaccinated, or the "worse for vaccination."

Silica .. Stool of hard lumps: scanty; difficult; after urging and straining till abdominal walls sore. Stool already protruded slips back ("bashful stool") (*Thuja, Sanicula*).

Much urging, but inability to expel (*Alum.*, no urging).

Straining with suffering and sweating head.

Silica is chilly; great want of self-confidence.

Head is apt to sweat in sleep (*Calc., Sanic.*).

Sanicula .. No desire for stool till a large accumulation.

Stool hard, impossible to evacuate; of greyish white balls (Comp. *Calc.*).

Stool, partly expelled, recedes (*Sil., Thuja*).

Odor of stool persists, despite bathing (*Sul.*).

Children, look old, dirty, greasy, brownish.

Head sweats profusely at night (*Sil., Calc.*).

Lycopodium .. No desire for days: yet rectum full, no urging.

Stool hard, difficult, small and incomplete.

Spasmodic constriction of anus preventing stool.

Lycopodium is always belching: distension of abdomen; has to loosen clothing.

Desire for sweets: hot drinks; < 4-8 p.m.

Magnesia mur. The keynote for *Mag. mur.* is *worse from salt*: salt food, salt baths, sea air.

Constipation at the sea side.

Stools dry: crumble at anus.

BRIEF POINTERS IN
ACUTE UNCOMPLICATED DIARRHOEA

(Compare Intestinal Conditions and Colic: also Cholera Infantum.)

Camphor   ..   A couple of drops of tincture on sugar, repeated in a quarter-hour, if necessary, will generally cure acute diarrhœa
N.B. — Keep Camphor away from other medicines.

Colocynth   ..   *Doubled up* with colic.
Pain only relieved by *bending double,* and *pressing into abdomen.*

Cuprum   ..   Diarrhœa associated with *cramps.* Cramps in abdomen, in fingers, calves, feet.

China   ..   *Painless* diarrhœa. Much flatulence.
Passes undigested food.

Veratrum alb. ..   Coldness.
COLD SWEAT.
Profuse evacuations with *profuse, cold sweat.*
Cold sweat on forehead.

Arsenicum   ..   After eating ices; or cold drinks when hot.
After *tainted meat and foods* or fruit.
Relentless vomiting and purging.
THE GREAT REMEDY FOR PTOMAINE POISONING

Carbo veg.   ..   Diarrhœa from bad food (like *Ars.*) but with more distension.

Podophyllum ..   Excessive evacuations, very offensive: with much flatus, and much colic.

Phos. acid   ..   Like *Podoph.* But not offensive, and no colic.

Aloe   ..   Stool urgent: at once after eating.

Dulcamara   ..   Diarrhœa from DAMP, OR DAMP COLD.

Baptisia   ..   Influenzal diarrhœa: very sudden onset: with prostration, drowsiness, putridity.

Pyrogen   ..   Rapidly curative in sudden, exhausting summer diarrhœa; profuse, watery, painless: extreme restlessness.

SOME MEDICINES OF ACUTE INTESTINAL CONDITIONS, COLIC AND DIARRHOEA

Aconite .. Abdominal conditions — *sudden* attacks — after exposure to violent cold: after being chilled.

Pressive weight in stomach — in hypochondria: swollen distended abdomen, like ascites.

Flatulent colic in hypogastrium, as if had taken a flatus-producing purgative.

Abdomen burning hot, tense, tympanitic, sensitive to least touch; cutting pains; fever; anguish.

Before or after diarrhœa, nausea and perspiration.

Stools white (*Calc.*): like chopped spinach: slimy, bloody, with tenesmus.

Catarrhal inflammatory troubles of all the viscera; hepatitis, *but "with the Aconite restlessness, awful tortures of anxiety, fear of death; red face, glassy eyes; great thirst."*

Belladonna .. Abdominal pains, violent; *come and disappear suddenly.* Are squeezing; clawing; as if gripped by nails; violent pinchings.

"Violent colic, intense cramping pain, face red as fire.

Frequent urging to stool, little or no result (*Nux*). Spasmodic contraction of sphincter ani.

Tenderness of abdomen, *worst least jar.*

Great pain in ileo-cæcal region: cannot bear slightest touch, even of bedclothes (early appendicitis. Local external applications to abort).

Typical *Bell.* has red, hot face; big pupils: is sensitive to pressure, draughts, jar.

Dulcamara .. Colic, such as is usually caused by *cold wet weather.*

Sudden attacks of diarrhœa in cold, wet weather.

Colic as if diarrhœa would occur.

Yellow watery discharge twice in a day, with tearing — cutting colic before every evacuation, as after taking cold.

Ætiology: *cold wet weather.*

Bryonia .. *Stitching* and bursting pains (*Kali carb.*) — as if stomach would burst — as if abdomen would burst. (*Aloe.*)

Effects of disordered stomach; taking cold; having been overheated: from cold drinks when heated. (*Ars.*)

Worse from pressure. (Everywhere else *Bry.* has relief from pressure: not in stomach or abdomen.)

Lies still, knees up to relax abdominal muscles.

Unable to move; breathing shallow; since movement increases the pain. (*Ars.* rolls about and is never still.)

Does not want to talk, or think.

Diarrhœa preceded by cutting in abdomen.

Nux .. Qualmishness: after eating.

Qualmish, anxious, nauseated, as after a violent purge. Cutting colic with qualmishness.

Pressure as from a stone in stomach. (*Bry.*)

Violent gastric symptoms.

Flatulent colic here and there in abdomen.

Better rest, sitting or lying.

Anxious, ineffectual desire for stool.

Frequent ineffectual desire for stool after evacuation.

Sensation after stool as if some remained behind.

Constipation: or, "The *Nux* diarrhœa consists of small, mostly mucous stools, with straining."

The *Nux* abdominal condition, pains and stools are due to *irregular peristalsis*. And here *Nux* cures.

Nux is irritable and hypersensitive. (*Cham.*)

Opium .. Violent griping in abdomen with constipation.

Cutting into abdomen.

Pain, pressive, as if intestines would be cut to pieces.

Almost unconquerable chronic constipation.

Constipation for weeks of small, hard dark-brown pieces.

No activity. Rectum fills with hard, black balls. (*Plumb.*)

Colocynth   ..   Violent griping, cutting, twisting, colic pains about umbilicus; frequent discharge of flatus, with relief.

Deep stitches, in right, or left flank.

Abdomen greatly distended, and painful.

Violent pain in abdomen, worst three fingers' breadth below umbilicus, *obliging him to bend over.*

Pinching pain as if bowels were pressed inwards, with distortion of face and eyes: *pain is only relieved by pressing on bowels and doubling up.*

Pinching, "Bowels squeezed between stones."

Very violent colic in paroxysms, obliging him to bend forward . . . "unexpressible colic."

Frequent excessive urging to stool.

Stannum   ..   Pains slowly increase till their acme, then slowly decrease: leaving a sensation of a hole.

Intestinal obstruction.

Magnesia phos.   Spasms of cramp in stomach, nipping, gripping, pinching, with belching which does not relieve (*Coloc.* which does not relieve).

Flatulent colic, forcing patient to bend double (*Coloc.*), *better from warmth* and rubbing.

Cramps in abdomen: violent cutting pains, has to scream out. Better bending double, pressing with hand (*Coloc.*), warmth.

Cannot lie on back stretched out.

Mag. phos. is worse cold air, cold water, touch: better heat, warmth, pressure, bending double (*Coloc.*).

Spasmodic conditions, > by heat and pressure.

(In relief from heat comp. *Ars. Ars.* has *burning* pains relieved by heat. *Mag. phos. cramping* (not burning) relieved by heat.)

Dioscorea   ..   Constant distress (umbilical and hypogastric regions), with severe cutting colic pains every few minutes in stomach and small intestines.

Griping in umbilical region: in lower bowels.

Rumbling in bowels and passing large quantities of flatulence.

Worse doubling up (op. of *Colocynth*).

Chamomilla .. Violent retching. Covered with cold sweat.

Cutting colic. Nightly diarrhœa with colic. Doubles up (*Coloc.*) and screams. *A wind colic.*

White slimy diarrhœa with colic; or painless green watery diarrhœa. Stool hot, smelling like rotten eggs. (*Cham.*)

Cham. is frantically irritable: impatient: oversensitive (*Nux*).

Uncivil irritability: snappish: admits it.

Excessive sensibility to pain.

Ailments from anger.

The colic of teething babies: want this and that, and then push it away.

China .. Flatulent colic (*Carbo veg., Lyc., Colch.,* etc.).

Abdomen feels packed full. not better by eructations. (Rev. of *Carbo veg.*)

Diarrhœa generally *painless;* watery with much flatus; *passes undigested food.* Very debilitating.

Cocculus .. Violent cramp in stomach.

Griping in upper abdomen; takes breath away.

Flatulent colic about midnight: wakened by incessant accumulation of flatus, which distends abdomen, giving oppressive pain here and there. Passed without much relief, while new flatus collects for hours.

Lies on first one side and then the other for relief.

Says, "Abdomen full of sharp sticks or stones." "Intestines pinched between sharp stones."

Worse for loss of sleep; night-nursing; overwork.

Worse for thought or smell of food. (*Colch., Sep., Ars.*)

Colchium .. Very great distension of abdomen: tympanitic; Griping pain. (Membraneous colitis.)

A *Colch.* keynote, very sensitive to smell of food. (In diarrhœa, etc.)

Nausea from smell of food (*Ars., Cocc., Sep.*).

Lycopodium .. Abdomen bloated: distension in epigastrium after a meal.

Flatulence after eating: fermentation, rumbling, rattling, relieved by discharge of flatus.

Incarcerated flatus, with pressure up and down with frequent urging to urinate.

Immediately p.c., full, distended and tense.

So full cannot eat. Hungry, but first mouthful fills him up.

Cannot bear weight or pressure of clothes (*Lach.*). *Must loosen clothing at waist.*

Always belching. (*Asaf.*) Colicky pains.

"*Lyc., Carbo veg.* and *China* are the most flatulent of remedies. *China* bloats whole abdomen," *Carbo v.* the upper part, and *Lyc.* the lower part.

Lyc. desires sweets and hot drinks: its bad hours are from 4-8 p.m. Suffers from anticipation.

Pulsatilla .. Eructations: of gas: tasting of food: of bitter fluid in the evening: like bad meat, or rancid tallow. With qualmishness.

Qualmish nausea, especially after eating and drinking.

Vomiting of food eaten long before.

Extremely disordered stomach.

Sensation of having eaten too much.

Food rises into mouth (*Phos.*) as if would vomit.

Pain, gnawing, scraping in stomach.

Colic, rumbling and gurgling in abdomen.

Flatus moves about in abdomen, rumbling and griping: worse in bed. Colic at night.

Cutting in abdomen: a stone sensation.

Diarrhœa green as bile at night, with movements in intestines before every stool.

Watery diarrhœa at night: discharge of green mucus.

Frequent evacuations of only mucus.

Typical *Pulsatilla* is tearful: must have air: is worse for heat — hot rooms.

(A curious symptom: one-sided sweat, face or body.)

Carbo veg. .. Great accumulation of flatus in stomach.

Distension. All foods turn to "wind."

Colic. Cramps in bowels and stomach.

Relief from belching. (Opp. *Lyc.* and *China.*)

Even headaches and rheumatic pains relieved by belching.

Argentum nit. .. Craves sugar: yet cannot digest it: it acts like physic and brings on diarrhœa.

Excessive flatulency.

Vomiting and purging at the same time: "gushing out both ways with great exhaustion." (*Ars.* also has this.)

Diarrhœa as soon as he drinks.

Kali carb. .. Severe pain in stomach. Will not tolerate the least amount of food: vomiting and fainting. Bloated.

Stomach as if cut to pieces.

Stitching in abdomen. (*Bry.*)

Violent cutting in intestines, must sit bent over pressing with both hands (*Coloc., Mag. phos.*) or lean far back for relief. (*Dios.*)

Colic, cutting pains with distension, doubling him up (*Coloc.*). Tremendous flatulence.

Great coldness with pains. (*Verat.*)

(For cases when *Coloc.* only relieves temporarily: in colics with periodicity: that recur.)

Kali carb.'s time aggravation is 3 a.m.

Plumbum .. Nausea. Constant vomiting.

Extremely violent pains, umbilical region; shoot to other parts of abdomen. Partly relieved by pressure.

At times so violent, patient almost wild, tosses about bed: presses fists into abdomen, says must go to stool.

Abdominal muscles forcibly retracted, till navel seems to press against spine (*Plat.*). Boat-shaped abdomen.

Violent colic: screams and assumes the strangest postures for relief.

Excessive pain in abdomen, radiates to all parts of body. Hyperæsthesia.

Stools hard and scanty: like balls. (*Opium.*)

Arsenicum .. Violent pains in abdomen. Rolls about on the floor and despairs of life.

Excessive pain in abdomen, causing *great anguish and despairs of life.*

Burning in intestines. Burning lancinations. Burning in intestines as from coals of fire.

Better from application of hot things: (the *Ars.* burnings are relieved by heat).

Vomiting of everything taken: *heat relieves:* temporary relief from hot drinks.

In the abdomen all the symptoms of peritonitis. Great distension — a tympanitic state. Cannot be handled or touched, yet cannot keep still. Great exhaustion.

Ptomaine poisonings.

Excessive vomiting and purging: often simultaneous. Tongue dry — even black.

Stools bloody — watery — or black and horribly offensive.

Veratrum alb. .. One of Hahnemann's three cholera medicines. Here the indications are: *Excessive vomiting and purging, excessive cold sweat, with exhaustion.*

Gastric catarrh, great weakness, cold, sinking feeling.

Cold feeling in abdomen, or burning, as from hot coals. (*Ars.*)

Coldness of discharges: coldness of body: coldness as if blood were ice-water. Internal chill runs from head to toes.

Profuse watery discharges

Cold sweat: especially cold sweat on forehead.

Abdomen distended: "intestines twisted into a knot."

"Flatulent colic: attacks bowels here and there, and the whole abdomen. The longer the flatus is retained, the more difficult its expulsion."

During profuse, watery stools chilliness and shivering, and extraordinary exhaustion.

"Forehead covered with cold sweat, coldness in spots over body: extremities cold as death. Full of cramps. Looks as if he would die."

Violent evacuations upwards and downwards.

Mercurius cor. Peculiar bruised sensation about cæcum and along tranverse colon. Tender to pressure.

Appendicitis. (*Bell.*)

Painful body discharges (from rectum) with vomiting.

Tenesmus, persistent, incessant, with insupportable cutting, colicky pains.

Diarrhœa — dysentery — *with terrible straining before, with, and after stool.*

Merc. cor. is almost specific for dysentry.

Very distressing tenesmus, getting worse and worse: nothing passed but mucus tinged with blood.

Cuprum .. Violent intermittent colic. Violent diarrhœa.

Violent pressure at stomach.

Spasmodic motions of abdominal muscles.

Abdomen tense, hot and tender to touch.

Cramps — start fingers and toes.

One of Hahnemann's *Cholera* medicines. (i.e. *Camphor, Cuprum, Verat. alb.*)

Camphor .. Everything vomited.

Tongue blue and cold: breath cold. (*Carbo veg.*)

Yet there may be internal burning — or cold sensation in stomach and abdomen.

Violent pain in stomach with anguished face (*Ars.*): feels he must die (*Ars.*).

In cold stage wants to uncover: in hot phase to be kept warm.

Baptisia .. Gastric and abdominal 'flu, with drowsiness.

Fullness in abdomen with rumbling and diarrhœa.

Sudden onset: rapid "typhoid" conditions.

Drowsy and stupid. *Putrid conditions and discharges: fetid, exhausting diarrhœa,* causing excoriation.

Lachesis .. Painful distension of abdomen. *Can bear no pressure,* the surface nerves are so sensitive.

Worse everywhere from pressure or constriction, throat, neck, chest, abdomen.

Lies on back with clothes lifted from abdomen.

Lach. sleeps into an aggravation.

Sulphur   ..   Inflation of the abdomen with wind.

Grumbling and gurgling in bowels.

Painless diarrhœa driving out of bed about 5 a.m.

Morning diarrhœa: must go immediately.

Anus red. Stool acrid.

Typical *Sulph.* patient, is starving about 11 a.m.

Hungry an hour before usual meal.

Burning soles at night, puts them out (*Cham., Med., Puls.*).

Loves fat and sweet things.

Worse after sleeping — eating — bathing.

Sulph. "a chronic remedy" is speedily curative in acute conditions in a *Sulphur* patient.

Aloe   ..   ..   Has to hurry to stool immediately after eating and drinking. (*Arg. nit.*)

Colicky pain in bowels from eating and drinking.

Diarrhœa from drinking beer.

Fullness: distensions as if abdomen would burst.

Loud rumbling, heard all over the room.

Gurgling and spluttering stools.

Early morning diarrhœa (*Sulph.*).

[A queer symptom, peculiar to *Aloe*: — may strain in vain, and presently a large formed stool slips out unnoticed.

Or, fæces involuntary after stool.]

"Jelly-fish stools." "Lumpy, watery stools."

Croton tig.   ..   Flatulence followed by urgent desire for stool.

Evacuations sudden: shot out of rectum: of a dirty green color and offensive. Worse least food or drink.

Swashing in intestines as from water.

Raphanus   ..   Post-operative intestinal stasis. Bits of intestine blown up here and there.

Paralytic ileus. (*Thuja.*)

Accumulation and retention of flatus, no relief up or downwards.

Thuja   ..   ..   Protrusion here and there as from a child's arm. "Something alive in abdomen." (*Crocus.*)

EPIDEMIC DIARRHOEA OF CHILDREN: CHOLERA INFANTUM:

Here Homœopathy, so rapidly curative in acute disease, gives splendid results. But, of course, the remedy must be, not only a "homœopathic remedy," but *homœopathic*. It must be a remedy not only of diarrhœa (every drug that can cause diarrhœa is that), but it must fit the peculiarities of *this* case of diarrhœa; otherwise there is nothing doing. One diarrhœa remedy will not do for another. A medicine, to cure, must be able to produce just the condition we seek to cure: outside that, no contact is made. Some people might express it, that the vibrations of disease and remedy must be identical — we seem to be approaching that idea. But, however that may be, and whether it is expressed in terms of electricity, or vibration, or Homœopathy, so urgent are these cases that one needs their remedies at one's finger-tips, or in portable form for easy reference.

But outside the giving of the remedy, the child should be kept warm, and, in desperate cases, when seen first at almost the last gasp, we must remember that the infant may have lost more fluid than it can afford to lose and live. Here fluid cannot be retained *per rectum,* and many a small life may be saved by slow absorption of warm saline, subcutaneously.

It is Hahnemann's teaching that not only do different cases of the same disease demand, by their peculiar symptoms, different remedies, but also that different epidemics of the same disease ask for different remedies. And here, in epidemic work, by carefully collecting the symptoms of several individual cases, the *genus epidemicus* may disclose itself in entirety, and may be fitted with a medicine which will be found to cure the majority of the cases, even where they do not all display the complete disease picture. But it is also found that in such epidemics the cases not covered by the epidemic remedy are often very difficult to match.

One remembers an epidemic when a number of children came to Out-patients with a diarrhœa that was painless, while the stools contained much indigested food. Here *China* quickly put matters right. *Colocynth,* with its agonies of abdominal pain, that double the victim up, again and again, and demand pressure, would have been useless. To discover the epidemic remedy, whatever it may be, makes prescribing easy and most satisfactory, until — which is possible! — the type changes — perhaps with the weather, when a fresh remedy has to be sought.

Mercurius cor.   Dysenteric, scanty stools with blood, and *incessant straining, not relieved by stool.*

Cuprum ..   Diarrhœa with *intense cramps.*

Ipecacuanha ..   Violent simultaneous vomiting and purging (*Ars.*).
Great nausea with pale face and clean tongue.
Stools like a mass of fermented yeast.

Podophyllum ..   Diarrhœa, *stools profuse, offensive,* gushing, seem to drain infant dry. Painless.
Stools larger than expected from food taken.
Desire for much water, none for food.
Marked gurgling.
Retching; vomits green froth or food.
Diarrhœa worse in the morning: in teething babies.
   Head sweats much during sleep.
Rectum may prolapse with soft stool.

China ..   Painless and undigested stools: copious: putrid.

Mercurius ..   Slimy, even bloody diarrhœa: with straining: followed by chilliness.
Profuse perspiration which does not relieve.
Mouth offensive. Salivation with intense thirst.
Tongue large, flabby, tooth-notched.
Worse at night: from warmth of bed.
Thighs and legs cold and clammy, esp. at night.

Phosphorus ..   Characteristic of *Phos.* thin stool oozes from open anus. Increased urine with diarrhœa.
Or stools large and forcible.
In the tall *Phos.* child: with fear alone — in the dark: thirst for cold water.

Pulsatilla ..   Colic and diarrhœa worse at night.
No two stools alike.
Relief from fresh air. Mild, weepy children.

Phosphoric acid   Long-continued diarrhœa, with cramps (*Cup.*).
Stools white (*Calc.*), watery, painless, profuse.
Pallid, weary, weedy children.

Sulphur ..   Intolerant of heat: kicks off the clothes: hungry: craves for fat.
Great hurry. Stool acrid. Leaves anus red.

Baptisia . .. Taken *suddenly* and frightfully ill. Sudden attack of diarrhœa and vomiting, with a rapidly typhoid condition.

Fœtid, exhausting diarrhœa, with excoriation.

Odor of stool putrid, penetrating.

Tongue swollen: dark: dry: yellow or brown center: cracked: ulcerated. (Comp. *Ars.*)

Drowsy, as if drugged, or intoxicated.

If roused, begins to speak, then fades back into stupor.

Dark, red, besotted countenance. Hot — flushed — dusky. Influenzal cases.

Veratrum .. *Diarrhœa with violent vomiting: stools — sweat very profuse.*

Thirst for much cold water, for acid drinks.

Exhaustion after each spell.

Cold sweat on forehead from last movement.

Carbo veg. .. Putrid, or bloody, offensive stools. Acrid.

Face pale, or greenish.

Abdomen distended: in lumps.

Emission of large quantities of flatus.

Skin, damp, cold: tongue and breath cold.

(The homœopathic veritable corpse-reviver.)

*   *   *

Aconite .. From *low temperature* in room.

From chill or fright.

Green, watery, frequent stools.

Dry heat of body: dry tongue, restlessness and fear.

Fear of death.

Bryonia .. Diarrhœa *from hot weather,* and the return of hot weather.

Vomits food immediately.

Colic, with thirst for big drinks, and lumpy diarrhoea.

Dry, parched lips.

Dulcamara .. Every *change of weather to cool,* brings diarrhœa.

(Rev. of *Bry.*) Exposure to cold, or damp.

Changeable stools.

Nausea with desire for stool.

Colic before and during stool. Prostration.

Croton tig. .. Yellow, watery stools, *come out like a shot,* while nursing, or immediately after.

Any food or drink starts this sudden stool.

A hand pressing on umbilicus produced protrusion of rectum.

Aloe .. .. Hurry to stool after eating or drinking.

Inability to retain — or to evacuate — stool.

(Straining may fail to produce stool, which presently slips out unnoticed.)

Ignatia .. Colic and diarrhœa in breast-fed infants, whose mothers are suffering from grief.

Kreosote .. Cholera infantum in teething infants, with *very painful dentition:* gums painful, spongy.

Severe cases, with incessant vomiting, and stools cadaveric-smelling.

Intensely irritable (*Cham.*).

(See Homœopathy, June, 1934, pp. 178-9.)

Chamomilla .. Watery, greenish stools: excoriating: smell like rotten eggs.

Very cross (*Kreos.*) . Must be carried.

Especially teething babies.

Cactus .. .. Bilious diarrhœa, preceded by great pain.

Great weight in anus; desires to pass a quantity, but nothing comes.

Belladonna .. Drowsiness (*Baptisia*) with dry, burning heat.

Pupils dilated.

Stools green, small, frequent.

Colic before stool: straining.

Child starts with every noise: twitches.

Colocynth .. Paroxysms of severe colicky pain precede stools. Immediately after eating.

Relief from doubling up and pressure.

Frothy stools. Stools watery, then bilious, then bloody; excoriating; frequent; not profuse.

Magnesia phos. Very like *Colocynth,* but urgently *demands heat as well as pressure.*

(A case in Hospital: *Colocynth* had helped diarrhœa, but the Resident thought the child would die. The only relief was from a warm hand pressed on abdomen. *Mag. phos.* saved the child.)

SEVERE URGENT CASES, WITH COLLAPSE.

Aethusa   ..   Intolerance of milk.

Face expresses anxiety and pain.

Linea nasalis — pearly whiteness on upper lip, bounded by a distinct line to angles of mouth.

Violent vomiting: of milk: after milk.

Stool undigested: thin: green: bilious.

Violent straining before and after stool.

Collapse — almost as bad as Ars. *only not restless.*

A remedy of violence — violent vomiting — violent convulsions — violent pains — violent diarrhœa.

Arsenicum   ..   Worse at night, 1 to 3 a.m.

Rapid emaciation; *exhaustion and collapse.*

Intense restlessness. (*Pyrog.*) (opp. of *Aeth.*)

Painless, offensive, watery stools.

There may be simultaneous vomiting and diarrhœa. (*Ipec.*)

After cold drinks; when heated; in older persons after ices.

Thirst for cold water, immediately vomited.

Coldness of extremities.

Pale cadaverous face.

Skin dry, wrinkled, toneless.

Camphor   ..   *Skin cold as marble* (*Carbo veg.*), *but child will not remain covered.*

Great prostration and diarrhœa.*

Pyrogen   ..   Extreme restlessness: has to keep on moving. Only momentary relief from moving, but has to move for that relief. (Comp. *Rhus.*)

Diarrhoea with frightfully offensive stools (*Bapt.*).

Profuse, watery, painless stools, with (?) vomiting.

(One has seen *Pyrogen* almost magic for sudden, very exhausting attacks of summer diarrhœa.)

---

* *Give a drop of the strong tincture on sugar. Repeat in 5 to 15 minutes if case urgent. Keep Camphor away from Homœopathic medicines.*

SOME REMEDIES OF ACUTE DYSENTERY

Mercurius cor.   Persistent straining before, during, and after stool
(rev. of *Nux*).
Scanty stools of bloody or shreddy slime.
Stools excoriate, burn. Burning in rectum.
"Never-get-done" sensation.
Straining to pass hot urine, drop by drop.
Merc. cor. IS ALMOST A SPECIFIC FOR DYSENTERY.
Tongue large, flabby, tooth-notched.
Mouth foul. Salivation.

Mercurius ..   Bloody, slimy stools with much straining: never-get-
done feeling (*Merc. cor.*); but *Merc. cor.* has a
more violent attack.
Stools followed by chilliness.
Rarely indicated where there is no slime.
Rarely indicated where the tongue is dry.
"Your first prescription should cure in epidemic dysentery, and if you work cautiously you will cure
every case." — KENT.

Aloe ..   ..   "Violent tenesmus, heat in rectum, prostration to
fainting and profuse clammy sweats."
Bloody mucus passes after urging and straining.
Rumbling, gurgling, sudden urge to stool.
Urine and fæces pass at the same time: cannot pass
one without the other (*Mur. a.*).
Curious symptom. Stools, even solid, pass unnoticed.
Sense of insecurity at anus.
Another curious verified symptom. On laying head
on pillow, as if a fine globe broke at base of brain,
fragments could be heard tinkling as they fell.

Nux ..   ..   Stools of slimy mucus and blood, but small and un-
satisfactory: *with relief, pro tem., after every stool*
(rev. of *Merc.* and *Merc. cor.*).
Irregular peristalsis.
Griping pains, now here, now there, in abdomen.
COLIC.
Nux is irritable, hypersensitive, offended.
Is chilly, with great aversion to uncovering.

Colocynth	..	With much colic, only *relieved by bending double,* and *pressing hard into abdomen.*

Sulphur   ..   Stools bloody with constant straining: with the *Merc.* "never-get-done" sensation.

Dysenteric stools, esp. at night, with colic and violent tenesmus.

"Follows *Nux,* esp. when worse at night: discharge of blood, slime, pus, with fever."

Pain so violent as to cause nausea and drenching perspiration.

Stools acrid: excoriate. Characteristic symptom, *redness about anus.*

Phosphorus   ..   Dysenteric stools oozing from an open anus.

Patient craves COLD DRINKS and food; ices.

Apis   ..   Stools with every motion of body as if anus constantly open (*Phos.*); oozes blood.

"Tomato-sauce" stools — blood, mucus, food.

Thirstless: can't bear heat — warm room.

Ipecacuanha   ..   Dysentery with *constant nausea.*

Sits almost constantly on stool and passes a little slime, or a little *bright-red blood.*

Tenesmus awful: pain so great that nausea comes on and he vomits bile.

Tongue clean with nausea.

Colchicum autumnale   Dysentery in the fall of the year, when days are warm and nights cold. (*Dulc.*).

Stools: shreddy and bloody like scrapings: thin, watery, but they cool to form a jelly.

Great meteoric distension (*Cargo veg.*).

Bloody discharges from bowels with deathly nausea.

The smell of food causes nausea to faintness.

Gelsemium   ..   Epidemic dysentery, malarial or catarrhal.

Acute catarrhal enteritis, mucous diarrhœa.

Discharges almost involuntary: intense spasmodic colic and tenesmus.

Fright, emotion, anticipation will produce diarrhœa (*Arg. nit.*).

Gels. has chills up and down back: trembling; and heaviness of limbs and eyelids.

Arsenicum .. RESTLESSNESS, ANGUISH, FEARFUL ANXIETY.
Worse after midnight.
Burning thirst for sips of cold water.
Internal, violent burning pain, with cold extremities.
Better heat, hot drinks. (Rev. of *Phos.*)
Great collapse and prostration.
Tongue dry, to brown, black.
Putrid stools: involuntary: with prostration: blood
and straining.
THE GREAT REMEDY IN PTOMAINE POISONING.

(N.B. — "Don't give *Ars.* in dysentery unless there
is the *Ars.* restlessness, anxiety, and thirst for frequent small drinks.")

Rhus .. .. Cases with *extreme restlessness* (*Ars.*).
Worse *damp weather: damp cold weather.*
Dry, dark-coated tongue: or triangular red tip.
Herpetic eruptions about mouth.
Copious, watery, bloody stools; drive him out of bed
(*Sulph.*) as early as 4 a.m.
"Diarrhœa with tearing pains running down back of
leg with every stool. Painful tenesmus with every
stool."

Aconite .. Stools of pure blood, with a little slime.
With anguish, cramp, terrible urging.
Or black, very fœtid stools.
Sensation, warm fluid escaping from anus.

Cuprum .. Frightful colic; > pressure.
Spouting stool of bloody, greenish water.
Cramps — abdomen, calves, soles, fingers, toes.
Strong metallic taste.

Podophyllum .. "Abdomen becomes tumultuous."
Gurgling: then sudden, profuse, putrid stools: generally painless: with perhaps prolapsus recti.

Psorinum .. Stools dark, gushing, horridly putrid.
Worse at night. Patient greasy, offensive.
Cases which do not respond to apparently indicated
remedy (*Tub.*).

Capsicum ..	Small frequent stools of blood and mucus.
	After stool tenesmus and thirst: but drinking causes shuddering. *Thirst after every dysenteric stool:* sudden craving for ice-cold water, which causes chilliness.
	Violent tenesmus in rectum and bladder at the same time (*Canth.*).
	Smarting and *burning* in anus and rectum.
	(*Caps.* burnings are like cayenne pepper.)
	Typical *Caps.* is plump, flabby, sensitive to cold: red, cold face: nose red and cold.
Cantharis ..	Stools like scrapings of intestines.
	Great burning: burning at anus.
	Tenesmus in rectum *and bladder* (*Caps.*).
	"It is a singular fact that if there be frequent micturition with burning cutting pain attending the flow, *Cantharis* is almost always the remedy for whatever other sufferings there may be."
Carbo veg. ..	"No matter what the trouble is, in *Carbo veg.* there is always burning."
	Diarrhœa, dysentery, cholera, with bloody watery stool. Watery mucus mixed with blood.
	Stools horribly putrid, with putrid flatulence.
	The more thin, dark, bloody mucus there is, the better the remedy is indicated.
	Anus red (*Sulph.*), raw, bleeding, itching.
	Cold breath, cold sweat, cold nose.
	Internal burning with external coldness.
	Coldness and collapse, with air hunger.
Veratrum alb. ..	Colic: burning, twisting, constricting, cutting. Distension, tenderness.
	Stools frequent; watery, greenish; blackish; bloody. Involuntary when passing flatus: from least movement of body.
	May be simultaneous stool and vomiting (*Ars.*).
	Sunken, hippocratic face. Characteristic symptom, *cold sweat on forehead.* (One of Hahnemann's great cholera medicines.)
	The straining is not marked in *Verat.*

SOME CHOLERA REMEDIES

HOMŒOPATHY won its first great world-wide laurels in the cholera epidemics some 100 years ago, reversing everywhere the mortality: i.e. where ordinary medicine lost three-quarters of its cholera patients, Homœopathy saved three-quarters — even in some localities and under certain doctors it lost *none*.

Hahnemann never having seen the disease, but knowing its headlong rush and symptoms, laid down the remedies that would be curative: and his disciples everywhere were absolutely masters of the situation.

His three great remedies were: *Camphor*, *Cuprum* and *Veratrum album*.

Camphor   ..   For early stage. Promptly curative.

       Dose   Give a drop of the strong tincture every five minutes on sugar, till warmth and rest are restored.

> (*The strong tincture is a saturated solution of camphor in rectified spirits of wine.*)
>
> (*A lump of camphor in a small bottle of whisky, etc., will make a saturated solution. The spirit dissolves only as much as it can.*)
>
> (*N.B. — Give Camphor on sugar. In water it nauseates and burns. Keep Camphor away from medicines.*)

Cuprum   ..   In the later stage of excessive vomiting and purging, and especially where CRAMPS are the feature of the case . . .

> (Copper poisoning and camphor poisoning are difficult to distinguish. Copper, a plate worn on the skin, is said to protect against cholera.)

"Workers in copper mines do not get cholera."

Veratrum alb. ..   For the cases with *very profuse evacuations, profuse vomiting and purging,* and *profuse, cold sweat.*

Repeat every hour or half-hour till warmth and rest are restored.

There has been the idea that *Camphor* (perhaps because of the need for frequent repetition) was not homœopathic to cholera; but that it was only proposed by Hahnemann for the treatment of cholera because of its destructiveness to the micro-organisms — which he sensed.

No greater mistake could be made. *Camphor* is *absolutely* homœopathic to cholera in its first stage — for which Hahnemann alone prescribed it. Later on, if the patient survived, *with the same organism,
but changed symptoms,* camphor was no longer indicated. *Cuprum* or
Veratrum alb., according to symptoms, would now be homœopathic,
and therefore curative.

Let us contrast the symptoms of cholera in its first stage with those of
camphor poisonings, and we shall see the absolute homœopathicity of
the drug.

CHOLERA SYMPTOMS — *First stage.*	CAMPHOR POISONING SYMPTOMS.
Giddy faint powerlessness.	Vertigo as if drunk. His senses leave him; he slides and falls to the ground.
Icy coldness of the body.	Icy coldness of body.
Strength suddenly sinks.	Great prostration and weakness. Could hardly be held upright Attempted to stand, but lay down again.
Expression altered.	Face pale, distorted, sunken.
Eyes sunk in.	Eyes staring, distorted, sunken, hollow.
Face bluish and icy cold.	Face and hands deathly pale — cold — blue.
Closure of jaws, trismus.	Closure of jaws, trismus.
Whole body cold.	Body quite cold. Skin cold. Extremities icy cold.
Hopeless discouragement and anxiety.	Great anxiety.
Dread of suffocation.	Suffocative dyspœna.
Burning in stomach and gullet.	Burning in throat and stomach.
Cramps in calves and other muscles.	Violent cramps.
On touching precordial region, he cries out.	Precordial anxiety. When spoken to loudly complained of indefinable distress in precordial region.

No thirst, no sickness, no vomiting or purging (as in the later stage).

And here, observe! Homœopathy can not only cure — abort —
prevent — give instant relief in acute sickness, even before it is possible
to make a diagnosis — but it can also lay down the remedy or remedies
that will be curative in an unknown disease, never seen, but whose
symptoms are known.

CONCERNING HOMOEOPATHY FOR CHILDREN

CHILDREN respond splendidly to the homœopathic remedy. And children's work is most fascinating: usually less complicated: the indications for the remedy are generally more clear; and the results more rapid of attainment.

Children are in the acute stage of life, rapidly growing and developing. The cell-life that clothes and binds them to earth is in a marvellous state of activity. They are hypersensitive to influences that normally exercise less power later on. They are subject to diseases that seldom attack adults. Besides which, with them, labelled diseases do not always run the same course as with their elders. For instance, what we call rheumatism — acute rheumatism — is a very different proposition, with widely different symptoms and outcome, in children and in "grown-ups".

The condition of high fever — profuse, sour sweating — tender, inflamed, painful joint or joints has very little in common with the, often trivial, *"growing pains"* — the *scarcely elevated temperature,* probably unnoticed till a thermometer is put into the mouth — the *no sweat* of the child; — where the heart is the subject of grave attack, and where extreme care and most skilful prescribing are essential if the condition is not to go on to a life-sentence of disability and suffering — to a dreary vista of cardiac break-downs, each one more damaging than the last.

Well, first — as elsewhere — one has to settle whether the ailment is acute or chronic; and, if the former, whether it occurs in a healthy or a diseased child. For a healthy child may be sick unto death, whereas a diseased child may be a museum of pathology and yet not "ill". In the latter case, treatment may have to be modified, or rather supplemented, in order to cover the whole case. A pneumonia in a child with T.B. glands or a T.B. family history, will probably not clear up till you give a dose of *Tub. bov.* And it is pathetic to find how often one has to come to *Lueticum* to make headway with the acutely sick hospital children.

In Homœopathy the essentials, — i.e. the symptoms so easy to get in the child, and so all-important, if marked, for a successful prescription, are, briefly,

(1) DISPOSITION; or, more important still, change of disposition due to illness.

(2) FEARS: habitual, or, more important, new to the child.

(3) SENSITIVENESS. One remembers a wee boy in our Children's Ward wandering about, just the right height to use the brass shields at

the foot of endowed cots as a mirror (his head and face were covered thickly with an eruption). He used to wail, "The children make such a *noise*!" — and the rattle of spoons on plates was, to him, torture. Such a symptom, in a child of his age, would be important, and must be considered when piecing together his disease-picture to be matched with the drug-disease-picture of a remedy.

(4) FOOD CRAVINGS AND LOATHINGS.

(5) THE GROSSER PATHOLOGICAL SYMPTOMS, when qualified by something that makes them rare and peculiar, and therefore diagnostic as regards the choice of the remedy.

Disposition. There is a broad distinction between the "child you want to spank" and the child you instinctively comfort and caress: and here one is at once shifted onto one or another of a totally different class of remedies. *Natrum mur.* and *Sepia* children are not amenable to sympathy. *Pulsatilla* children are weepy, but engaging little mites that claim attention and love. Then there is the heavy, lethargic, rather dull *Calcarea* type: the restless, suspicious, anxious *Arsenicum* type: the defiant, obstinate, passionate, sensitive, irritable *Nux* type: while *Chamomilla* demands a thing only to hurl it away, and cannot be placated . . . and so on. Whatever the disease, these things must be taken into consideration, if the prescription is to be successful.

Then *fears.* One little child will wander alone in the dusk through extensive school buildings where her parents are caretakers: another, put to play in the garden, hugs the window, and wants to be assured that his mother is on the other side of the glass, within call. Fears of the dark — of wind — of thunder — of strangers — of falling — of a bath.

The third useful point in determining a remedy for a child, is appetite: — *cravings and aversions.* One child craves fat, and will gnaw raw suet: another hates and is nauseated by the least morsel of fat, which has to be carefully cut off its meat (*Sulph.* has both of these). You must put the salt on a high shelf, out of reach of some children (*Nat. mŭr., Phos.,* etc.) while the next will steal sugar, and cries for "sweeties". Some children will eat earth, chalk, and crunch slate-pencils (*Alum.*). Some cannot be made to swallow meat.

This wee girl is greedy — always hungry — "will eat anything": while her delicate little brother can hardly be induced to eat enough, so it would seem, to keep body and soul together.

There is the untruthful child; the shy child, in terror of strangers, a bit difficult for a doctor. But — children are very susceptible to flattery. Tell a child that it is opening its mouth splendidly, — "now, *just a little wider!*" and you may see its throat. The same in breathing, when you want to listen to a chest. Or you may establish relations by expressing interest or admiration for a bracelet, buttons, scraps of embroidery: or, when nothing helps, "Ta-ta!" will abruptly suspend the sobs.

"With children, lunatics, and liars you have to observe for yourself": — and you have to "keep your eyes skinned" where children are concerned. There is the child that always kicks the clothes off; that never will be covered at night (*Sulph.*): that is found with its feet on the pillow and the bedclothes on the floor. There is the infant of only a few weeks that will wriggle over to lie on its face, till the mother is in terror lest it suffocate. But it may be kept right side up by a dose of *Medorrh.* — one has seen that.

The "dirty-nosed child", with nostrils always running, and red, and sore, is easy to prescribe for (*Sulph., Kali iod.*). The puny boys that won't grow or thrive (often *Sanic.*). . . .

Then the diseased, — or the children with heritage of poor resistance to tubercle — they are some of the joys of prescribing: children of eight years, who have never, in all their lives, been without bandages about their necks; with glands, sinuses and scars left by cuttings, and scrapings, and aspirations: — how they respond to Homœopathy to *Tuberculinum — Silica — Calcarea — Drosera — Sulphur,* according to their make-up and the symptoms they represent. It is to Homœopathy alone that these tuberculous gland and bone cases respond so magnificently! and it is here especially that the homœopathic physician tastes triumph.

SOME REMEDIES OF DENTITION

Calcarea . .	Fat, fair, flabby, perspiring.
	Fontanelles remain open (*Sil., Calc. ph.*). Deformed extremities.
	Deficient, or irregular bone development.
	Profuse perspiration: soaks the pillow (*Sil*).
	Sour sweat: sour diarrhœa: sour vomit.
	Flabby; FAT: lax muscles; bones that bend.
	Can't learn to walk: won't put feet to ground.
	Milk crust and eruptions in the *Calcarea* child.
	Teething cough or diarrhœa: in the *Calcarea* child.

Calcarea phos. . . Slow dentition with emaciation (reverse of *Calc.*).
Fontanelles remain open.
Soft thin skull, crackles when pressed upon.
Can't hold head up: it must be supported.
Flabby, emaciated: doesn't learn to walk.
"Great desire to nurse all the time."
Cough with rattling chest.
The *Calc. phos.* child is more wiry; less fair; without the sweating head of *Calc.*
Diarrhœa, stools green and spluttering.
Child shrunken and anæmic (*Sil.*).

Chamomilla . . Painful dentition.
Oversensitive to pain, which maddens.
Very irritable: snaps and snarls (*Cina.*).
Excessive uneasiness, anxiety, tossing, (*Acon.*).
Only to be quieted by being carried about.
Drowsiness with sleeplessness.
Sweats with the pain.
One cheek red and hot, the other pale and cold.
Wants this or that, only to push it away.
Turmoil in temper. *Chamomilla* is frantic: "cannot bear it!"
Dentition diarrhœa (*Calc., Kreos.*). Stools green: odour like rotten eggs: colicky pain.
Draws the legs up. Abdomen bloated.

Kreosotum . . "Child suffering from *very* painful dentition: won't sleep at night unless caressed and fondled all the time." (*Cham.,* unless carried up and down the room.)
Gums painful, dark-red or blue: teeth decay as soon as they come.
May have constipation, or diarrhœa.
Cholera infantum during teething: very severe: vomiting incessant, with cadaveric-smelling stools.

Aconite . . Feverish. Fever. Dry hot skin (*Bell.*). Child gnaws its fists; frets and cries.
Sleepless; excited; tosses; heat; startings and twitchings (*Bell.*) of single muscles.
Convulsions of teething children (*Bell.*).
Costive, or dark, watery stools.

Coffea   .. Wakeful: constantly on the move.
Not distressed: happy: but sleepless.
Remarkable wakefulness.
Over excitement of brain.

Belladonna   .. Red, hot face. Dry skin. Dilated pupils.
Starts and wakes when just falling asleep.
Twitchings and jerkings.
Quickness of sensations and emotions. Sudden pains, suddenly gone.
Convulsions.
The delirium of *Bell.* bites, strikes, wants to escape.
Acute attacks in *Calcarea* children.

Zincum   .. "Brain troubles during dentition.
Child cries out in sleep, rolls head from side to side: face alternately red and pale."
Incessant, fidgety feet, must move them constantly.

Podophyllum .. *Pod.* has a great desire to press the gums together during dentition.
Cholera infantum, stools profuse and gushing: larger than could be expected from amount of food taken: offensive.

Sulphur   .. The *Sulphur* baby will not remain covered.
Rough skin and hair: red lips and eyelids.
Redness around anus, hot palms and soles.
Acrid stools (*Calc.*) that irritate and inflame wherever they touch the skin. (The *urine* of *Lyc.* irritates the parts.)

Then the nosodes must not be forgotten in delayed dentition. Burnett proved the value of *Tuberculinum* in tardy development of all kinds, where there was a family history of deficiency of reaction to tubercle. One has seen a case of delayed dentition in a girl well on in her teens, where, after a dose of *Tub. bov.,* she erupted eight teeth in a couple of weeks.

And one would think of *Luet.* where the days are happy, but the nights a terror (*Lyc.*): or *Medorrhinum,* where the infant rolls over to sleep on its stomach (*Cina*), or a child can only sleep in the knee-elbow position: or the mother has had an evil discharge.

RICKETS

The same remedies, largely, apply to both difficult dentition and rickets, yet it may be well to more or less repeat, otherwise the picture will be incomplete.

Calcarea carb. .. For the fat, fair, lethargic type of child, with profusely sweating head, especially in sleep (*Sil., Sanic.*): with soft, fat, flabby, inadequate limbs that bend under its weight: with big abdomen.

The child of plus tissue of minus quality.

Calcarea phos. ... Like *Calc.* head large, fontanelles long open; but less sweating. Bones of skull thin.

Thin — even emaciated.

Sunken, flabby abdomen (reverse of *Calc.*).

Spine too weak to support body: thin neck, too weak to support head.

Child pale and cold. Seems stupid.

"Even cretinism may be developed by the continued use of *Calc. phos.*" (i.e. think of *Calc. phos.* in cretinism).

Silica .. Pale, waxen, earthy face.

Head large (the *Calcs., Sulph.*), fontanelles open.

Body small and emaciated, except the plump abdomen.

Bones and muscles poorly developed: i.e. slow in learning to walk.

Worse from milk: infant unable to take any kind of milk. (*Aeth.*)

Diarrhœa from milk.

Offensive sweat, head, neck, face, feet.

Sanicula .. *Sanicula aqua* contains *Calcarea, Silica,* etc. and combines many of the symptoms of these remedies. Invaluable remedy for unflourishing, ill-developing children.

Defective nutrition.

Thin and old-looking. Dirty brownish skin.

Stubborn and touchy.

Cold, clammy hands and feet.

Profuse sweat, occiput and neck.

Sulphur	..	Large head (like the *Calcareas*).
		Tendency to rickets. (*Calc. c.*)
		Voracious appetite, defective assimilation.
		Hungry yet emaciated. (*Iod.*)
		Shrivelled and dried up, like a little old man.
		Skin hangs in folds, yellowish, wrinkled, and flabby.
		(See Dentition — *Sulph.*)

Chamomilla	..	Intensely sensitive. Intensely irritable.
		Changeable: never satisfied.
		Wants to be carried: can't keep still.
		"The *Chamomilla* child can't be touched."
		Painful gums, painful teething: will hold cold glass against its gums.
		Pain — colic: doubles up and screams. Kicks.
		Diarrhœa. Grass green stool.
		One cheek red, the other pale.
		Coughing or ailments from anger.
		Sleepy but can't sleep.

Arnica	..	Tender to touch.
		Does not want to be disturbed, or irritated, or handled.
		Worse from heat.
		Especially if there has been any injury at birth or otherwise.

SCURVY RICKETS

Manganum	..	General aching, soreness, tenderness (*Arn.*).
		Bones ache, especially tibiae.
		Sickly face, anæmic.
		Constantly whining; fretful.
		Everything better lying down.
		Worse cold, damp weather.

Arnica	..	(See above.) *A great remedy here.*
Phosphorus	..	Bruising: extraversation. Gums bleed.
		Especially in nervous, slender children.
Kreosotum	..	Gums bleed and ulcerate.
		Offensive odours, mouth, etc.
		The *Cham.* temperament (see above) but *offensive and bleeds.*

THE COMMONER REMEDIES OF MAL-NUTRITION, WASTING MARASMUS

WITH DIAGNOSTIC SYMPTOMS

Calcarea .. COLDNESS.

Profuse sweats, head (*Sil.*) at night (*Sil.*).

Cold, damp feet: cold legs with night-sweats.

Milk disagrees. (*Calc. ph., Nat. carb., Mag. carb., Aeth., Sil., Lac. c.*)

Big head, with large, hard abdomen. (*Sil.*)

Stomach swollen, distended even with the rest of body emaciated.

"A big-bellied child, with emaciated limbs and neck." (*Sil.*) (Opp. of *Calc. ph.*)

Malnutrition, glands, bones, and skin.

Faulty bony development: late teething: rickets.

Fat, flabby, deficient bones, deficient teeth.

"Bones stop growing, and child goes into marasmus."

"Enlarged glands, emaciation of neck and limbs, while the fat and the glands of the belly increase."

Flabby: feeble: tired.

Sourness of sweat, of sweating head. Sour stool. Sour vomit.

White stools: constipation with white stools.

"Wormy babies", pass and vomit worms.

Chew and swallow, or grit teeth in sleep (*Cina*).

Cross and fretful: easily frightened.

Calc. phos. .. Vomits milk. (*Calc., Nat. carb., Mag. carb.*)

Stools green, slimy, lienteric, with foetid flatus.

Face pale. White; sallow.

Neck cannot support head.

Marasmus: shrunken, emaciated, and very anaemic.

Tall scrawny children with dirty, brownish skins.

Peevish, restless, fretful.

Flabby, sunken abdomen (opp. of *Calc. carb.*).

Phosphorus ..   Tall, slender, delicate: grow too rapidly.

"Children emaciating: rapidly: going into marasmus. Tendency to consumption."

Delicate: waxy: anæmic. Hectic blush.

Bleed easily: bruise easily. Sensitive to cold.

Love to be touched: rubbed.

Fear that something will happen: of thunder: of the dark: of being alone.

Indifferent.

"The sickly, sunken, earthy face of consumption, or of those going into consumption."

Desire for cold water: ices: salt: savouries.

May complain of a hot spine.

Chilly patient, yet stomach and head better for cold: chest and limbs better for heat.

Better for sleep — for short sleep. (*Sep.*)

One of the great vertigo medicines. (*Con.*)

Tuberculinum   "Deep-acting; long-acting: affects constitutions more deeply than most remedies (*Sulph., Sil., Dros.,* etc.)."

"*Tubercular taint:* debilitated and anæmic: here give *Tub.* on a paucity of symptoms."

Hopelessness: desire to travel: to go somewhere.

"Closely related to *Calc.,* to *Sil.* All go deep into life: interchangeable, i.e. one may be indicated for a while, then the other" (KENT).

Sensitive: dissatisfied. Fear of dogs.

Aversion to meat: craves cold milk.

"Gradual emaciation — increasing weakness — fatigue."

Excessive sweat in chronic diarrhœa.

Driven out of bed with diarrhœa.

Air-hunger: suffocated in a warm room.

Better riding in a cold wind. Worse damp cold.

"When at every coming back of the case, it needs a new remedy."

Old dingy look.

Very red lips (*Sulph.*) and very blue sclerotics suggest *Tub.*

Sulphur .. Farrington says, of marasmus of children,
"Ravenous, especially at 11 *a.m. Heat vertex: with cold feet. With these three symptoms Sulphur will never fail you."*
Wakes screaming.
Great voracity: puts everything into its mouth.
Or, "drinks much and eats little".
Thirsty, wants much water.
Craves fat: will eat raw suet.
"Slow, lazy, hungry, and always tired."
Red lips, nostrils, eyelids, anus.
Stool offensive, excoriating.
Frequent, slimy diarrhœa, or obstinate constipation. Screams before large stool.
"*Sulphur* children have the most astonishing tendency to be filthy."
Fear of bath: hates bath: worse from bath.
Limbs emaciate, with distended abdomen.
Muscles wither, even abdominal, with much distension of abdomen itself.
Emaciates with good appetite. (*Iod.,* etc.)
Eruptions: itching: worse at night. Boils.

Psorinum .. Pale, sickly, delicate children. Look unwashed (*Sulph.*).
Have a filthy smell, even after a bath.
Dread the bath (*Sulph.*).
Kent says, *"Offensive to sight and smell."*
Very chilly: worse open air: also worse warm bed.
Stools fluid, fetid.
Works miracles in these amazingly offensive (perhaps consumptive) children. One has seen it!

Sepia .. "No ability to feel natural love." *Indifference.*
Absence of joy. "Never happy unless he is annoying someone."
Comprehension difficult.
Progressive emaciation. Skin wrinkled.
Child looks like a shrivelled, dried-up old man.
Freckled, esp. across nose and cheeks, "the *Sepia* saddle".
Child wets the bed *in its first sleep.*
Damp cold legs and feet: (*Calc.*).

Silica   ..   Child weak, puny, from defective assimilation.

Big abdomen from (?) mesenteric disease.

"Large head, body small, emaciated, except abdomen which is round and plump.

Face pale, waxy, earthy or yellowish.

Pinched and old-looking. Limbs shrunken.

Bones and muscles poorly developed, for that reason late walking.

Coldness: chilliness.

Head sweats profusely: in sleep (*Calc.*).

Offensive sweat head and face.

Feet sweat: offensive foot sweat (*Bar. c., Petr.*).

Little injuries fester: poor healing (*Hep.*).

Boils and pustules, and sepsis.

Want of self-confidence.

Natrum mur. ..   Nutrition impaired. Eats and emaciates all the time (*Iod.*), neck particularly. (*Sars.*)

Emaciation, weakness, nervous prostration, nervous irritability.

Skin shiny, pale, waxy, as if greased; or,

Skin dry, withered, shrunken.

An infant looks like a little old man (*Iod., Abrot., Arg. nit., Sanic., Sars., Op., Ars.*).

Collar-bones become prominent and neck scrawny: but hips and lower limbs remain plump and round. (Opp. of *Abrot. Lyc.* also emaciates downwards.)

Children with *voracious appetite, yet emaciate.* (*Iod., Sulph.,* etc.)

One of the few "mapped-tongue" remedies.

Gets herpes about lips.

Terrible headaches.

Craving for salt. Hates bread and fat.

Weeps easily: but not amenable to sympathy.

Abrotanum   ..   Emaciation mostly of legs. Ascending (rev. of *Nat. mur., Lyc.,* etc.).

Bloated abdomen.   Cross irritable children.

Pale, hollow-eyed, old face (*Iod., Nat. mur., Sulph.,* etc.). Wrinkled.

Appetite very great: *ravenous while emaciating.* (*Iod.,* etc.)

In marasmus: skin flabby; and hangs loose.

Iodine   ..   *General emaciation: wants to eat all the time.*
                        While the body withers, the glands enlarge.
                        "Withering throughout the body, muscles shrink,
                            skin wrinkles, and face of child like a little old per-
                            son, *but glands under arms, in groins, and belly,
                            enlarged and hard. (Arg. nit., Abrot., Nat. mur.)*
                        Always hungry: eats between meals, and yet is hungry.
                        Better eating. Emaciates with an enormous appetite.
                        Excitement: anxiety: impulses. Worse trying to keep
                            still.
                        Worse heat: better cold. (*Lyc.*) (opp. to *Sil.*, etc.)
                        Always too hot.

Sanicula   ..   Child looks old (*Arg. nit.*, etc.), dirty, greasy, and
                            brownish.
                        Progressive emaciation.
                        Kicks off clothing in coldest weather. (*Sulph.*)
                        Sweats on falling asleep, mostly neck. Wets clothing
                            through. (*Calc., Sil.*)
                        Cold clammy sweat occiput and neck.
                        Child craves meat, fat bacon, *salt.* (*Nat. mur., Arg.
                            nit., Nit. ac.*)
                        Child wants to nurse all the time, yet loses flesh.
                        After intense straining the stool, nearly evacuated,
                            recedes (*Sil.*).
                        Body smells like old cheese.
                        Foul footsweat, chafes toes (*Sil.*).

Sarsaparilla   ..   Neck emaciates (*Nat. mur.*): skin lies in folds
                            (*Abrot.*).
                        Weakness of mind and tissues.
                        Marasmus of children from heredity.
                        Emaciation about the neck. (*Nat. mur.*)
                        Dry, purple copper-like eruptions.
                        No assimilation.
                        Children emaciated: face looks old. (*Nat. m., Arg.
                            nit.*, etc.)
                        Big belly: dry, flabby skin.
                        Screams when about to urinate. Or, *at close of urina-
                            tion gives an unearthly yell.*

Lycopodium ..	Emaciates from above downwards (*Sanic., Nat. mur.*).
	Lower limbs fairly nourished.
	Flatulent: distended like a drum (*Arg. nit.*), can hardly breathe. So full, he cannot eat.
	Wakes "ugly". Worse 4-8 p.m.
	No self-confidence (*Sil.*): miseries of anticipation (*Arg. nit., Ars., Sil.*).
	Cries when thanked: when receiving a gift.
	Withered lads with dry cough; headache.
	Better from cold. Worse warm room (*Iod.*).
	Red sand in urine: "red pepper deposit."
	Craves sweets (*Arg. nit.*) : hot drinks.
	One foot hot, one cold (characteristic).
	Sickly wrinkled face with contracted eyebrows.
Argentum nit.	Child looks dried up, like a mummy (*Op., Ars.*).
	Old-looking, pale, bluish face.
	Progressive emaciation.
	Craves sweets (*Lyc.*) which disagree.
	Craves salt (*Phos., Nat. mur.*).
	Wants cold air (*Lyc.*), cold drinks (opp. of *Lyc.*).
	A most flatulent remedy (*Lyc.*) distended to bursting (*Lyc.*).
	Emotional diarrhœa: from anticipation (*Gels.*).
	Examination funk. Fear of high places.
Opium ..	"Shrivelled little dried up old man."
	Painlessness: inactivity: torpor: —
	Or, sleeplessness: inquietude, nervous excitability.
	Lack of reaction to well-selected remedy. (*Sul.*)
	Fear and fright.
	Constipation from painless paresis of bowels.
Arsenicum ..	Atrophy of infants.
	Marasmus. "Dried-up mummy" child.
	Face pale, anxious, distorted.
	Skin harsh, dry, tawny.
	Rapid emaciation: sinking of strength.
	Least effort exhausting. Chilliness.
	Diarrhœa as soon as begins to eat or drink.
	Stools undigested: offensive.
	Restlessness: constant distress.
	"*Ars.* has *anxiety, restlessness, prostration, burning and cadaveric odours.*"

Hepar   ..   Sour smell (*Calc.*): white (*Calc.*) fœtid evacuations: undigested stools.

Seems better after feeding. (*Nat. mur.*)

"Does not play: does not laugh."

Chilly: oversensitive: to cold: to dry cold; to draughts (*Nux., Sulph.*); to touch.

Mind also oversensitive: every little thing makes him angry, abusive, impulsive (*Nux*).

Quarrelsome (*Nux*).

Little injuries fester (*Sil.*) are fearfully sensitive. Ears discharge: threatening mastoid.

Lax, chilly, sweats all night.

Worse cold: better warm: wrapped up (*Sil.*).

Nux   ..   "Oversensitive: irritable: touchy: never satisfied. Violent temper: uncontrollable."

"Jerks things about: tears them up."

Very chilly: cannot uncover (rev. of *Sulph.*).

"Always selecting his food, and digesting almost none."

Yellow, sallow, bloated face.

Constipation: alt. diarrhœa and constipation.

Irregular peristalsis: i.e. contents of intestine driven both ways: i.e. fitful or fruitless urging to stool.

Natrum carb. ..   Nervous withered infants: cannot stand milk: diarrhœa from milk. Aversion to milk.

"A nervous, cold baby, easily startled."

Better for eating: eats to keep warm.

All-gone feeling and pain in stomach, which drives him to eat; constantly "picking".

Abdomen hard and bloated: much flatus: loud rumbling.

Worse and esp. hungry at 11 p.m. and 5 a.m.

Headache from any mental exertion.

Ankles "turn" — weak.

Magnesia carb.   Puny and sickly from defective nutrition.

Milk refused: causes pain. Passed undigested.

Griping colic. Limbs drawn up for relief.

Stools sour, green, like frog-spawn on pond: or with lumps like tallow. (*Coloc.*, but has not the green, slimy stool).

Petroleum   ..   Emaciation, with *diarrhœa by day only.*
Hunger immediately after stool.
Aversion to fat, meat and open air.
"Coldness (*Calc.*) and sweating in single parts."
Offensive feet and axillæ (*Sil.*).
Dirty, hard, rough and thickened skin.
Skin fragile, cracks deeply (*Graph.*).
Eruptions worse in winter, better summer.
Hands crack and bleed: worse in winter.
Chilblains, sea and train sickness.
"Constant hunger with diarrhœa, but can't eat without pain: emaciation: eruptions: unhealthy ragged fingers that never look clean: can't wash them, as this chaps them."
"'Hands and feet burn: wants palms and soles (*Sulph., Cham., Puls., Med.*) out of bed."
("Don't be too sure of *Sulph.* because soles burn, or too sure of *Sil.* because feet sweat." —KENT.)

Baryta carb.   ..   "Dwarfishness: mind and body. Mental dwarfishness, and dwarfishness of organs."
"Suspends development that makes child into man or woman." (*Baryta mur.*)
"Emaciation in those who have been well nourished." (*Iod.*, etc.)
"Enlarged glands: enlarged abdomen: emaciation of tissues, emaciated limbs and dwarfishness of mind. You have there the whole of *Baryta carb.* marasmus."
Shy, bashful. Easily frightened.

Other disease products may have to be considered, in cases that make no progress, such as

Lueticum   ..   Dwarfish (*Bar. carb.*). Marasmic.
Worse at night.
Impulse to wash hands.
Where Syphilitic taint is the bar to progress.

Medorrhinum ..   Sycotic taint blocks progress. Poor reaction.
Lies on abdomen: sleeps in knee-elbow position.
Fiery-red, moist, itching anus (*Sulph.*).
Worse by day (opp. of *Luet.*).

TUBERCULOSIS DISEASE, GLANDS AND BONES

THE homœopathic treatment of "T.B." glands and bones in children is pure joy. One has seen children of 6 or 8 years of age, "eaten up" with tubercle, who from babyhood have been "never without a bandage" and subject to repeated operations, where homœopathic treatment has not only promptly stopped further progress of the disease but has closed the wounds; while long-suffering and feeble existence are replaced by new energy and health.

One remembers a dusky child, riddled with tubercle. She had lost the phalange of one finger, was crowded with hideous scars all round her neck, on chest also — and arm — and leg. Here a couple of years' treatment not only closed wounds and sinuses, but arrested the disease.

Many of our remedies are of great service in T.B. gland and bone, but in our experience, DROSERA EXCELS THEM ALL.

Drosera   .. Drosera has been proved *to break down resistance to tubercle in animals said to be immune; therefore, homœopathically it should, and does, raise resistance to tubercle.* Tubercular manifestations, or a strong family history of tuberculosis, put up a strong plea for the consideration of *Drosera* in any disease. Under the influence of *Drosera* glands of neck, if they have to "break", produce only very small openings; old suppurating glands soon diminish in size, and close. Old cicatrical tissue yields and softens; deep, tied-down scars relax, and come up, so that deformity is greatly lessened. While the improvement in health, in appearance, in nutrition, where *Drosera* comes into play, is rapid and striking.

Drosera has also great use in the diseases of joints and bone (in persons with a T.B. history), even when these are not tuberculous: quickly taking away pain, and improving health and well-being.

Hahnemann urged that *Dros.* should be given in infrequent doses, and the 30th potency. This, *"one of the most powerful medicinal herbs in our zone"* still (as he then said) "needs further proving".

357

Silica   .. Hardened glands, especially about the neck: "Scrofulous glands."

A deep remedy for eradicating the tuberculous tendency when symptoms agree.

Worse in wet, cold weather, better in dry, cold
weather, but very chilly.

Tendency to swelling of glands, which suppurate.

The *Silica* child is timid, lacks confidence, "grit".

Head sweats in sleep (*Calc.*).

For nearly all disease of bone.

Fistulous openings: discharges offensive: swollen;
pouting round them hard, swollen, bluish-red.

Sweat of feet, often offensive feet.

Symphytum   .. A case of necrosis of lower jaw, after an accident.
Sil. and *Tub.* failed to effect improvement. Then
Symph. was given, with the expulsion of a seques-
trum, whereupon it healed. But *Symph.* has its
"schmertz-punct" in that situation — left lower jaw,
and is an outstanding remedy for BONE. (*Dros.,
Phos.*)

Sepia   .. A case of T.B. bone, with a sinus on each side of the
right middle finger, one above and one below the
first joint. Also other T.B. manifestations; in a
woman who had nursed her husband dying of
phthisis. *Sil.* and *Tub.* failed to help, even with
three weeks at a Convalescent Home. At long last,
she was given *Sepia*, BECAUSE HER INDIVIDUAL SYMP-
TOMS DEMANDED SEPIA; whereupon the finger got
well in spite of the fact that it was all day long in
dirty water, scrubbing and cleaning in the public-
house in which she worked. It is sometimes difficult
to remember that *it is the remedy called for by the
individual symptoms of the patient, that will stimulate him to put his house in order, and get well.*
One is too apt to stress the disease and treat that!

The typical *Sepia* patient is indifferent: overburdened:
dull. Has axillary sweats, offensive (*Sil.*), hates
noise and smells: only "wants to get away alone and
be quiet".

Sulphur   ..   "Prince of remedies in scrofula — in caries in early childhood.

"Voracious appetite: greedily clutches at all that is offered, edible or not, as if starved.

"Shrivelled and dried up like a little old man."

Tuberculinum .. Patients with a T.B. family history, or with T.B. manifestations, glands, etc.

A deep-acting, long-acting remedy.

Closely related to *Calc.*: one may be indicated for a while, then the other. (*Sil., Dros.*)

Always wanting to go somewhere — to travel.

Feeble vitality: tired: debilitated: losing flesh.

Emaciation, with hunger (*Iod.*).

Worse in a close room, in damp weather; better cold wind, open air.

Desire for alcohol, bacon, fat ham, smoked meat, cold milk, refreshing things, sweets.

Calcarea   .. Affects the glands of neck and all the glands.

Glands of abdomen become hard, sore, inflamed.

Useful in T.B. formations, calcareous degenerations.

But in the *Calc. child:* i.e. the child of plus quantity, minus quality: with large, sweating head, especially at night. Phlegmatic; the "lump of chalk" child, fair, pale, fat.

Necrosis of bone in such children.

Very useful in T.B. abdomen — when symptoms agree: which they generally do. (*Psor.,* when odour of child is very offensive.)

Phosphorus   .. Like *Dros.* appears to break down resistance to tubercle, since workers in match factories have been esp. liable to consumption, and have suffered from caries and necrosis of bone.

Phos. helps to cure not only bone troubles, but "scrofulous glands", but always in the typical slender *Phos.* children, who grow too rapidly: delicate, waxy, anæmic.

Bruise easily: easy bleeders: with

Thirst for cold water, hunger for salt: love of ices.

Are nervous alone — fear the dark, rather apathetic and indifferent.

Iodium .. Scrofulous swellings and induration of glands: large, hard, usually painless.

"Iodine is torpidity and sluggishness. The very indolence of the disease suggests *Iod*."

Cross and *restless*. Impulses.

Anxiety: the more he keeps still, the more anxious.

Always too hot.

Eats ravenously yet emaciates.

Dark hair and complexion. (*Brom*. fair and blue eyes.)

"Enlargement of all the glands except the mammæ: these waste and atrophy."

Compelled to keep on doing something to drive away his impulses and anxiety, (*Ars*.). But *Iod*. is warm-blooded, and wants cold: *Ars*. is cold and wants heat — warm room, warm clothing, etc.

Bromium .. Very useful in enlarged glands with great hardness without any tendency to suppurate.

Glands take on tuberculosis, and tissues take on tuberculosis.

Glands that inflame for a while begin to take on a lower form of degeneration.

"It is very similar to those enlarged, hard, scrofulous glands that we often find in the neck . . ."

Swelling and induration of glands is a strong feature of the remedy.

Those needing *Brom*. for chronic glands, etc. will have a "grey, earthy colour of the face. Oldish appearance".

Or plethoric children, with red face, easily overheated.

Left-sided remedy.

Worse dampness.

Weak and easily over-heated, then sweaty and sensitive to draughts.

Glands in persons of light complexion, fair skin and light blue eyes (distinguishes from *Iod*.).

Tonsils deep-red, swollen, with net-work of dilated vessels.

Cistus can.   ..   Scrofulous swelling and suppuration of glands of
throat.

Scrofulous hip disease, with fistulous openings leading
to the bone, and ulcers on the surface, with night
sweats.

A curious *Cistus* symptom, which has led to the cure
of chronic colds and nasal catarrh, is *great desire
for cheese.*

Theridion   ..   "Has an affinity for the tubercular diatheses."

Has been used with success in caries and necrosis of
bone. "It appears to go to the root of the evil and
destroys the cause" (DR. BARUCH).

Theridion is hypersensitive, especially to noise: shrill
sounds penetrate the teeth.

Nausea from motion, and from closing the eyes.

Baryta carb.   ..   Glands swell, infiltrate, hypertrophy: sometimes suppurate.

Dwarfish children, late to develop: with dwarfish
minds.

Slow, inept: mistrustful of strangers. Shy.

Affected by every cold.

Cold, foul footsweat. (*Sil.*)

Tearing and tension in long bones: boring in bones.

Mercury   ..   A curious, but useful symptom, "sensation of shivering in an abscess", or in a sinus from diseased bone.

COMMON REMEDIES OF MEASLES

Aconite . . Catarrh and high fever: before rash clinches diagnosis.
Redness conjunctivae: dry, barking cough.
Itching, burning skin: rash rough and miliary.
Restless, anxious, tossing: frightened.

Gelsemium . . Chills and heats chase one another. Sneezing and
sore throat: excoriating nasal discharge.
Severe, heavy headache: occipital pain.
Thirstlessness is the rule with *Gels.* (*Puls.*)
Drowsy and stupid. Lids heavy: eyes inflamed.
Face dark-red, swollen, besotted (*Bapt.*).

Belladonna . . Rash bright-red: skin hot and dry — such cases as
suggest scarlet fever.

Euphrasia . . Cases with great catarrhal intensity.
"A wonderful medicine in measles. When symptoms
agree will make a very violent attack of measles turn
into a very simple form. . . .
"Streaming, burning tears; photophobia; running
from nose; intense throbbing headache, dry cough
and rash." — Kent.
Copious *acrid* lachrymation, with streaming, *bland*
discharge from nose (rev. of *Allium cepa,* which has
acrid discharge from nose, but bland from eyes).

Sulphur . . "Measles with a purplish appearance. *Sulphur* to
modify the case when the skin is dusky and the
rash does not come out."
"The routinist can do pretty well in this disease with
Puls. and *Sulph.,* occasionally requiring *Acon.* and
Euphrasia." Kent.
Convalescence makes tardy progress, and the patient
is weak and prostrate.

Acon. and *Puls.* have an old reputation for measles, but
Pulsatilla . . "If much fever, *Puls.* will not be the remedy."
Catarrhal symptoms: profuse lachrymation.
Dry mouth, but seldom thirst.

Kali bich.	..	"Is like *Puls.* only worse." Follows *Puls. Puls. in the mild cases.*

It has a rash like measles, with catarrh of eyes.

Measles with purulent discharge eyes and ears. With pustules on cornea.

Salivary glands swollen: catarrhal deafness.

Kali bich. has stringy, ropy discharges.

Morbillinum .. Said to be prophylactic.

TARDY OR SUPPRESSED ERUPTION: BRAIN AFFECTED

Bryonia .. Rash tardy to appear.

Hard, dry cough with tearing pain.

Little or no expectoration.

Or rash disappears and child drowsy: pale, twitching face, chewing motion of jaws (*Zinc.* grits teeth).

Any motion causes child to scream with pain.

Mild delirium, "Wants to go home," at home.

Or, instead of rash, bronchitis or pneumonia, with *Bry.* symptoms.

Apis .. .. Rash goes in and brain symptoms appear.

Stupor with stinging pains, extorting cries (Crie cerebrale)

Thirstless: worse from heat, hot room, hot fire.

Better cool air. Urine scanty.

A great remedy for œdema and effusions.

Cuprum .. Symptoms violent. Starts up from sleep.

Spasms: cramps: convulsions.

Cramps of fingers and toes, or start there.

Helleborus .. "When entire sensorial life is suspended, and child lies in profound stupor."

Zincum .. Where child is too weak to develop eruption.

Rash comes out sparingly. Body rather cool.

Lies in stupor gritting teeth. (*Bry.* chews.)

Dilated pupils: squinting and rolling eyes.

Fidgety feet.

Stramonium .. Rash not out properly. Child hot, bright-red face.

Tosses, cries as if frightened in sleep.

Convulsive movements.

SCARLET FEVER

Belladonna for scarlet fever affords such a beautiful example of Homœopathy in the common cases of epidemic scarlet fever, and shows such startling results, not only for the disease (when properly prescribed, i.e. when the symptoms agree), but also as a prophylactic, from the days when Hahnemann discovered its use here, and wrote about it, and forced its acceptance on the Government of his day, that one need not say much about it.

Cases where it has been used as a prophylactic, or used suitably on its indications, abort, or run a very mild course, leaving no sequelae, and are practically (as so many report) not even infectious.

Belladonna ..	Bright red, hot face. Glossy, scarlet skin: intense heat: "burns the hand."
	"In the true Sydenham scarlet fever, where the eruption is perfectly smooth and truly scarlet."
	Bell. everywhere, is HEAT, REDNESS, BURNING.
	Eyes red; injected: pupils later very dilated.
	Lips — mouth — throat, red, dry, burning.
	Strawberry tongue.
	For eruptions like roseola and scarlet fever, with fever, sore throat, cough and headache.
	Twitching, jerking; possibly wild delirium.
	(Here *Apis* wants to be cool, uncovered; *Bell.* wants to be warm. *Bell.* also has more thirst.)

SCARLET FEVER: PROPHYLAXIS AND SEQUELAE

Hahnemann writes of *Belladonna*:

"The remedy capable of maintaining the healthy uninfectable by the miasm of scarlet fever, I was so fortunate as to discover. I found also that the same remedy given at the period when the symptoms indicating the invasion of the disease occur, stifles the fever in its very birth; and more-over is more efficacious than other known medicaments in removing the greater part of the after-sufferings following scarlatina that has run its natural course, which are often worse than the disease itself. . . ." He talks about this "divine remedy" as a preservative and a curative in scarlet fever.

SEQUELAE

And he also says: "*Belladonna* displays a valuable and specific power in removing the after-sufferings remaining from scarlet fever. . . . *Most medical men have hitherto regarded the consequences of scarlet fever as at least as dangerous as the fever itself and there have been many epidemics where more died of the after-effects than of the fever*": and he enumerates them.

And he gives one interesting hint, "where ulceration has followed scarlet fever and where *Belladonna* is no longer of service," *Chamomilla* "will remove in a few days all tendency to ulceration: and the suffocating cough that sometimes follows the disease is also removed by *Chamomilla,* especially if accompanied by flushing of the face, and horripilation of limbs and back." "Protection against scarlet fever" (*Lesser Writings*).

Apis .. .. Thick rose-coloured rash, feels rough. Or,
When rash does not come out, with great inflammation of throat, with scarlet fever in family.
Throat sore, swollen, œdematous: with stinging pain.
Convulsions when rash fails to come out (compare *Cup., Zinc., Bry.,* as given, under MEASLES).
Worse from heat: wants covers off: a cool room: (reverse of *Bell.* which needs heat).

Ailanthus .. Scarlet fever; plentiful eruption of bluish tint.
Eruption slow to appear, remains livid.
Irregular, patchy eruption of a very livid colour.
Throat livid, swollen, tonsils swollen with deep ulcers.
Pupils widely dilated (*Bell.*).
Semi-conscious, cannot comprehend.
Dizzy: can't sit up. Restless and anxious: later, insensible with muttering delirium.
Tongue dry, parched, cracked.
"Malignant scarlet fever."

Mercurius .. May follow *Bell.* for sore mouth, throat, tonsils, with ulceration and excessively foul breath.
Perspiration which aggravates the symptoms.

Rhux tox.   ..   "Useful in scarlet fever with coarse rash. Or rash suppressed with inflammation of glands and sore throat" (KENT).

"You may rely on *Rhus* whenever acute diseases take on a typhoid form, as in scarlet fever, when no other remedy is positively indicated" (FARRINGTON).

"*Rhus* supplants *Bell.* when child grows drowsy and *restless.*"

Fauces dark-red, with œdema (*Apis*).

Tongue red (? smooth) with triangular red tip.

Ammonium carb.   Malignant scarlatina (*Ail.*) with somnolence.

Body red, as if covered with scarlatina.

Dark red and putrid throat. External throat swollen.

As if forehead would burst.

State like blood poisoning: with patchy surface; great dyspnœa; face dusky and puffy.

Lachesis   ..   Advanced stages: malignant scarlet fever.

A purple face belongs to *Lachesis.*

Worse for heat (reverse of *Bell.*).

Bursting, hammering pains in head.

Throat worse left side: may extend to right.

Jealousy and suspicion suggests *Lach.*

Impelled to talk: loquacious delirium.

Lach. sleeps into an aggravation.

Terebinthina   ..   Albuminuria and uræmia following Sc. fever.

Intoxication: confusion: better profuse urination.

Often indicated in dropsy after scarlet fever.

Hæmaturia: urine cloudy and smoky.

"Hæmaturia: dyspnœa: drowsiness."

Tongue dry and glossy.

N.B. — NIT A., *Phos.*, or one of many other drugs might be needed in difficult cases, or in cases first seen later on in the disease and with complications; but all according to the symptoms and make-up of the patient.

For SUPPRESSED or RECEDING eruption, see under MEASLES.

TYPHOID SCARLATINA

Writing of AILANTHUS, in *"typhoid scarlatina with eruption plentiful of a bluish tint"*, Kent says:

"When you go to the bedside of scarlet fever you should not call to mind the names of these remedies you may have heard recommended for scarlet fever; let the appearance of the patient bring to mind such remedies as appear like *this* patient, regardless of whether they have been associated with scarlet fever or not.

"When you see the rash perhaps you will say that it looks like an *Aconite* rash, but there is such scanty zymosis in the nature of *Aconite* that it is no longer thought of. *Belladonna* is not suitable, for in that remedy the rash is shiny and smooth, the typical Sydenham rash. On the other hand you will say, *Pulsatilla* has a measly rash, and often associated with a low form of fever, but not so low as the typhoid state, so *Pulsatilla* goes out of your mind. You now think of the remedies that are typical of all zymotic states: the prostration, the aggravation after sleep, general stupor and delirium, and almost at a glance you see *Lachesis,* the type of such forms of disease. Its picture comes into your mind speedily. You see another case of scarlet fever where there is a scanty rash, the child before you keeps on picking the skin from the lips and nose, lies in a state of pallor and exhaustion, no rash to speak of, urine nearly suppressed; almost in a moment you think of *Arum triph.* It is the aspect of things that will call the remedy to mind. In another case you have all the purple appearance I have spoken of in this remedy (*Ailanthus*); the horrible fœtor, a good deal of sore throat, and the child cannot get water cold enough, wants a stream of water running down the throat all the time; you may safely trust to *Phosphorus.*

"In these low types of sickness there is always something to tell the story if you will only listen, study, and wait long enough."

WHOOPING-COUGH

"Most cases of whooping-cough, in the care of a homœopathic physician will get well in a week or ten days under a carefully selected remedy. When allowed to run, they continue a long time, gradually increasing for six weeks, and then declining according to the weather. If it is in the Fall the cough will sometimes keep up all winter, so whooping-cough furnishes an opportunity for the homœopathic physician to demonstrate that there is something in Homœopathy." — KENT.

Drosera .. HAHNEMANN says: "A single dose (of the 30th potency, and not repeated) is quite sufficient for the homœopathic cure of epidemic whooping-cough, according to the indications given by symptoms" (which he enumerates).

Impulses to cough follow one another so violently, that he can hardly get his breath.

Oppression of the chest, as if something kept back the air when he coughed and spoke, so that the breath could not be expelled.

When he breathes out a sudden contraction in hypogastrium, which makes him heave and excites coughing.

Crawling in larynx which provokes coughing.

The cough makes him like to vomit. (*Kali carb.*)

On coughing he vomits water, mucus and food.

When coughing, contractive pain in the hypochondria. Cannot cough on account of the pain, unless he presses his hand on the *scrobiculus cordis* ("hollow of the epigastrium").

The region below the ribs (hypochondria) is painful when touched and when coughing, must press his hand on the spot to mitigate the pain.

Spasmodic cough, with retching and vomiting. Caused by tickling or dryness in throat.

Kali carb. .. Convulsive and tickling cough at night.

Cough so violent as to cause vomiting.

Cough at 3 a.m., repeated every half-hour.

Whooping-cough, worse at 3 a.m.; gagging and vomiting.

Bag-like swellings between the upper lids and the eyebrows; often puffy face also.

"One of the most violent coughs of all the medicines. Face racked."

"Dry, hard, racking, hacking cough."

Bryonia .. "Child coughs immediately after eating and drinking and vomits, then returns to the table, finishes his meal, but coughs and vomits again." — Lilienthal.

"Dry spasmodic cough: whooping cough, shaking the whole body." Cough makes him spring up in bed — Even *Bry.!*

Carbo veg.   ..   Cough, mostly hard and dry: or sounds rough: apt to occur after a full meal.

Every violent spell brings up a lump of phlegm, or is followed by retching, gagging and waterbrash.

Pain in chest after cough: burning as from a coal of fire.

Craving for salt. (This determined the remedy in a case that promptly recovered.)

"One of the greatest medicines we have in the beginning of whooping-cough. Gagging, vomiting and redness of face." — KENT.

Paroxysms of violent spasmodic coughing; with cold sweat and cold pinched face after attack.

Belladonna   ..   Weeping (*Arn.*) and pains in stomach before coughing. Feels head will burst.

Dry spasmodic cough, worse at night; lying.

"Spasms of larynx which cause cough and difficulty of breathing." — KENT.

Kent says, "The *Bell.* cough is peculiar. As soon as great violence and great effort have raised a little mucus there is peace, during which larynx and trachea get dryer and dryer and begin to tickle, then comes the spasm and the whoop, and the gagging." Especially after exposure to cold.

Arnica   ..   "A wonderful whooping-cough remedy."

Violent tickling cough if child gets angry:

Begins to cry before cough (*Bell.*): knows it is coming and dreads it.

Antimonium tart.   ..   Cough when child gets angry, and after eating. Ends in vomiting. "Chest full of rattles." Thirstless: coated tongue.

Carolium rub. ..   Smothering before cough. Exhaustion after it.

Bromium   ..   *With sensation of coldness in throat.*

Larynx as if covered with velvet, but feels cold.

"Whooping cough in spring, towards hot weather." Worse hot weather.

Carbo an.   ..   *With feeling of coldness in chest.*

Severe dry cough, shakes abdomen as if all would fall out; must support bowels (*Dros.*).

Kali sulph. .. Whooping-cough, with retching, without vomiting. Yellow, slimy expectoration.

Tongue coated with yellow mucus.

Hot and sweating. *Hates* cough and weeps (*Bell.*).

Looks "fat, fair and forty" even as a child!

Coccus cacti. .. Worse at night, when hot in bed.

Better lying in cool room without much covering: wants room cold.

If mother can get to it quickly enough with a drink of cold water she can ward off the paroxysm.

Child holds its breath to prevent coughing.

"Wakes in morning with paroxysm of whooping-cough, which ends in vomiting ropy mucus, which hangs in long strings from mouth — great ropes. Here *Coccus c.* will cut short the disease." ("*Kali bi.* stringy but yellow: *Coccus c.* clear" or white.)

Cuprum .. Better by swallowing cold water. (*Coccus c.*)

Uninterrupted paroxysms till breath completely exhausted. Gasps with repeated crowing inspirations till black in the face. Mucus in trachea and spasms in larynx.

Cramps beginning in fingers and toes.

Thumbs tucked in during cough.

Mephitis .. Whooping of any violent cough: very violent, spasmodic, as if each spell would terminate life.

Frequent paroxysms especially at night.

Desire for salt (*Carbo veg.*).

Worse lying down. Child must be raised.

Magnesia phos. Violent spasmodic attacks of cough, with face blue and turgid. Ends in a whoop.

(Schuessler's remedy for cramps and spasms.)

Ipecacuanha .. Stiffens: goes rigid, loses breath: grows pale: then relaxes and vomits phlegm with relief.

Convulsions in whooping-cough, frightful spasms especially of left side.

Cina .. .. The same rigidity, with clucking sound down in oesophagus as it goes out of paroxysm.

Not relieved by eating: stomach bloated, yet hungry. Grits teeth.

Lobelia .. *Cough ends with violent sneezing.*

SOME REMEDIES FOR MUMPS

A NUMBER of remedies are set down as being useful in mumps:

PILOCARPINE

But Dr. Burnett's homœopathic remedy for mumps seems to surpass all the rest, i.e. PILOCARPINE. And ever since one came across that fertile hint, mumps has been easy to deal with, and so far as one has observed, painless. *Pilocarpine* acts very quickly. It has always seemed to finish up the cases promptly, *besides taking away the pain,* which means a great deal to the sufferer. (*Phyto.*)

Moreover, *Pilocarpine* has a reputation for the metastases in which mumps excels, whether to testes or mammæ; when the swelling suddenly subsides, as the result of a chill, and other — worse — troubles supervene.

Pilocarpine also acts as a prophylactic. Of course *Pilocarpine* (Jaborandi) causes a very rapid swelling of all the salivary glands, and its action here is specific.

Aconite .. For the *Acon.* fever with restlessness and anxiety.

Belladonna .. Inflammation of *right* parotid with bright redness and violent shooting pains.
Glowing redness of face. Sensitive to cold.

Phytolacca .. Inflammation of sub-maxillary and *parotid* glands with stony hardness.
Pain shoots into ear when swallowing.
Worse cold and wet.
("Rheumatoid arthritis has been cured, when accompanied by swelling of the parotids").

Mercurius .. Mumps, especially *right* side. Farrington says, "especially left, where it is dark red" (*Merc. i. f.*)
Offensive salivation.
Foul tongue, and offensive sweat. (*Merc. cor.*)

Lycopodium .. Begins *right* side, and goes to left.
It has not the offensive mouth and salivation of the *Mercs.*
Desires warm drinks.

Bromium   ..   Parotids, especially *left* affected: especially after scarlet fever.

"Swelling and hardness of left parotid: warm to touch."

Swelling of all glands about throat.

Slow inflammation of glands, with hardness.

Brom. especially helps those who are made sick by being overheated: but when attack comes on, sensitive to cold and draughts.

Worse damp, hot weather.

Lachesis   ..   Especially *left* side parotid, enormously swollen: sensitive to least touch; least possible pressure — severe pain; shrinks away when approached: can scarcely swallow.

Throat sore internally. Face red and swollen. Eyes glassy and wild.

There is not the offensive mouth and dirty tongue of the *Mercs.*, but more throbbing; with the usual *Lachesis* horrible tension.

Rhus tox.   ..   Parotid and sub-maxillary glands highly inflamed and enlarged.

Mumps on *left* side.

Worse cold: cold winds: cold wet.

"Always with herpes on lips."

Pulsatilla   ..   Lingering fever, or metastases (*Carbo veg.; Abrot.*).

"If in mumps the patient gets a cold, the breasts swell in a girl: in boys it is testicle. *Puls.* is the common remedy for enormously swollen testicles from mumps."

"*Puls.* breaks up complaints that flit about."

Carbo veg.   ..   Parotitis. Face pale, cold.

"When mumps change their abode, and go in the girl to the mammary glands and in the boy to the testis, *Carbo veg.* is one of the medicines to restore order: will often bring the trouble back to its original place and conduct it through in safety."—KENT.

Baryta iod.   ..   In the *Baryta* child: backward — shy — "deficient".
or *mur.*

DIPHTHERIA

THE temptation to less experienced homœopaths is to follow the line of least resistance and to administer antitoxin which, whether it be best or no for the patient, puts the doctor right with the powers that be, and in the event of an adverse issue silences carping friends perhaps inimical to Homœopathy; but which never gives anything like the good results of the correct homœopathic remedy.* All our good prescribers (and we have had the same experience) have again and again seen cases of diphtheria where swab and culture were swarming with Klebs-Loeffler bacillus, and where a second culture twenty-four to forty-eight hours later was sterile; and this, mind you! with none of the distresses — sufferings — even dangers of antitoxin. Patients treated homœopathically simply get well. And not only this; one must realize how, with a rapidly sterile throat, the chance of spreading the disease must be greatly lessened or averted. Disease, convalescence and quarantine are reduced to their minimum

In a rapid and dangerous disease like diphtheria, one needs to be on the spot with its remedy; and, as elsewhere, one drug will not do for another. But, as will be seen, their indications are very definite and should not be missed. In diphtheria, as in all diseases, it is *only the "like" remedy that will cure; and the curative remedy in each case is to be picked out only by the methods of Hahnemann.* Routine prescribing, even with a drug like *Merc. cy.* will only cure the *Merc. cy.* cases, leaving the rest untouched, and here, the routinist will come to the conclusion that "Homœopathy has failed" — whereas it never *was* Homœopathy.

Mercurius cy. is one of the greatest of diphtheria remedies — since it has produced such a good imitation of the real thing, that in one recorded case the patient was notified, certified and buried as diphtheria, and it was only exhumation that showed the case to be one of poisoning by the cyanide of mercury. We once saw a beautiful proving by one of our residents which demonstrated that *Merc. cy.* does produce a membrane mistakable for dipththeria. This young doctor got the wind up, after

*A case was quoted in 'HOMOEOPATHY,' July, 1934, when a child of six, seen in Casualty with a "throat" and a patch on left tonsil, tongue clean, got Lach. cm., two doses, and was practically well next day, when he only needed Arnica for a fall. But when the Laboratory report came to hand it read: "Klebs-Loeffler bacillus with pneumococcus and Vincent's angina;" and a child in the house had had diphtheria. Diphtheria cured in 24 hours, and the child remained well.

recklessly infecting her lips when doing a tracheotomy on a case that she had not suspected of being diphtheria, but where the P.M. showed the membrane in throat, trachea and bronchi. Thereafter she carried *Merc. cy.* about with her, and took a dose every time her fears got the upper hand, till she actually produced, and retired to bed with an apparent *"diphtheria membrane in her throat,"* which rapidly disappeared when the drug was discontinued.

One has seen *Merc. cy.* rapidly curative also in *Vincent's angina.* In one case, with the tongue extensively ulcerated away on one side, with filthy saliva, with apparent infiltration towards the cheek, and where the provisional diagnosis was "epithelioma of tongue — possibly complicated with syphilis" it turned out to be a *Vincent's angina;* and what was left of the tongue rapidly healed while the mouth returned to normal with a few doses of *Merc. cy.* 200 (or 30, one forgets which).

Think of *Merc. cy.* then, where there is a thick, greyish membrane on throat; early, rapid, and extreme prostration, and putridity. Or again, in ulcerations of mouth or throat, with salivation, and extreme offensiveness.

There is another drug which has, in provings, produced what appeared to be diphtheritic patches on the throat "pronounced" (Dr. CLARK says) " 'severe diphtheria', but they soon got well," and *Lac caninum,* in consequence, has won fame as a curative and prophylactic remedy against diphtheria — symptoms agreeing.

Merc. cy.   ..   Fairly rapid onset, with prostration.
One or both sides of throat affected.
Membrane spreads rapidly over entire throat.
Colour white, yellow, or greenish.
Tongue thickly coated, moist: salivation.
Odour always putrid. Hot sweats.
Tepid liquids better swallowed than hot or cold.
Patient (generally) worse late evening and night.

Lycopodium   ..   Patient worse from 4 to 8 p.m.
Starts in nose (*Kali bic.*) or right side throat, spreads to left.
Warm drinks more easily swallowed: but reverse sometimes the case.
Movement of nostrils.
Diminished urine or copious sediment of urates, or fine red sand.

Lachesis   ..   Membrane starts left side, spreads to right.

Face and throat look cyanotic. Choking.

Cold things more easily swallowed than hot.

Great sensitiveness of neck and throat, so that patient cannot stand the touch of bed clothes, and pulls neck of night attire open.

General and local aggravation from heat, and all symptoms are worse after sleep. The longer the sleep, the worse he is on waking.

Mental characteristics of *Lach.* are loquacity and suspicion.

Phytolacca   ..   Frequently indicated.

Membrane grey or white, may start on uvula.

May spread from right tonsil to left (*Lyc.*). But, unlike *Lyc.*, the pain is worse from heat.

Fauces dark-red: complains of lump in throat; or as if red-hot ball had stuck in throat.

Pain goes to ear.

Lac caninum   ..   Patients nervous, imaginative, highly sensitive.

Skin hypersensitive (*Lach.*). Touch unbearable, though hard pressure gives no pain.

Membrane pearly, or silver white.

Milky coating on tongue.

Characteristic feature is *alternation of sides*.

Pain will jump from side to side, and back; alternations of sides anywhere.

Arsenicum   ..   Membrane looks dry, shrivelled; with the *Ars.* anxiety, restlessness and prostration.

Worse at night: at 1 a.m.

Chilliness: incessant thirst for small quantities.

Kali bichrom. ..   Nasal diphtheria: ropy discharges.

Exudation tough and firmly adherent.

Baptisia   ..   Putridity: with dull red face; drowsiness; patient as if drugged.

Membrane dark: dry brown tongue.

Apis   ..   Throat bright-red, puffy, "varnished". Uvula long; œdematous. Nothing must touch throat (*Lach.*).

DIPHTHERINUM

Dr. H. C. Allen (*Keynotes*) has much to say about *Diphtherinum*. His symptoms are "cured" symptoms, verifications which he had found guiding and reliable for twenty-five years. "The remedy is prepared, like all nosodes and animal poisons, according to the Homœopathic Pharmacopœia, and is, like all homœopathic remedies, entirely safe when given to the sick."

Like all the nosodes, it is practically worthless below the 30th, while its curative virtues increase with the higher potencies. It should not be repeated too frequently. He has used it for twenty-five years as a prophylactic and never known a second case to occur in a family after it had been administered.

Diphtherinum	When the attack from the onset tends to malignancy.
	Painless diphtheria. Symptoms almost, or entirely objective.
	Patient weak, apathetic. Stupor.
	Dark-red swelling of tonsils and throat.
	Breath and discharges very offensive (*Merc. cy.*).
	Membrane thick, dark-grey or brownish black.
	Temperature low, or subnormal. Pulse weak and rapid. Vital reaction very low.
	Epistaxis, or profound prostration from the onset. Collapse almost at the very beginning.
	Swallows without pain, but fluids are vomited or returned through nose.
	Laryngeal diphtheria; post-diphtheric paralysis. (*Caust., Gels.*)
	When the patient from the first seems doomed, and the most carefully-selected remedies fail to relieve, or permanently improve.
	"It will cure every case that crude antitoxin will: and is safe: and easy to administer."
	To remove persistent diphtheria-organisms, in "carriers".

POST-DIPHTHERIC PARALYSIS

Gelsemium . .	With regurgitations through nose (*Lyc., Caust., Cocc.*).

376

COMMON REMEDIES OF SMALL-POX*

Variolinum .. Probably the most potent of all, having the complete picture of the disease from which it is prepared.

Dullness of head.

Severe pains in back and limbs, which became quite numb.

Chills, followed by high fever.

Violent headache.

White-coated tongue.

Great thirst.

Severe pains and distress in epigastric region with nausea and vomiting, mostly of greenish water.

In many cases profuse diarrhœa. In some, despondency.

Small-pox pustules on different parts of the body, mostly abdomen and back. Pustules perfectly formed, some umbilicated, some purulent.

"Given steadily the disease will run a milder course. It changes imperfect pustules into regular ones, which soon dry up. Promotes suppuration and desiccation. Prevents pitting." — LILIENTHAL.

Antimonium tart. Long held by Homœopaths to be specific for small-pox.

Pustules with red areola, like small-pox, which leave a crust and form a scar.

Pains in back and loins.

Violent pain in sacro-lumbar region: slightest movement causes retching and cold sweat.

Violent headache: < evening; < lying; > sitting up; > cold.

Variola; backache, headache; cough with crushing weight on chest; before or at beginning of eruptive stage; diarrhœa, etc. Also when eruption fails.

LILIENTHAL says: "Tardy eruption with nausea, vomiting, sleeplessness, or suppression of eruption. Putrid variola with typhoid symptoms (*Bapt.*) especially typhoid pneumonia, etc."

* Protect the patient from light, or exclude actinic rays.

"If the use of *Ant. tart.* was long continued after it had produced an eruption like small-pox, the pustules got large, full of pus, deepened in the centre and became confluent, with great pains: crusts were formed leaving great scars."

Sarracenia .. (Drug of the North American Indians) seems to have done marvelous work in aborting and curing small-pox.

Crotalus hor. .. Pustular eruptions. After vaccination.
Eruptions, boils, pustules, gangrenous conditions, when fever is low and parts bluish.
Hæmorrhagic cases.

Lachesis .. Hæmorrhagic cases. (*Crot. h.*)
Characteristics: — Worse after sleep.
Dusky or purplish appearance, with excessive tenderness to touch.

Hamamelis .. Hæmorrhagic cases (*Crot. h.*)oozing of dark blood from nose; bleeding gums; hæmatemesis, bloody stools. (All *Crot. h.*)

Thuja .. Which will cause the pustules of vaccination to wither and abort, should be one of the great remedies of small-pox also.
LILIENTHAL says, "pains in arms, fingers, hands, with fullness and soreness of throat.
"Areola round pustules marked and dark red.
"Pustules milky and flat, painful to touch; give especially during stage of maturation, where it may prevent pitting."

Aconite .. To modify first stage and early second stage:
High fever: great restlessness. Fear: of death.

Belladonna .. First stage: high fever and cerebral congestion.
Intense swelling of skin and mucous membrane.
Dysuria and tenesmus of bladder.
Delirium and convulsions. Photophobia.

Hyoscyamus .. Eruption fails to appear, causing great excitement, rage, anguish, delirium in paroxysms. Wants to get out of bed, and uncover.

Cuprum sulph.	Cerebral irritation, where eruption fails to appear. Convulsive phenomena.
Mercurius ..	Stage of maturation: ptyalism. Tendency of blood to head. Moist swollen tongue with great thirst. Diarrhœa or dysentery with tenesmus, especially during desiccation.
Sulphur ..	Tendency to metastasis to brain during suppuration. Stage of desiccation: or occasionally intercurrent, where others fail.
Phosphoric acid	Confluent, with typhoid conditions. "Pustules fail to pustulate; degenerate into large blisters, which leave raw surface." Stupid: wants nothing; not even a drink. Answers questions but does not talk. Subsultus tendinum: restlessness. Fear of death. Watery diarrhœa.
Baptisia ..	Typhoid symptoms: fetid breath. Pustules thick on arch of palate, tonsils, uvula, in nasal cavities; but scanty on skin. Great prostration with pain in sacral region. Drowsy; comatose; limbs feel "scattered."
Phosphorus ..	Hæmorrhagic diathesis. Bloody pustules. Hard dry cough: chest raw. Hæmorrhage from lungs. Back as if broken: faintings. Great thirst.
Rhus tox. ..	"Eruptions turn livid and typhoid symptoms supervene." Dry tongue. Sordes lips and teeth. Wants to get out of bed. Great restlessness (*Ars.*). Confluent: great swelling at first, afterwards eruption shrinks, and becomes livid.
Apis	Erysipelatous redness and swelling, with stinging-burning pains, throat and skin. Absence of thirst. Urine scanty — later suppressed.

Anthracinum .. Gangrenous cases, with severe burning.

Arsenicum .. Great sinking of strength.
Burning heat: frequent small pulse.
Great thirst. Great restlessness.
Rash irregularly developed with typhoid symptoms.
Hæmorrhagic cases, or when pustules sink in, and areolæ grow livid.
Metastasis to mouth and throat.
Worse cold. (*Apis* worse heat.)

VACCINATION

Vaccination for most of us comes far more within the sphere of "practical politics" than does small-pox.

Homœopathy has a very great *antidote to vaccination, and remedy for the after effects of vaccination, in* THUJA. See "VACCINOSIS AND HOMŒOPROPHYLAXIS," by the late Dr. James Compton Burnett, which everybody should read.

At times babies, and "grown-ups" are made very ill indeed by vaccination, and here *Thuja* promptly puts them right — one has to see it to believe how promptly! — while the maturing pustules wither and leave no scar. At other times, persons are *simply blasted by vaccination*. Encephalitis is now recognized as one of the sequelæ of vaccination, resulting in some poor children in "Parkinson's disease," or in others, moral defects, which are probably never recovered from.

Therefore knowing that vaccine *pus,* may prove terribly destructive to health and well-being, it is well to have a drug at our command wherewith to antidote and restore — so far as restoration is possible.

But short of actual tragedies, perhaps irreparable, numbers of persons date their ill-health of skin, or nerve, — their years of headache, asthma, epilepsy, etc., to vaccination — or these may be found to date from vaccination — perhaps repeated — probably unsuccessful. For it is just the cases that do not "take" (i.e. react superficially) that seem more particularly to vitiate health. Burnett's "VACCINOSIS" must be reckoned with, as one of the Chronic Diseases which we have to treat.

For the ill-effects, acute or chronic, of vaccination, KENT (Repertory) gives: *Apis, Ars.,* MALAND., SIL., SULPH., THUJA.

Thuja ..   .. A direct antidote to the vaccinial poison.
            In acute cases, wipes out the fever and eruption, and causes the pustules to disappear.
            In chronic diseases, it may be impossible to cure many conditions of skin — nerve — etc., without *Thuja.* It acts like all the chronic remedies; and where symptoms improve to a point, and then always recur, while the disease can be traced back to a vaccination, or vaccinations, *Thuja* will generally supply the deep stimulus that leads to cure.

Malandrinum .. Nosode, prepared from "grease" in horses. Very like *Thuja* in symptoms and effects.

CLARKE says, "Burnett's indications are — Lower half of body: greasy skin and eruptions. Slow pustulation, never ending."

Silica .. .. The *Sil.* patient is feeble, lacks "grit," shrinks from responsibility.

Is chilly: sensitive to draughts, but enervated with very hot weather.

Head sweats at night. (*Calc.*) Sweaty, offensive feet.

Sulphur .. Warm patient. Hungry for everything: for fats.

Intolerant of clothing and weight of clothes.

Kicks off bedclothes: puts feet out. Eruptions of every kind.

Arnica .. Must not be forgotten. It does not destroy the vaccination like *Thuja* and *Maland.* but it has amazing power of taking away pain, swelling, and all inconveniences, while the process goes on to completion.

———

CHICKEN-POX

Aconite .. Early cases, with restlessness, anxiety and high fever.

Antimonium tart. Delayed or receding, blue or pustular eruptions.

Drowsy, sweaty and relaxed; nausea.

Tardy eruption, to accelerate it.

Associated with bronchitis, especially in children. (*Ant. crud.*)

Belladonna .. Severe headache: face flushed; hot skin.

Drowsiness with inability to sleep.

Rhus tox. .. Intense itching.

"Generally the only remedy required; under its action the disease soon disappears."

Mercurius .. "Should vesicles suppurate."

SHINGLES (HERPES ZOSTER)

Since Herpes Zoster seems to have some intimate connection with chicken-pox, it may as well come in here.

Ranunculus bulb.   One has over and over again seen shingles clear up rapidly with 2 or 3 doses of *Ran. b.* in high potency — 10*m*.
  Vesicles filled with thin, acrid fluid.
  Burning-itching vesicles in clusters.
  Worse from touch, motion, after eating.
  Severe, neuralgic pains, especially intercostal.

Variolinum   ..   BURNETT says: *Variolinum,* for him, has wiped the condition out, pain and all — and one has seen this also.

Mezereum   ..   With severe neuralgic pains.
  Itching, after scratching, turns to burning.
  Worse from touch: in bed.
  Vesicles from a brownish scab.

Rhus   ..   ..   "Probably no remedy oftener found useful in herpes zoster than this." — NASH.
  Especially when it occurs after a wetting.

  Case, "Golfer, got very wet, and a violent attack of shingles. *Rhus* cleared it up in a couple of days."

Arsenicum   ..   Confluent herpetic eruptions with *intense burning* of the blisters.
  Sleepless after midnight.
  Nausea and prostration: weakness.
  Worse from cold of any kind, better from warmth.
  "Herpes having a red, unwholesome appearance."

Apis   ..   ..   Burning and *stinging* pain, much swelling.
  Vesicles large, sometimes confluent.
  Comes out in cold weather.
  Ulcerate with great burning, stinging pain.
  Worse warmth: better cold applications (reverse of *Ars.*).

COMMON REMEDIES IN ERYSIPELAS
WITH INDICATIONS

Aconite   ..   Sudden violent onset after exposure to cold wind. Intense fever, with restlessness, and *fear of death*.

Belladonna   ..   Swelling, smooth, bright-red, streaked red; or, from intensity, deep, dark red.
Not much tendency to œdema or vesication.
Pains are throbbing; throbbing in brain.
Brain affected. Cases with delirium.
Jerking of limbs.
Belladonna is acute, *sudden,* and violent.
Belladonna is red, and intensely hot, dry.

Apis   ..   May be in patches. Great tumefaction.
High degree of inflammation, with *stinging, burning,* and *œdema* and vesication.
Eyelids like sacs of water.
Amelioration from cold: aggravation from heat.
Fidgety, nervous, fretted: sleepless.

Lachesis   ..   Purple, mottled, puffy: "not bloated, puffy."
"A marked remedy for erysipelas and gangrene.
"When the cerebral condition does not yield to *Belladonna.*" *Bell.* is red: *Lach.* gets *less red and more blue.*
Especially affects the left side.
Lachesis, typically, is worse after sleep: is loquacious — suspicious — jealous.
Is hypersensitive to touch, esp. on throat: wants face free, or suffocates.

Veratrum viride   "One peculiar symptom — characteristic — I have verified in a very severe case of erysipelas, which was accompanied by great delirium, is *a narrow, well-defined red streak right through the middle of the tongue.*" — NASH.
"Phlegmonous erysipelas of face and head." — CLARKE.

Rhus .. .. Erysipelas of the vesicular variety, accompanied by
restlessness.

Erysipelas of face with burning; large blisters, rapidly
extending: becomes very purple and pits on pressure.

Often extends from l. to r. across face.

Rhus is worse from damp: from cold: relieved temporarily, at least, by motion.

Cantharis .. Erysipelas of face with large blisters.

Burning in eyes: whole atmosphere looks yellow:
scalding tears.

Like *Rhus,* but when very violent, *Canth.* will be
indicated.

"*Rhus* has the blisters and the burning, but in *Canth.*
between your two visits the erysipelas has grown
black: it is a dusky rapid change that has taken
place, looks as if gangrene would set in. Burning
like fire from touch: as if the finger were a coal of
fire. Not so in *Rhus.*

"The little blisters, if touched, burn like fire. *Eruptions burn when touched.*" — KENT.

Erysipelas of eyes, with gangrenous tendency.

"Unquenchable thirst with disgust for drinks."

Euphorbium .. Vesicular erysipelas: erysipelas bulbosum.

*Red inflammatory swelling, with vesicles as large
as peas, filled with yellow liquid.*

Red, inflammatory swelling, with boring, grinding,
gnawing from gums into ear, followed by itching
and tingling.

Vesicles burst and emit a "yellow humour."

Shuddering and chilliness.

Temporary attacks of craziness.

Croton tiglium "*Erysipelas that itches very much.*"

"Eruptions that itch very much; but cannot bear to
scratch, as it hurts. A very slight scratch, a mere
rub, serves to allay the irritation." — GUERNSEY.

Sensation, "Insects creeping on face."

"Cough disappears and the eruption comes; then
eruption goes and cough comes back."

Mercurius   ..   *With salivation:* bitter or salt taste.

With offensiveness: breath, sweat.

Erysipelas with sloughing: with "brown mortification." With burning: ulceration.

Chilliness and heat alternately: or heat and shuddering at the same time.

Creeping chilliness: in single parts: in places of pus formation, or ulceration.

Worse at night.

Crotalus hor.   ..   Frequently recurring erysipelas of face.

General local phlegmonous, phlectenous or œdematous erysipelas. Skin bluish-red; low fever.

Gangrene: skin separated from muscles by a fetid fluid. Black spots with red areola and dark, blackish redness of adjacent tissues.

Crotalus is yellow, and hæmorrhagic.

"*Crotalus* is indicated in disease of the very lowest, the most putrid type, coming on with unusual rapidity, reaching that putrid state in an unusually short time." — KENT. (*Bapt.*)

Baptisia   ..   *Drowsy, dusky, comatose;* face dark-red, with besotted expression. May be roused, but falls asleep answering.

Typhoid conditions, in the course of disease.

Acts very rapidly; rapid collapse, and rapid restoration. (*Crot. h.*)

Arsenicum   ..   "Sudden inflammatory conditions like gangrenous and erysipelatous inflammations."

A sudden inflammation that tends to produce malignancy in the part, belongs to *Ars.*"

The secretions of *Ars.* are acrid.

Characteristic, *burnings relieved by heat:* intense *anxiety, restlessness* and prostration.

Secale   ..   Gangrenous erysipelas: competes with *Ars.* The only distinguishing feature between the two remedies may be that *Secale* wants cold and *Arsenicum* wants heat.

Burning: "sparks of fire" falling on the part.

Formication: "mice creeping under the skin."

Hippozæninum (Glanders)	"Malignant erysipelas, particularly if attended by *large formation of pus, and destruction of parts.* Ulcers with no disposition to heal, livid appearance." — CLARKE.

Thuja .. .. Œdematous erysipelas of face.

Cases that occur in the much vaccinated may need *Thuja,* or cases that occur *after vaccination.*

A curious, characteristic symptom, profuse sweat only on uncovered parts.

Cuprum .. Erysipelas of face disappears suddenly.

Eruptions "strike in" and cramps, spasms, convulsions supervene. To bring the eruption back, with relief.

Cramps begin characteristically in fingers and toes.

LESS SEVERE CASES

Arnica .. "Erysipelas of face, with *soreness,* and sore *bruised feeling* all over the body: you need not wait longer before prescribing *Arnica.*"

"Bed feels too hard; must move to get into a new place." "*Rhus* moves from restlessness and uneasiness, cannot lie still: *Arnica,* to ease the *soreness* by gettting into a new place." — KENT.

Pulsatilla .. Erysipelas in the *typical Pulsatilla patient.*

Mild, but irritable: changeable: weeps: craves sympathy.

Craves open air: cool air: worse for heat.

Not hungry or thirsty.

Graphites .. "Eruptions oozing out a thick, honey-like fluid . . . erysipelas sometimes takes this form, and in such cases recurs again and again." (*Sulph.*)

Erysipelatous, moist, scurfy sores.

Or, "Thin, *sticky,* glutinous, transparent watery fluid." — GUERNSEY, *Keynotes.*

Sulphur .. Recurrent attacks of erysipelas. (*Graph.*)

Much burning: worse from heat of bed or room. Purplish appearance. (*Lach.*)

"For erysipelas, as a name, we have no remedy, but when a patient has erysipelas and his symptoms conform to those of *Sulphur,* you will cure him with *Sulph.*" — KENT.

"When symptoms agree, *Sulph.* will be found a curative medicine in erysipelas."

The typical *Sulph.* patient is hungry, especially at 10 to 11 a.m. Loves fat, "Eats anything."

Kicks off the clothes at night, or puts feet out. Craves, or hates, or is worse for fats.

His eruptions itch; are worse for heat, for warm room, for warm bed: worse for washing.

Worse at night. Skin cannot bear woollens.

The untidy, ragged philosopher. Selfish.

"*Sulphur* may be given on a paucity of symptoms."

Ammonium carb. "Erysipelas of old, debilitated persons.

Eruption faintly developed, or has seemed to disappear, from weakness of patient's vitality to keep it on the surface.

With cerebral symptoms, simulating a drunken stupor." — NASH.

"Eruption comes out, and does not give relief to the patient."

"Erysipelas of old people when cerebral symptoms are developed."

Defective reaction.

Hepar .. .. Any trouble occurring on the skin, when there is *great sensitiveness to the slightest touch.* (Comp. *Canth.*)

Extreme sensitiveness runs through the whole remedy: to the slightest draught of air: to the slightest noise: and also mental sensitiveness and irritability — almost to murder, when angered.

SOME REMEDIES OF TYPHOID CONDITIONS
IN FEVERS: TYPHOID

Baptisia .. Typhoid fever. Typhoid conditions in fevers.
Rapid onset. Rapid course.
Abdomen distends early.
Odour horrible. Delirium.
Besotted condition: purple, bloated face.
Answers a word or two, and is back in stupor.
Feels there are two of him. Is scattered.
Tries to get the pieces together (*Pyrog.*).
In typhoid, "*Bapt.* vies with *Pyrog.* and *Arn.*"
N.B.—*In recent provings of* Bapt. *on examination of the blood, the typical typhoid agglutination was found to occur.*

Pyrogen .. (BURNETT's great remedy for typhoid.)
Bed feels hard (*Bapt.*).
Great restlessness: must constantly move (*Rhus*), to relieve soreness of parts (*Arn.*).
Tongue (typically) clean, smooth, fiery-red; or dry and cracked.
Horribly offensive diarrhœa (*Bapt.*).
Sense of duality (*Bapt.*).
Pulse quick: or out of proportion to temperature.

Rhus .. .. "Fevers take on the typhoid type: triangular red-tip-ped tongue and restlessness."
Cannot rest in any position (*Pyrog.*).
Slow and difficult mentation. May answer correctly. Talks to himself.
Refuses food and medicine. Fears poison (*Hyos., Lach.*).
Dreams of strenuous exertion.

Arnica .. Says she is "So well!" when desperately ill.
Can be roused, answers correctly, then goes back into stupor (*Bapt., Phos. a.*).
"I am not sick: I did not send for you: go away!"
Foul breath — stool. Hæmorrhagic tendency.
"Bed feels so hard" (*Bapt., Pyrogen*).
"So sore," can only lie on one part a little time: restlessness *from this cause.*
Involuntary and unnoticed stools and urine.

Taraxacum ..	Restlessness of limbs with tearing pain. "Like *Rhus* only *mapped tongue*."
Bryonia ..	A most persistent remedy: develops slowly.
	Lacerating, throbbing, jerking headache.
	Nausea and disgust, whitish tongue.
	Bitter taste. Thirst for large draughts of cold water (*Phos.*).
	"Nervous, versatile or cerebral typhoid."
	Sluggishness, then complete stupefaction.
	When roused, is confused: sees images.
	Thinks he is away from home and wants to be taken home.
	Irrational talk: *prattles of his business:* worse after 3 p.m.
	Delirium apt to start about 9 p.m.
	Wants to be quiet. Pain, limbs, when moving.
	Tongue dry.
	Easily angered.
	Faint if sits up.
Arsenicum ..	Rapid sinking of strength: great emaciation.
	Least effort exhausts.
	Great restlessness: constantly moves head and limbs: trunk still, because of extreme weakness. Tongue dry, brown, black.
	Face distorted, hippocratic, sunken, anxious.
	Rapid sinking of forces: extreme prostration.
	ANXIETY: RESTLESSNESS: EXHAUSTION.
	Thinks he must die. (*Arn.* says he is "not ill.")
	Worse 1 — 2 a.m. and p.m.
	Cadaveric aspect: cadaveric smelling stools.
	Thirst for cold sips (rev. of *Phos., Bry.*).
Phosphorus ..	Abdomen distended, sore, very sensitive to touch (*Lach.*).
	Worse lying left side: better, right.
	Stools offensive, bloody, involuntary. *The anus appearing to remain open* (*Apis.*).
	Burning in stomach: burning thirst for cold water. Ices: ice cream (*Ars.* burns, > heat).
	Fear alone: in the dark: of thunder.
	Especially useful in typhoid pneumonias.
	Suspicious. (*Lach*),

| Lachesis | .. | Loquacity: delirium with great loquacity. |

Lachesis .. Loquacity: delirium with great loquacity.
Face puffy, purple, mottled.
Much rumbling in distended abdomen.
Clothing cannot be tolerated: must not touch abdomen or throat.
Tongue swells (*Crot. h.*): difficult to protrude.
Suspicious. "Trying to poison her!" (*Rhus.*).
Worse after sleep: sleeps into aggravation.
Cold, clammy (*Crot. h.* cold, dry).
Stool with dark blood.

Terebinth .. Tongue bright-red, smooth, glazed (*Pyrog.*).
Extreme tympanitis (*Phos. acid, Phos.*).
Thick scanty urine: mixed with blood, or cloudy, smoky, albuminous.
Diarrhœa with blood intermixed.
Fresh ecchymoses in great numbers (*Arn.*).

Crotalus hor. .. Typhoid with decomposition of blood and hæmorrhages — anywhere.
Intestinal hæmorrhage; blood dark, fluid, non-coagulable.
Tongue fiery-red, smooth, polished (*Pyrog.*), intensely swollen.
Yellowness of skin is an indication for *Crot. h.*
"*Lach.* cold and clammy: *Crot. h.* cold and dry."
Attacks that come on with great rapidity (*Bapt., Hyos*).
Rapidly increasing unconsciousness. Besotted appearance (*Bapt.*).
Typhoid when it becomes putrid.
"Diseases of the very lowest, the most putrid type, coming on with unusual rapidity."

Phosphoric acid "One of our best remedies in typhoid."
Simultaneous depression of animal, sensorial and mental life from the start.
Slowly increasing prostration.
Advanced typhoid.
Lies in stupor, unconscious of all that goes on: but if roused is fully conscious (*Arn., Bapt.*).
Glassy stare, as if slowly comprehending.
Prostration. Tympanitic abdomen.

Phos. acid (cont.)	Dry brown tongue (*Ars.*). Dark lips. Sordes.
	Bleeding; nose, lungs, bowels (*Crot. h.*).
	Jaw drops: "as if must die of exhaustion."
Hyoscyamus ..	Fevers rapidly become typhoid (*Bapt., Crot. h.*).
	Sensorium clouded.
	Staring eyes: Carphology. Picks bedclothes.
	Teeth covered with sordes.
	Tongue dry, unwieldy, rattles in mouth, so dry.
	Involuntary stool and urine (*Phos., Arn.*).
	Subsultus tendinum.
	Mutters, or says no word for hours.
	Mentally very suspicious: refuses medicine, thinks you will poison him (*Rhus., Lach.*).
	Jealous (*Lach.*). Alternately mild and timid, then violent. Will scratch, and try to injure.
	Exposes person (*Phos.*). Wants to be naked.
	Talks to imaginary people: to dead people.
	Illusions: hallucinations; talking, with delirium, then stupor.
	Busy with wall paper, or imaginary things which he puts in rows, and leads like toys.
	Early can be roused: later complete unconsciousness.
Muriatic acid ..	"Also one of our best remedies in typhoid."
	Tongue dry, leathery, shrunken (*Hyos., Ars.*).
	Muscular prostration comes first, mind remains long clear (reverse of *Phos. acid*).
	Lower jaw drops. Slides down in bed from excessive weakness. (*Phos. acid*).
	Cannot urinate without the bowels also moving.
	"Nearer to *Carbo veg.* than any other remedy."
Carbo veg. ..	"A sheet-anchor in low states of typhoid, in the last stages of collapse; where there is coldness, cold sweat, great prostration; dyspnœa — wants to be fanned. Cold tongue."
	"Desperate cases. Blood stagnates in the capillaries."
	Blueness — coldness — ecchymoses.
	Can hardly breathe, air-hunger. Says "Fan me! Fan me!"
	Hæmorrhages, dark, decomposed, unclotted (*Crot. h.*).
	Indescribable paleness face and body."

SOME REMEDIES OF VERTIGO
WITH INDICATIONS

Conium   ..   A very great remedy of vertigo — *of its kind*.

Vertigo, *turning or moving head, turning eyes*.

Sensation of turning in a circle.

Lying, *as if bed turned in a circle*. Vertigo on turning eyes when lying.

Vertigo turning in bed: looking around: —

When rising from a seat: —

When watching moving objects.

Cannot endure the slightest alcoholic drink.

Curious symptom: sweats, day and night, on closing eyes.

Sanguinaria   ..   Dizzy: *cannot turn quickly* without fear of falling.

Vertigo with long-continued nausea and headache: then spasmodic vomiting.

With sensation of some hard heavy substance in stomach.

Vertigo on quickly turning head: looking up: lying down: during sleep.

Rush of blood to head with dizziness; feels sick and faint: would fall if she rose from sitting.

(One of the "sick-headache" remedies.)

Vertigo in cold weather.

Aconite   ..   Vertigo: *on rising up from lying;* red face becomes deathly pale; or, becomes dizzy, falls: and fears to rise again; with nausea.

Vanishing of sight, or unconsciousness.

Vertigo from fall or concussion: after a fright: anxious as if dying: must lie down.

Vertigo from congestion, as in the sun (*Bell.*): on stooping: staggers to right.

Ailments with anxiety and restlessness.

"Aconite is a great storm and soon over."

"A woman runs up suddenly against a dog and becomes violently dizzy. Vertigo that comes on from fear: from sudden fear."

Bryonia   ..   Vertigo, rising; from a seat, or from lying.

Dizzy and faint from raising head.

Worse from least motion.

Vertigo and confusion on least motion.

Typically, tongue dry: constipation with hard dry stools.

Thirst for large drinks. White tongue: irritable. Better left alone.

Curious symptoms, sinking with, or through bed. (Comp. *Thuja.*)

Tendency to run backwards. (Comp. *Camph. monobrom.*)

Nux   ..   Vertigo: *rising from seat or bed.* (*Acon.*, etc.): or raising head (*Bry.*).

Vertigo with vanishing of sight and hearing:

At night, wakes him from sleep.

After stooping: when looking up: must clutch something to avoid falling.

Objects seem to move round him.

Falls forward — to one side — backward.

As if brain turning in circle: room whirling.

Reeling in a.m.; after dinner; red, hot face, vision obscured: staggering.

From digestive disturbances; constipation; sedentary habits; alcohol; smoking; smell of flowers, gas; from mental over-exertion. (Comp. *Phos.*)

Nux, typically, is irritable: oversensitive: drowsy p.c. Chilly if uncovers or moves.

Better for sleep. Red face.

Belladonna   ..   A remedy of *suddenness*: of *violence.*

Has quickness of sensation: of motion.

Pains come and go suddenly.

Blood goes to head, with vertigo.

Vertigo with pulsations in head, dilated pupils, nausea.

As if being rocked: when lying down: *as if bed bounced her up and down.*

When stooping: at night: turning in bed: with every change of position.

As if sinking with, or through bed (*Bry.*, comp. *Thuja*).

Belladonna (cont.)   Tends to fall to left, or backwards.
Objects sway to and fro.

Phosphorus   ..   Vertigo: *looking upwards, downwards.*
On rising from a seat: on moving head.
Sensation, as if looking down.
Chair seems to rise with him.
Sensation, as if would fall forwards.
Staggers while walking. Everything turns.
Worse lying on left side.
Worse mental exertion: smell of flowers (*Nux*).
Typical *Phos.* tall, thin; craves cold drinks: ices: salt.
Fears thunder, the dark: being alone.

Natrum   Vertigo *with flickering before eyes.* Objects turn
   muriaticum ..   round.
Tends to fall forward.
After coffee, tea, alcohol, tobacco (*Nux*).
From straining eyes or close study.
Typical *Nat. mur.* weeps, but no one must see: sad,
   reserved. Craves salt.

Opium   ..   Great vertigo *compels him to lie down.*
As if *all went round in a circle with him.*
Giddy intoxication: staggers hither and thither.
Vertigo from injuries to head: after fright.
As if flying or hovering in air (rev. of *Bry.*, etc.).
Fainting turns with vertigo, rising from bed: with
   return of animation on lying down.

Secale   ..   Vertigo: constantly increasing: stupefaction.
Reeling: inability to stand upright.
Head, esp. occiput, feels light (*Gels.*, rev. of *Tabac*).
   Unsteady gait.
Typical *Secale* is emaciated, withered, wrinkled; with
   unhealthy skin.
Externally icy-cold; yet burns internally.
Numbness; tingling; crawling; cramping.

Onosmodium ..   *Fears to look down,* lest she fall down (Comp. *Gels.*)
   that she might fall into fire: "in spite of all his will
   power, did fall into fire."
Inco-ordination. Misjudges distances.
Staggering. Feels as walking on cotton.
Curious symptom: *headache worse in the dark.*

Camphor
  monobromide
Feels he is journeying in one direction when actually
  moving in the opposite.
Imagines that he is turned round, going north instead
  of south.
Feels he is going in wrong direction: though house
  numbers show he is not.

China   ..
Dizziness and fainting after loss of blood.
Vertigo, head tends to sink backwards: worse moving
  and walking: better lying down.

Salicylicum
  acidum   ..
Vertigo, tends to fall to left side, while surrounding
  objects seem falling to right.
Auditory nerve vertigo. (Menière's disease.)
Comes and goes from no known cause.
Noises in ear. (?) deafness.

Lycopodium ..
Nausea: *everything turning round*: dreads falling.
Vertigo while drinking: *in hot room* (*Puls.*): rising
  for seat: from bed. Reels back and forth.
Gets hot, face reddens, eyes dim and watery.
Flatulence and distension: has to loosen clothing
  about waist. Worse cold drinks.
Lyc. has the 4-8 p.m. aggravations.

Dulcamara   ..
Momentary vertigo, with darkness before eyes.
At noon, before eating, while walking, giddy, *as if
  all objects remained standing* before him, and as if
  it became black before eyes.
On rising, almost fell: with weakness and trembling.

Tabacum   ..
Vertigo: *excessive heaviness of head* (rev. of *Secale*).
Qualmishness stomach: deathlike paleness of face:
  weakness, to loss of consciousness.
Better in open air, and by vomiting.
Vertigo on rising, and looking upwards.
From immoderate smoking of cigars (*Nux*).
Excessive vertigo *with copious* (*cold*) *sweat*.
Deathly nausea with violent vomiting: worse least
  movement. Worse opening eyes.

Gelsemium . .	*Head feels light and large,* with vertigo.

Dizziness with blurring of vision: gradually increasing. Spreads from occiput over head: pupils dilated (*Bell.*); sight dim: from heat of sun, or summer.

Seems intoxicated when trying to move.

Worse from smoking (*Nux*).

Giddiness, with loss of sight, chilliness, quick pulse: double sight.

Muscles refuse to obey will: giddy: confused; loss of co-ordination.

Sensation of falling. Child clings to nurse, or crib: screams with fear of falling (*Borax*).

(Case: child with this fear of falling: must hold to something firm — not even to her mother.

After *Gels.* she was climbing trees.)

Ferrum . . Face fiery red (Comp. *Bell.*), feet cold: with vertigo *worse rising from lying or sitting* (*Acon.*).

From walking over a bridge, or by running water, or riding in car or carriage.

Argentum metallicum . . Crawling and whirling in head, as if drunken.

When *looking at running water,* is giddy.

Or when crossing running water. (Comp. *Con.*).

Argentum nitricum . . Vertigo *looking at high buildings.*

Has great fear of high places.

Craves sugar and sweets, which disagree.

Pulsatilla . . Excessive — violent vertigo like intoxication: as if one had turned round in a circle a long time: with nausea.

Worse sitting; lying. Better walking in open air: — or the opposite, "as a secondary or alternating state" (rev. of *Sulph.*).

Vertigo caused by indigestion: with vomiting p.c.

Vertigo when turns eyes upwards: as if would fall: as if dancing. Better in cold room.

Stooping: could scarcely raise herself again.

Typical *Puls.* is changeable, weepy, exacting, irritable — the *wind-flower*.

"A remedy of many uses (polycrest)."

Ceanothus am.   Violent vertigo, on lying down and then turning over to right side.

Everything turning violently to right: has to cling to sides of bed.

Chelidonium ..   Vertigo: with bilious vomiting: with pain in liver.

With confusion: stumbling, as if to fall *forwards*.

On closing eyes, as if *everything turned in a circle.* (Comp. *Con., Apis.*) On sitting up in bed.

With shivering, upper part of body.

On attempting to rise. Keeps him in bed.

Giddiness on waking, with indigestion.

Typical *Chel.* has *pain under angle rt. scapula.*

Tongue coated thickly yellow with red edge: tooth-notched.

Desire hot drinks: hot milk. (*Phos.* cold.)

Apis   ..   Vertigo *on closing the eyes*: worse sitting than walking, extreme when lying and closing the eyes (*Chel.*).

Typical *Apis* is intolerant of heat: thirstless: has relief from cold.

Ailments from jealousy, fright, rage.

Silica   ..   Vertigo: to fainting: with nausea.

Vertigo *creeping up spine into head*.

Tends to *fall forward*: worse motion: looking up. Staggering.

Worse closing eyes (*Chel., Apis*): lying on right side (*Phos.* worse lying on left).

Vertigo *during sleep*.

On closing eyes all things turn with him: passes off on opening them.

Vertigo as if moving to and fro in head.

Vertigo with retching: water comes from mouth.

Better riding in open air: worse back in room.

"As if head were teeming with live things whirling around it."

Silica patients lack "grit"—"Sand".

Are worse for cold: head and feet sweat—ailments from suppressed foot-sweat (? foul).

Sulphur ..	Much troubled with dizziness. When *he goes into the open air,* or *when he stands* any length of time, he becomes dizzy.

On rising in the morning his head feels stupid, and on getting on his feet he is dizzy.

Not rested by sleep: "things go round". "Takes time to establish an equilibrium."

Worse from sleep and from standing.

Vertigo lying on back.

After lying a quarter of an hour, whirling vertigo, as if would faint.

Typical *Sulphur* is the "ragged philosopher": unkempt: argumentative.

Agaricus .. "Vertigo and confusion of mind are mixed up."

Vertigo when walking *in open air (Sulph.)*: reeling: great sensitiveness to cold air.

Objects whirling: tends to fall forward.

Better by quickly turning the head (rev. *Con.*).

Cannabis indica .. Vertigo on rising, with *stunning pain back of head,* and he falls

Heavy pressure on brain, must stoop.

(Typically) *Cann. ind.* has exalted sensations: with exaggeration of time and distance.

Sensation of calvarium opening and shutting: as if brain boiling over and lifting cranium like lid of tea-kettle. (Comp. *Cocc.*)

Cocculus indicus .. Vertigo: *things go round: whirl from right to left;* with confusion; with nausea.

Whirling vertigo: worse *rising from lying.*

Nausea to fainting with severe vertigo.

Sick-headache with vertigo and nausea: from riding in carriage, boat, train, car.

(Sea-sickness *Tab.*)

Head, abdomen, chest "empty and hollow".

Hot, flushed face.

Extreme aversion to food: nausea from smell of food (*Colch., Sep., Ars.*) but with hunger.

Inco-ordination: tremor: prostration.

"Occiput opens and shuts" (Comp. *Cann. ind.*).

Petroleum   ..   Vertigo: *in occiput*: as if intoxicated: like sea-sickness.

Obliges him to stoop: more violent when standing than sitting (Comp. *Puls.*). Goes all over him, makes him numb and stiff.

Digitalis   ..   Vertigo from cardiac weakness (*Ars., Hydrocy. acid, Camph., Verat.*).

Severe vertigo *with very slow pulse.*

With anxiety, as if she would faint.

On rising from sitting: limbs weak.

Constant dizziness with ringing in ears.

·   "As if heart would stop if she moved" (*Gels.* must move to keep it beating).

Pulse full, irregular, slow and weak; intermits.

Cyclamen   ..   A curious *"transparent vertigo"* — to coin an expression.

On waking in a.m., or on rising, looking ahead, any object — say a wardrobe — is seen whirling unsteadily, and flickering away to the side (? right side); while all the time, through the whirl, the same object is seen standing solid and immovable.

Cycl. has promptly cured.

Sensation of brain moving within cranium.

Vertigo: *objects turn in a circle,* or about her, or make a see-saw motion: when walking in open air.

"Visual effects, or vertigo."

Baptisia   ..   A *rapid* septic state.

Stupid: prostrated: looks besotted.

Swimming sensation: worse stooping and noise.

Confusion as if drunk.

Vertigo with paralysis of eyelids.

Feels scattered about: can't get the pieces together (*Pyrog., Petr.*).

Ailanthus   ..   Dizzy: face hot: cannot sit up: drowsy but restless and anxious. In malignant scarlet fever, diphtheria, etc.: with stupidity and mottled skin.

SOME COMMON REMEDIES FOR HEADACHE

*Natrum
muriaticum*

"One of our best remedies for chronic headaches."

"The headaches are awful: dreadful pains: bursting, compressing as in a vice: as if skull would be crushed in."

"Little hammers in the head as soon as moves: on waking in a.m."

May begin at 10 or 11 a.m., last till 3 p.m. or evening. *Periodic,* every day, or third or fourth day.

Better sleep: must go to bed and be perfectly quiet (*Bry.*). Intermittent fever headaches, *after much malaria and quinine.*

Relief from sweating: or relief to all but head from sweating. (*Gels.* has > from copious urination.)

May begin with fiery zigzags (*Sep.*).

Beware of *Nat. mur.* when acute and violent: it may needlessly increase the suffering: give its "acute" *Bry.*: and after the paroxysm, *Nat. mur.*

Characteristics. Weepy (*Puls.*) but no one must see. Emotional to pathetic things, books, plays. Worse, or anger from consolation. Aversion to bread, fats: desire for salt. A crack in middle of lower lip (*Sep.*).

Sepia .. ...

Headaches nervous, bilious, periodic, violent.

Better lying and quiet: often cured by sleep, even a short sleep (*Phos.*).

Relief from lying down, or from violent motion (slow *Puls.*). Long walk in open air that warms her, relieves.

Worse stooping, coughing, jarring, light, thinking. Better hard exercise or a tight bandage, or applied heat: but worse hot room.

Occipital headaches, loathing of food: then nausea and vomiting: then sleep and wakes without it. Headache with nausea: worse smell of food. Fiery zigzags (*Nat. mur.*).

In the *Sepia* patient: characteristically sallow with brown patches. Indifferent: wants to get away and be at peace. Hates fuss.

Aconite .. "The headaches can scarcely be described, they come with such violence.

"Tearing, burning in brain, in scalp, *with fear, with fever, with anguish.*"

Fullness and heaviness in forehead, as if an outpressing weight there: as if all would be forced out at the forehead. (Compare *Sulph., Bell.,* down one nostril *Borax.*)

Throbbing in left forehead with strong beats in right side by fits.

Skull constricted by a ligature (*Sulph.*).

Acon. is sudden: wild: worse from cold winds; with restlessness, anguish, fear.

Belladonna .. Headaches of great violence.

Congestion: red, hot face: dilated pupils.

Violent throbbing in brain . . . and carotids.

Violent shoots and cutting stabs.

Jerking headache: worse walking, going up stairs. At every step jerked downwards like a weight in occiput.

Cutting knife-stabs and shoots.

Bursting pain: as if brain would be pressed out: worse stooping, as if brain would fall out, push forward: or eyes would drop out.

Worse noise, jar, motion, light, lying: better pressure.

Rush of blood to head.

Violent headaches, *better for drawing head back.*

Headache with dizziness: worse stooping.

Headache from washing the head.

Bell. headaches come suddenly, last an indefinite time, and depart suddenly.

CASE. — A little maid would come down at night, "Oh! my head! my head!" — frantic with pain: her hands held out quiveringly before her. A dose of *Bell.* and, in a few minutes, suddenly, "It's gone!" and off she would go happily to bed. (A case of cerebral tumour, as it turned out: but showed the wonderful palliative action of *Belladonna.*)

Another case: — boy, after exposure to a very hot sun, got a terrific headache, with very high temperature. *Bell.*: and well by next day. (Compare *Glon.*)

Glonoin .. Very like *Bell.*: perhaps "more so".

Upward rushes of blood (*Bell.*).

Waves of terrible, bursting, pulsating headache. ("A tempestuous remedy.")

Worse bending head back (*reverse* of *Bell.*).

A great remedy for sunstroke (*Bell.*).

Worse for having hair cut (*Bell.*, head washed).

Can't bear heat about head.

Throbbing head: holds it with both hands.

Brain too large: full: bursting: throbs at every jar, step, pulse (*Bell.*).

Head hot: face flushed — purple or bright red.

"Skull too small: brain will burst it."

Waves of pain: and brain seems to move in waves.

CASE. — Youth, after an appalling smash (motor bicycle) skull fractured: terrific, unbearable pain in head for which he implored morphia. Got *Glonoin* instead, and never asked for morphia again. Its effect was magic.

Melilotus .. Congestion to brain equal to *Bell.* and *Glon.*

Intense redness of face: throbbing carotids.

Better for profuse epistaxis.

Lachesis .. Violent congestion to head: with vomiting and loss of sight. Almost delirious with headache.

Throbbing, bursting pains in head (*Bell., Glon.*) as if all the blood of body had gone to head.

Sun-headaches, of the more chronic type (*Bell., Glon.* for the very acute violent "sunstroke" headache). Chronic headaches whenever exposed to the sun. Worse heat.

Pressure on vertex: relieved by pressure: often extending to root of nose.

Sleeps into the headache: dreads to sleep, as wakes with such a distressing headache (*reverse* of *Phos.* and *Sepia*). Headaches from suppressed discharges — nasal, uterine, etc. Relief from their reappearance.

Characteristics. Loquacity; or great slowness. Intolerance of pressure, especially on throat and abdomen. Left-sided ailments; may cross to right side.

Cocculus ind. ..   Headache as if skull would burst: or like a great valve opening and shutting.

Sick-headaches with vertigo.

Thought or smell of food nauseates (*Ars., Sep., Colch.*): makes the patient gag.

"Train sickness" with nausea and vertigo.

Effects of night-nursing and loss of sleep.

On motion, eyes as if being torn from sockets: or head empty and hollow: or constriction.

Pulsative pains, vertex or temples.

Headache, occiput and nape, pain as if opening and shutting like a door.

Worse eating, drinking, sleeping: better rest indoors.

Slow in answering.

Least jar unbearable (*Bell.,* etc.).

Crotalus
   cascavella ..   Skull compresses brain like an iron helmet.

Something alive walks in a circle in the head.

Head and chest compressed by iron armour.

A red-hot iron stuck into vertex.

Acute lancinations right temple (many of the pains are lancinating).

Shocks in head, almost throw her off balance.

Headache after sleep (*Lach.*).

Headache, epistaxis and great excitement, caused by starting from sleep.

Great coldness: icy feet.

Crot. casc. has peculiar hallucinations.

"This terrible serpent . . . whose poison acts with frightful intensity."

Gelsemium ..   Congestive headache: most violent in occiput.

Every pulsation, "a hammering base of brain".

Lies high, exhausted and paralyzed with pain.

Later, whole head congested. One grand pain too dreadful to describe; lies bolstered up in bed, eyes glassy, pupils dilated, face mottled, extremities cold.

Or, neuralgic headache, temples and over eyes, with nausea and aggravation from vomiting.

Relieved by copious urination, i.e. urine, scanty, becomes free, and headache subsides.

A great influenza medicine.

Phosphorus .. Congestive and throbbing headaches.
Better from cold: worse from heat. Worse motion; better rest; but worse lying down.
Phos. is chilly and worse from cold; yet needs cold for his stomach and head: craves ices or quantities of ice-cold water.
Headaches most violent; with hunger, or preceded by hunger. With red face: scanty urine.
Violent neuralgic pains also; darting, tearing, shooting.
Periodic headaches: from mental exertion: with stiffness of face and jaws.
Worse noise, light; becoming heated.

Pulsatilla .. Throbbing, congestive headaches.
Head hot, better for cold applications.
Better slowly walking in open air.
Headaches connected with menses: or from suppressed menses.
Periodic sick headache: vomits sour food.
Headache from over-eating: from ice cream.
Thirstless: easily weeping: changeable.
Must have air; better motion. Worse heat.

Apis .. .. Pain, occiput, with occasional sharp shrieks.
Pains like bee-stings, with the thrust and the burning pain following.
Brain affections of children with sudden sharp shriek (*Crie cerebrale*). Bends head back, or bores in pillow.
Thirstless: sweat without thirst: scanty urine: piercing screams sleeping or waking.
"Bruised all over," sensitive to touch.
Worse heat: warm room: hot bath. Better cold room: cold air: cold applications.
"Alternately dry and hot, then perspiring."

Chamomilla .. A little headache seems an enormous thing.
Congestive headaches.
Pressing, bursting pain, worse thinking of it.
Irritable: capricious: over-sensitive to pain. *"Cannot bear it."*
Face red and hot on one side, pale the other.

Mercurius   ..   Congestion, head: feels it will burst: fulness of brain: constricted by a band: as if in a vice, with nausea: worse at night.

Burning in head, especially left temple: worse at night.

Headache over nose and round eyes, as if tied with a tape, or tight hat pressing.

Sensitive to air: worse cold, damp: violently worse in a draught.

Better in room: worse in cold or warm room.

Wants to be covered, but worse from heat.

Dirty offensive tongue and mouth: offensive sweat.

Catarrhal, rheumatic or syphilitic headaches.

China   ..   ..   Congestive headaches: extremities covered with cold sweat.

Stitches from temple to temple.

Pain from one temple to the other: from occiput over whole head.

Intense throbbing headache;

Brain beats in waves against skull (compare *Glon.*).

"As if head would burst" (*Glon.*).

After loss of fluids, hæmorrhages, etc.

Ringing in ears.

Worse draught; open air; sun; touch; better from hard pressure.

Nux vomica   ..   Headaches connected with gastric, hepatic, abdominal or hæmorrhoidal troubles.

"Congestive and abdominal headaches."

A nail driven into brain (*Thuja, Ruta*): stitching pains with nausea and sour vomiting.

"As if skull would split" (*Cocc.*).

Headaches on waking: on rising: after eating: in open air: on moving eyes.

Headaches of sedentary persons: after coffee.

Irritable, vehement disposition.

Oversensitive and touchy.

Better head wrapped up: covered: lying down: warmth and heat (Compare *Sil.*): warm in bed: in damp warm weather.

Iris versicolor .. "One of our best remedies for sick-headache."

Sick-headaches of gastric or hepatic origin: always begin with a blur before eyes.

Nausea and vomiting: burning of tongue, throat, œsophagus and stomach.

Profuse secretion of ropy saliva. (Compare *Kali bich.*)

Vomit ropy, hangs like strings from mouth.

Watery stools: anus feels on fire.

Vomiting spells *every month or six weeks*.

Sanguinaria .. Sick-headaches (*Iris.*).

Pain starts occiput, spreads over head to right eye (*Sil.; Spig.,* left) with nausea and vomiting.

Periodic sick-headache: *every seventh day* (or third).

Sun-headache, starts morning, increases all day, lasts till evening.

With chills, nausea, vomiting of bile.

Feels head must burst (*Merc., Chin., Glon., Bell.*).

Better lying down in the dark: better sleep.

Vomits bile, slime, yesterday's food, then relief and sleep.

Palms and soles burn: puts feet out of bed (*Sulph., Puls., Cham., Medorrh.*).

Circumscribed redness of cheeks.

Sulphur .. Burnings: vertex: palms: soles. Everywhere.

Heaviness in head, stooping, moving, even when sitting and lying.

"Tight hat" sensation. And headache from pressure of hat; better head uncovered.

Throbbing, beating, hammering: rush of blood to head, and pressure, as out of eyes.

Periodic sick headaches: congestive: with stupefaction, nausea and vomiting.

Sick-headache once a week or two weeks — the characteristic *seven-day aggravation*.

"The Sunday headache of working men."

Worse motion, eating, drinking.

Red engorged face, eyes red, engorged.

The characteristic *Sulph.* patient is hungry: starving about 10 a.m.; loves fat; cannot stand long; untidy: argumentative.

Cedron   ..   Attacks of headache occur with *clock-like regularity*.
        Head felt as if swollen.
        Sick-headache every other day at 11 a.m.

Arsenicum   ..   *Periodic headaches:* every other day — every fourth
        day — seventh day — fourteenth day. Malarial head-
        aches.

        Ars. is very chilly and needs warm clothing, but *with
        congestive headache* wants body warm and head
        bathed in cold water; "blankets to the chin, and
        head out of the window". (Compare *Phos.*)

        But *Ars. neuralgic headaches* need to be wrapped up
        and kept warm.

        Head, and physical symptoms alternate.

        Congestive headaches, throb and burn, with restless-
        ness and anxiety: hot head and relief from cold.

        Headaches with nausea and vomiting. Sick-headaches
        of the worst sort; with thirst for little and often.

        Dreadful occipital headaches; stunned and dazed:
        they start after midnight, or from excitement.

        With head symptoms, head in constant motion.

        Ars. is *restless: anxious; prostrate,* and characteristic-
        ally, very fastidious (*Nux*).

Argentum met.   *Precisely at the hour of noon* many troubles come on.
        Headaches, etc.

        Violent neuralgias one side at a time, deep in brain,
        involving one half of brain.

        Painful sensation of emptiness in the head.

        Pressing, burning pain in skull, *every day at noon*.

        Gradually the pain gets more violent, then *ceases sud-
        denly.* (*Bell.* sudden onset and sudden cessation.)

        Often, old history of suffering from heat of sun (*Nat.
        sul.*).

        "All the nervous excitement that is possible in rem-
        edies comes up in this remedy."

Spigelia .. "Sun-headaches." Start every morning with sunrise: get worse till noon: gradually decrease till sun sets: —this even on cloudy days.

Pains from occiput to eyes, especially left, which waters (*Sang.; Sil.,* to right).

Worse from all movement (*Bry.*): noise: jar.

Stitching, shooting, burning pains: like hot needles (*Ars.*).

Very violent neuralgia, followed by soreness.

Very violent heart-action is characteristic of *Spigelia.*

Intolerable pain in eyeballs: feel too large for orbits (*Lycopersicum*); sensitive to touch.

Stitching pains.

Bryonia .. *Worse from any motion.* Cannot bear any disturbance, mental or physical.

Cannot sit up in bed.

Bursting, or splitting, or heavy crushing headache: worse any movement.

Fronto-occipital headache.

Nausea or faintness rising or sitting up: better lying still.

Irritable: thirsty: dry lips and mouth.

Vehement and quarrelsome.

Pain in head from coughing: grasps head when going to cough. Worse straining at stool.

Headache after washing with cold water when face was sweating: "from ironing".

Rush of blood to head. Epistaxis.

Worse from slightest motion: after eating.

Eupatorium perf. Sick headache: on waking: lasts all day.

Pain and weight occiput: must use hand to raise head. "Terrible sick headaches."

Pains throbbing, shooting, darting, thumping.

Painful soreness of eyeballs.

Malarial and influenzal headaches, with aching and breaking sensations in bones and joints.

Eupatorium promptly cured a case of influenza, with soreness in bones and a headache so intense that she dared not move a hand, as the slightest movement made the pain intolerable (*Bry.*).

Silica .. .. Chronic sick-headaches with nausea, even vomiting.
Begins nape of neck, goes forward over vertéx to eyes,
especially right eye (left, *Spig.*).
Better pressure: better lying: *wrapping head up
warmly*: tying head up tightly. *Better applied heat.*
Better profuse urination. (*Gels.*)
Silica is chilly, yet sweats much, especially face and
feet. Offensive foot sweat.

Calcarea .. *Icy coldness in and on head:* on vertex.
Heaviness in forehead.
Stunning, pressive pain in forehead.
Tearing headache above eyes down to nose.
Semilateral headaches with empty risings.
Head numb, as if wearing a cap (*Sulph.*).
But in the *Calc.* patient "Fat blondes who sweat easily:
especially head, neck, chest, during sleep."
Cold, damp feet (*Sep.*).
Chilly: lax muscles.
Profuse head-sweats during sleep (*Sil.*).
Worse milk.

Veratrum alb. .. *Head feels as if packed in ice. Feels as if ice lay on
vertex and occiput.*
Troublesome neuralgic headaches of great violence.
Violent pains drive to despair: great prostration, fainting, cold sweat and great thirst.

CASE. — Elderly woman with violent, unendurable pains in head.
Almost out of her mind: utterly changed in appearance and mentality.
Sensation of *ice on vertex* suggested *Verat. alb.,* which gave rapid relief
and cured.

Heloderma .. Very violent headaches: pressure as if skull too full
(*Bell., Glon., China, Merc., Sang.*): as of a tumour
forming and pressing inside skull.
Burning in brain: or sensation of a cold band round
head.
Characteristic. *Intense, arctic coldness:* internal coldness, *as if being frozen to death from within outwards.* Coldness at heart, as if being frozen to death.
Cold rings round body: cold waves.

Arnica .. .. Burning in head — in brain, the rest of the body being cool.

Aching pain over eyes, to temples; as if integuments were spasmodically contracted.

Great shoots in head from coughing, sneezing.

Cutting in head, as from a knife; then coldness.

Effects of injuries to head; of concussion.

After cerebral hæmorrhages.

Arn. feels *bruised and beaten*; says "bed too hard".

Epiphegus .. Headache when "tired out". Better for a good sleep (*Phos., Sep.*)

Characteristic: constantly wants to spit: saliva viscid.

Argentum nit. Constitutional headaches from brain fag.

Hemicrania. Feeling of expansion, as if head were enormously enlarged.

Better tied up tight.

Wants cold air, cold drinks, cold things.

Craving for sweets: sugar, which disagree.

Strange notions and impulses.

Psorinum .. Always hungry during headache. (Compare *Phos.*), but the antithesis of *Phos.* in appearance.

"*Hungry headaches*" may alternate with cough.

If goes without a meal, has a headache.

Fulness vertex as if brain would burst out.

Not room in forehead for brain, in a.m.; better after washing and eating.

A chilly edition of *Sulph.* Typically, looks dirty: "offensive to eye and smell". "No amount of washing will make him look clean."

Anthracinum .. Headache, "as if a smoke with a heating pain was passing through head" (*Fumee de douleur chaude*).

Head is affected in an indescribable manner.

Dullness: confusion: dizziness: loss of consciousness.

If conscious complain of great pain in head.

Rhus .. .. Headache, as if stupefied: as if intoxicated.

As if brain loose and falls against skull.

Weight in head: stooping, a weight falls forward into forehead, drawing head down.

Must hold head up straight to relieve this.

On waking and opening eyes gets violent headache: first occiput then occiput-temples.

Brain loaded, loose, torn, fluctuating; as if much blood shot into it when stooping.

Worse from wetting head (Bell.), from cold; damp: getting wet when perspiring (Dulc.).

Thuja .. .. As if a nail were driven into vertex: into right parietal bone: into left frontal eminence (*Rumex*).

Severe stitches in left temporal region.

Boring-pressing in head.

Pulsation in temples.

Heaviness in head: cross and disinclined to speak.

Dull, stupefying headache: worse stooping: better bending head back.

Worse from tea: from onions.

Has cured the most severe and chronic headaches, after repeated *vaccinations*.

THE MORE COMMON REMEDIES IN APOPLEXY
WITH INDICATIONS*

Arnica   ..   "Chief remedy, because of its great power to produce absorption of extravasated blood."

Stupor with involuntary stool and urine.

Paralysis — especially left side.

Pulse full and strong.

Head and face hot: body cool.

Falls into a deep stupor while answering.

Sore, as if bruised. Restless because bed feels so hard. Bedsores form rapidly.

Characteristic symptoms. Horror of instant death, especially at night (*Acon.*).

Says he is "well" when desperately ill (*Opium.*).

Fear of being touched.

Aconite   ..   Congestion, often apoplectic. Apoplexy.

Head hot. Pulsation of carotids. Pulse full, hard, strong (*Arn.*).

Especially after fright or vexation: or in cold dry weather (high barometer).

Dry hot skin. Arterial tension.

Often, one cheek red and hot, the other pale and cold. Looks frightened (*Stram.*).

Burning headache, as if brain agitated by boiling water. Fullness, as if everything would push out of forehead.

If conscious, terror, anxiety, agonizing fear.

Glonoine   ..   "Throbbing headache *seems to arise from neck* is characteristic: no mere sensation — visible in carotids. The vessels are full to bursting, and if walls unhealthy, there is danger of apoplexy." — NASH.

"Violent pulsations, upward rushes of blood. Waves of terrible bursting pulsating pain in head." — BOGER.

Worse heat: shaking: jar (*Bell.*).

Throbbing in front of head.

Pressure and throbbing in temples.

"Skull too small: brain trying to burst it."

* *Grouped for intensity or for comparison.*

413

Belladonna ..   Apoplexy: flushed, hot, bloated face: dilated pupils; a fixed, threatening look. Nausea. Threatening apoplexy: rush of blood to head (*Glon.*). Pulsation of cerebral arteries: THROBBING inside head.

The pain worse leaning forward, better bending back. Worse stooping: light: JAR.

"Head will burst!"

Pressure, especially in forehead: eyes as if starting from their sockets.

Pain comes suddenly, lasts indefinitely, ceases suddenly.

First stage apoplexy where severe congestive symptoms are present; or later, when extravasation causes inflammatory reaction. Violent delirium with intense redness, burning. Especially in plethoric, vigorous intellectuals.

"The more congestion in *Bell.*, the more excitability: the more the congestion in *Opium*, the less the excitability." KENT.

(*Bell.* craves lemons, *Stram.*, > vinegar.)

Opium ..   Comatose sleep, with rattling and stertor.

Red, bloated face.

Eyes blood-shot and half open. Jaw drops.

Skin covered with hot sweat.

Cheeks blow out with every expiration.

There is no response to light, touch, noise or anything else, except the indicated remedy, which is *Opium*. NASH.

Characteristics: Abnormal painlessness. (Compare *Arn.*, *Stram.*)

Bed feels so hot, cannot lie on it. (*Arn.*, bed so hard.)

Veratrum viride   Congestive apoplexy: cerebral hyperæmia.

Sudden cerebral congestion. Intensely congestive headaches.

Becomes stupid: thick speech; slow, full, *hard* pulse.

Convulsions from intense congestion of brain.

Ringing in ears: bloodshot eyes: dim vision, with nausea and vomiting.

Millefolium .. All the blood seems to ascend to head.

Nose bleed; excessive congestion to chest and head.

Confused: especially in evening: knows not what he is about.

At night a stream from chest to head, like a gust of wind, with nose bleed.

Apoplexy.

Violent headache: strikes head against wall.

Worse stooping. (Compare *Bell*.)

Red face (? without heat).

Bryonia .. Rush of blood to head: heat in head.

Fullness, heaviness, forehead, as if brain were pressing out.

Worse moving head, or eyes: better closing eyes: *better pressure*.

Vertigo and confusion on slightest motion.

Nose bleed.

Apoplexy.

Natrum sulph. As if forehead would burst: especially p.c.

Brain feels loose, when stooping: as if it fell towards left temple.

Base of brain as if crushed in a vice: something gnawing there.

Especially after injuries to head.

Indescribable pain vertex, as if it would split.

Worse from damp.

Natrum carb. Head feels too large: as if forehead would burst (*Nat. sul.*).

Headache from slightest mental exertion.

Worse from sun: heat.

Chronic effects of sunstroke.

Strontium carb. Threatened apoplexy with violent congestion of head. Thickened arteries.

Hot, red face every time he walks.

Exertion increases circulation towards head.

Smothering sensation, heart.

Cannot rest.

Better wrapping head, cannot bear least draught of air.

Headache, better wrapping head warmly (*Sil.*).

Nux .. Apoplexy in drunkards: of high livers.

Falls unconscious: tends to fall backwards.

Face pale: head hot: automatic motions of right hand to mouth.

Whole left side paralysed and motionless (*Lach., Arn.*).

Mouth distorted: loss of speech: stertor.

Jaw drops. Legs cold, without sensation.

Attack preceded by vertigo: buzzing in ears: nausea, urging to vomit.

Attacks after a hearty dinner; abuse of liquor or coffee: of high livers, leading an easy life.

Paralysis, especially of lower limbs.

When spoken to open eyes, stutters, and sinks again to sleep. Eyes muddy, with purulent matter in canthi.

Pulse quick, hard, or full, sluggish.

Organs of deglutition and lower limbs completely paralyzed. Maxilla right side relaxed.

Crotalus horridus   Apoplectic convulsions.

Apoplexy in hæmorrhagic or broken down constitutions; or in inebriates.

Softening of brain, etc., or apoplexy following toxæmic states.

Fevers from septic absorption.

Hæmorrhages from every part of body.

Yellow colour of whole body.

Broken-down constitutions.

Occipital ache, in waves from spine. (Comp. *Glon.*)

Right side, and worse lying on right side.

Lachesis .. *Purple, puffy face*, with convulsive movements. Blowing expiration (*Op.*). Paralysis *especially of left side.*

Preceded by absence of mind: rushes of blood to head: throbbing, burning: worse vertex.

Face spotted, or purple: eyes engorged: looks suspicious (*Hyos.*).

Suffocation and strangling: cannot bear touch on throat, or anything near mouth.

Rouses from sleep with suffocation, dyspnœa, violent pain back of head. Worse heat, *worse sleep,* loquacity, suspicion, belong to *Lachesis.*

Cocculus .. Headache as if skull would burst: or like a great valve opening and shutting. (Comp. *Actea*.)

Pain as if opening and shutting in occiput and nape.

Apoplexy: violent headache, from vertex to left forehead and nose.

With nausea and inclination to vomit.

Whirling vertigo.

Inco-ordination. Numbness.

Loathing of food — thought, smell of food.

"Attack preceded by vertigo, nausea, convulsive motions of eyes, paralysis, especially of lower limbs, with insensibility."

Actea racemosa Brain as if too large: pressing from within outwards.

Rush of blood to head: brain feels too large for cranium.

An opening and shutting sensation, when moving head and eyes. (Comp. *Cocc.*)

Top of head as if it would fly off, worse going upstairs.

"Vertex opens and lets in cold air." (Comp. *Cocc.*)

Aurum met. .. Rushes of blood to head with violent palpitation.

Sparks before eyes: glossy, bloated face.

Intense pain in head: especially in syphilitic patients.

The *Aurum* patient looks on the dark side: is weary of life: loathes life: suicidal.

Absolute loss of enjoyment in everything.

Ipecacuanha .. "Apoplexia nervosa et serosa: vertigo: drooping of lips: impaired speech; dribbling of saliva: paralysis of extremities.

"Headaches, as if bruised all through bones of head, down to root of nose, and roots of teeth, with nausea and vomiting.

"Nausea, distressing, constant; not relieved by vomiting.

"Loose rattle in chest.

"No thirst.

"*Ipec.* is a great stopper of bleeding." KENT.

Phosphorus .. Apoplexy: suddenly fell unconscious. Life apparently extinct: pulse and resp. lost.

Face red, but, like body, cool to touch.

Irresponsive to all stimuli.

Apoplexy: grasps at head: mouth drawn to left.

Heaviness, dullness, confusion in head.

Hyperæmia of brain: heat, vertex: buzzing and throbbing in head: swelling under eyes.

Congestion up spine to head: burning, stinging, pulsations; begin in occiput.

Thirst for cold drinks.

Worse lying left side: alone: in twilight and in the dark.

Sees "things coming out of corners".

Stramonium .. Apoplectic seizures: paroxysms of syncope, with stertor. Bloody froth at mouth. Dark brown face. Lies on back with open, staring eyes. Fetches breath with great difficulty. Paralysis after apoplexy: spasmodic drawing of head to either side. One side twitches, the other paralysed. (Compare *Hell*.)

"An absolute stand-by in renal convulsions."

"*Stram.* has more violent delirium. *Hell.* is more stupid."

Helleborus .. Stupor complete or partial. Unconsciousness.

Lies on back, eyes partly open: or wide open and insensible to light.

Rolling head: bores into pillow.

Automatic motion of one arm and leg. (Compare *Stram*.)

Answers slowly, if at all: appears semi-idiotic.

Greedily swallows water: bites the spoon.

Chewing motions of mouth.

Apoplexy followed by idiocy.

Gelsemium .. Threatened or actual apoplexy with stupor, coma, and nearly general paralysis.

Intense passive congestion to head.

Headaches with nausea, giddiness, staggering.

Brain tight: eyelids and limbs heavy.

Great weight and tiredness, body and limbs.

Face purple, mottled. "The trembling remedy."

Speech incoherent, stupid, forgetful.

Pulsatilla   ..   Throbbing, pressive headache, worse pressure. (Better pressure, *Bry*.)

Congestion of blood to head: stinging pulsation in brain, especially when stooping (*Bell*.).

Puls. is worse from heat: craves fresh cool air.

Weeps. Craves sympathy.

Sulphur   ..   An old homœopathic doctor, who had recovered from several cerebral hæmorrhages, used to say, "Mind! first *Arnica* and then *Sulphur,* for apoplexy." The *Sulphur* patient is lean, lank, hungry, dyspeptic.

Rush of blood to head: burning vertex with cold feet.

Nux moschata   Stupor and insensibility. Comatose condition.

Apoplexy: A case: woman of 80. Comatose condition for nine weeks, after thrombosis. Coma increased till it was almost impossible to feed her. *Nux mosch*. 200, promptly brought back consciousness; she went on to complete recovery — and lived another five years, in full possession of her senses.

Zincum   ..   Followed *Nux mosch*. in the above case, and seemed to quickly re-establish the reflexes, and restore motion to the paralyzed limbs.

Kent says: "When reflexes are abolished then *Zinc*. comes in."

Causticum   ..   "Paralysis from apoplexy: not for immediate results, but for remote symptoms when, after absorption, paralysis persists on opposite side of body."

Baryta carb.   ..   Complaints of both ends of life.

Especially adapted to apoplexy of old people, or tendency thereto. Mental and physical weakness. In persons addicted to alcohol.

Serious apoplexy, loss of speech, trembling limbs.

Absent minded.

Has no clear perception.

SOME COMMON REMEDIES FOR SLEEPLESSNESS
WITH INDICATIONS

Aconite   Restlessness: excitement: tossing: fear: anguish: fear of death. Sudden chill in cold, dry weather.

Especially useful after chill: shock: fright: operation. But in any illness the *Aconite* condition may come on at night, when *Acon.* will give peace and sleep.

Chamomilla   Sleepy, but cannot sleep (*Bell.*). Restless.

If he sits down by day, wishes to sleep, but if he lies down, is unable to sleep.

Pain that comes on at night, so violent that he cannot keep still: in a child, it wants to be carried: an adult, gets up and walks the floor.

Pains that drive him out of bed at night, with twitchings of limbs.

As soon as bedtime comes, is wide awake: is sleepless and restless, especially early night.

Chamomilla is irritable; capricious; uncivil. Frantic with "cannot bear it!" — in adults and *teething babies.*

Staphisagria   "Doctor, if I ever have a dispute with a man, I come down with nervous excitement, sleeplessness: headache."

Child wakes, pushes everything away, and wants everybody to go away: restless, as from frightful dreams; calls for mother often.

Calcarea   Sleepless from many thoughts crowding mind: or mind turning on same thought: from mortification at trifles.

The same disagreeable idea always rouses the sick as often as they fall into a light sleep.

Cold feet at night in bed.

Head sweats in sleep, wetting the pillow.

"Especially helps the real leucophlegmatic constitutions, with large head, large features, pale skin with chalky look and, in infants, open fontanelles:" (and delayed dentition).

Coffea   ..   The kind of lively sleeplessness some persons experi-
                    ence after drinking coffee.

                      Sleeplessness from coffee: — also:

                      Simply wide awake. Unusual activity of mind and
                    body. Full of ideas, i.e. cannot sleep.

                      From sudden emotions, pleasant surprises, exciting
                    or bad news. (Comp. *Cypreped.*)

Cyprepedium ..   Sleeplessness: with desire to talk, or with crowding
                    of pleasant ideas.

                      Children wake and are unnaturally bright and play-
                    ful, with no desire to go to sleep again.

Pulsatilla   ..   "Sleep before midnight is prevented by a fixed idea: as
                    a recurrent melody."

                      Wide awake in the evening, does not want to go to
                    bed; first sleep restless: sound sleep when it is time
                    to get up. (Compare *Nux.*)

                      Sleepless from orgasm of blood: after late supper, or
                    eating too much; from ideas crowding in mind.

                      Weeping because she could not go to sleep.

                      Characteristic: Sleeps with arms over head.

                      The *Pulsatilla* patient is changeable: weepy: mild and
                    yielding. (Reverse of *Nux.*)

Nux   ..   Insomnia after mental strain: abuse of coffee, wine,
                    alcohol, opium or tobacco.

                      Sleeplessness from excessive study late at night.

                      Sleepy in the evening, hours before bedtime: awakes
                    at 3 or 4 a.m.; ideas crowd on him: then falls into
                    a dreamy sleep at daybreak from which he is hard
                    to rouse: wakes tired.

                      All complaints worse from morning sleep.

                      Nux is irritable and hypersensitive.

Sulphur   ..   Irresistibly drowsy by day: wakeful at night.

                      Sleepy in evening; but night full of unrest.

                      Tosses, nervous, excitable; orgasm of blood.

                      Cannot go to sleep for great flow of thoughts with
                    inclination to perspire.

                      Wakes at 3, 4, 5 a.m., and cannot sleep again. If
                    does sleep later, cannot be roused. Gets his best and
                    soundest sleep late in morning.

                      Soles burn at night: puts feet out (*Cham., Puls.,
                    Med.*). Worse warmth of bed (*Merc.*).

Arnica   .. Too tired to sleep.

Bed feels too hard: and part laid on too sore; must move to try for relief.

After exertion and strain, physical or mental.

Cocculus   .. From vexation, grief, anxiety, and prolonged loss of sleep.

Worn out and exhausted, and when the time has come for sleep cannot sleep.

Ill-effects from long nursing and from night watching. Slightest loss of sleep tells on him.

Extreme irritability of nervous system.

Rhus   .. Restless at night: has to change position frequently. (Comp. *Arnica*.)

Sleepless: could not remain in bed.

Sleepless *from pain*: has to turn often for ease.

Arsenicum   .. Sleeplessness after midnight.

Sleeplessness with restlessness and moaning.

Tossing: uneasiness: anguish (*Acon*.).

Attacks of anxiety drive him out of bed.

Despair of life: fear of death: thinks it near.

Sleepless from anguish, restless: tossing: worse after midnight.

From climbing mountains, or other muscular exertion: want of breath, prostration, cannot sleep.

Nocturnal sleeplessness, with agitation and constant tossing.

Ars. is anxious, restless, usually chilly; fastidious. Constant thirst for small sips.

Thuja   .. Persistent sleeplessness.

Restless sleep, with frequent rising from bed, and much talking. < by moonlight (*Sil*.).

If he slumbers for a moment he dreams about dead people.

Sees apparitions on closing eyes, disappear when they are open, reappear as soon as they are closed (*Spongia*.).

After vaccination, or re-vaccination.

Spongia .. Very short sleep, with many dreams. Wakes at midnight, but cannot sleep again on account of restlessness; whenever he closes his lids the most vivid pictures would immediately arise before his vision, while waking: it seemed to him as if a battery of guns were discharged, or as if everything were in flames; again scientific objects forced themselves upon his mind: in short a mass of subjects crossed each other in his imagination, disappearing at once when he opened his eyes, but reappearing so soon as they were closed.

Awakens in a fright and feels suffocating (*Lach.*).

Lachesis .. Has some of its most characteristic symptoms in regard to sleep.

All symptoms are worse after sleep.

Afraid to go to sleep; or the mother afraid to let the child sleep (croup, convulsions, etc.).

As soon as he goes to sleep, the breathing stops; cannot go clear off to sleep, because just on the verge of it he wakes catching for breath (*Spong.*).

Sleeps into an aggravation.

Awakens at night and cannot sleep again.

Could not sleep on account of strangulation.

Persistent sleeplessness. Sleepless from anxiety.

Afraid to go to sleep for fear he will die before he wakes.

Wakes in a fright: worse after sleep.

Nothing must touch throat: bedclothes must be lifted from abdomen at night.

["I once had a very obstinate case of constipation . . . he was at last taken with very severe attacks of colic. The pains seemed to extend all through the abdomen, and always came on at night. After trying various remedies until I was discouraged, he let drop this expression: 'Doctor, if I could only keep awake all the time, I would never have another attack.' I looked askance at him. 'I mean', said he, 'that I sleep into the attack, and waken in it.' I left a dose of *Lachesis* 200. He never had another attack of the pain, and his bowels became perfectly regular from that day and remained so. I could give more cases where this symptom has led me to the cure of ailments of different kinds." NASH.]

Silica   ..   Sleepless from ebullitions, orgasm of blood.

Night sweats.

Somnambulism: esp. at new and full moon.

Argentum nit.   Prevented from falling asleep by fancies and images.

Wakes wife or child, for someone to talk to.

Arg. nit. has irresistible desire for sweets and sugar, which disagree.

Feels the heat. Full of weird apprehensions.

Belladonna   ..   Sleepy yet cannot sleep.

Uneasy sleep before midnight: child tosses, kicks and quarrels in sleep. Twitches.

Restless sleep with frightful dreams.

Skin dry and hot to touch: face red. Dilated pupils. Quick sensations and motions.

Fear of imaginary things: sees ghosts, animals, hideous faces. (Comp. *Thuja, Spong.*)

Stramonium   ..   Sleep full of turmoil and dreams.

Sleepy, but cannot sleep (*Bell., Cham., Opium*).

Desires light and company: cannot bear to be alone: worse in dark and solitude.

Cannot go to sleep in the dark: but soon falls asleep in a lighted room.

Hyoscyamus   ..   Intense sleeplessness of excitable persons from business troubles; often imaginary.

From nocturnal, spasmodic cough: < lying down, > sitting up. Diseases with increased cerebral activity, but non-inflammatory.

"The sleep is a great tribulation to this nervous patient: times of sleeplessness: then again, profound sleep."

Sleepless: or constant sleep. . . .

Lying on back suddenly sits up, looks all round, wonders what terrible thing he has been dreaming about. Sees nothing: lies down again. He keeps doing that all night.

Starts up: jerks: cries out: grits teeth: laughs in sleep.

Hyocyamus is jealous and suspicious (*Lach.*) and has much delirium.

Opium .. .. Sleepy but cannot sleep. (*Bell., Cham.*)

Sleepless, *with acuteness of hearing*. Distant clocks striking and cocks crowing keep him awake.

Bed so hot she cannot lie on it: moves to find a cool place (*Sulph.*). (Bed too hard, moves to relieve soreness of parts lain on, *Arn.*)

Sleepless, full of unwelcome fancies and imaginations . . . as in delirium.

Capsicum .. Sleepless from emotions, *homesickness,* cough.

Great drowsiness after eating.

Characteristic: — "Homesickness: with red cheeks and sleeplessness."

Bryonia .. Restless: could hardly sleep for half an hour; and when slumbering was continually busy with what he had read the previous evening.

Sleeplessness before midnight, with thirst, heat, ebullitions: with frequent shivering sensation of one arm and foot: then sweat.

Delusion, "away from home and wants to go home".

Cactus .. .. Sleeplessness from suffocative constriction (*Lach.*) and palpitation.

Ignatia .. Sleepless from grief, care, sadness.

Baptisia .. Restless from 3 a.m. Tosses about. Head and body feel scattered about the bed.

Abies nigra .. Sleepy by day: sleepless at night.

Indigestion with sensation of undigested hard boiled egg in stomach.

Allium sat. .. Sleep prevented by *thirst.*

Selenium .. Sleeps in cat-naps: (*Sulph.*) Wakes often: roused by slight disturbance.

Hungry in the night.

Plumbum .. Sleepiness by day: sleepless at night: from colic.

Inclined to take strangest attitudes and positions in bed.

Phosphorus .. Sleepy all day, all night restless: awakened by vivid dreams.

Sleeplessness before midnight.

Sleeplessness with drowsiness.

Phos. has fears alone, in the dark, of something creeping out of the corners.

Sepia .. .. A great remedy for sleeplessness in the *Sepia* patient: dull and indifferent: chilly, yet craves air. Hates sympathy and fuss. Often, with weariness and sagging of internal organs.

Mercurius .. Sleepless at night; on account of anxiety, ebullitions and congestions; from itching: from seeing frightful faces. Frequent waking.

Falls asleep late: wakeful till 3 a.m.

As soon as he went to bed, pains recommenced and banished sleep.

Night sweats.

Lueticum .. Sleepless nights: dreadful nights. All the sufferings are *worse at night*.

INDICATIONS FOR THE CHIEF REMEDIES IN
COLLAPSE

Carbo veg. . . *An almost "corpse-reviver"* (as one has seen).

Lack of reaction after some violent shock, some violent attack, some violent suffering.

After surgical shock, collapse; and danger of dying of shock.

Air-hunger: desire to be fanned: must have more air.

Cold:—Knees cold: breath cold: tongue cold: cold sweat: cold nose.

Nose and face pinched; cadaveric.

Face: very pale: greyish-yellow; greenish; corpse-like.

May be distension of stomach and abdomen (*Colch.*).

Veratrum alb. . . . Wonderful coldness: coldness of discharges: coldness of body.

Profuse cold sweat: cold sweat on forehead.

Fluids run out of body; produces watery discharges.

Lies in bed, relaxed and prostrated, cold to finger-tips: blue, or purplish: lips cold and blue: face pinched and shrunken: sensation as if the blood were ice-water (*Ars.*).

Head packed in ice: ice on vertex.

One of Hahnemann's great cholera medicines.

Opium . . From fright. Shock from injury (*Arn.*), severe cases.

Rapid breathing: every breath a loud moan: face livid or pale; lips livid. Cool clammy skin: eyes fixed unequally:—or,

Long, slow expirations; cheeks blown out: or mouth wide open.

Coldness, extremities; or burning heat of perspiring body.

Characteristics: "painlessness, inactivity and torpor".

Increased excitability of voluntary muscles with decreased excitability of involuntary muscles.

Arnica .. From mechanical injuries (*Opium*). Concussion, with unconsciousness, pallor, drowsiness.

Cold surface; depressed vitality from shock.

Stupor with involuntary discharges.

Characteristic: — While answering falls into a deep stupor before finishing.

Camphor .. Coldness, blueness, *scanty sweat*. Scanty discharges (rev. of *Verat.*).

"*Camph.* is cold and dry. Cold, with profuse discharges, *Verat.*"

"*Camphor* is heat, wants to be covered up: his coldness is relieved by cold: wants more cold.

"A troublesome patient to nurse: the more violent the suffering, the sooner he is cold, and when cold must uncover and be in a cold room: then a flash of heat, and he wants covers on, wants hot bottles: and while this is being done, is cold again, and wants windows open, and everything cool.

"Here the camphor bottle has established a reputation*": but potentized camphor will do far more, and will put him into a refreshing sleep." KENT.

Arsenicum .. The collapse of *Ars.* is marked by restlessness, and fear. *Prostration with awful anxiety.*

"The prominent characteristics of *Ars.* are *anxiety, restlessness, prostration, burning,* and *cadaveric odours.*

"In bed, first moves whole body; as prostration becomes marked, can only move limbs. At last so weak, he lies quiet, like a corpse.

"Every symptom is *Arsenic*: he looks like it, acts like it, smells like it, and *is* it.

"Mouth black, parched and dry.

"Ceaseless thirst for small quantities often.

"With his violent chills and rigors, says the blood flowing through his veins is like ice-water (*Verat.*) then fever comes, and he feels that boiling water is going through his blood-vessels." KENT.

* N.B. — *Camphor* may need to be repeated every five minutes in desperate cases, till reaction is established. A couple of drops on a lump of sugar is the best way to administer it — or in potency.

Aconite   ..   Agonized tossing about. Excessively restless.

Extreme anxiety (*Ars.*). Expression of fear and anxiety; especially *fear of death*.

Condition *sudden and violent*.

After exposure to cold, dry, wind.

Sits straight up and can hardly breathe: grasps throat: wants everything thrown off.

Anguish with dyspnœa.

As if boiling water poured into chest: warm blood rushing into the parts. (Comp. *Ars.*)

Compare *Ars.* all through: but *Ars.* comes far on in the condition, with *terrific exhaustion,* instead of *terrific violence.*

Antimonium tart. Asphyxia: from mechanical causes, as apparent death from drowning, from pneumonia, capillary bronchitis, etc., from accumulation of mucus which cannot be expectorated.

Impending paralysis of lungs.

Drowsiness or coma, pale or dark-red face; blue lips: delirium; twitchings.

Thread-like pulse.

Ammonium carb. Skin mottled, with great pallor. Face dusky, puffy.

Lack of reaction: livid, weak and drowsy.

Increasing shortness of breath: better cool air. Rattling in chest, but gets up little.

Weak heart, causing stasis, dyspnœa, etc.

Cold sweat: tendency to syncopy.

"One of the best remedies in emphysema."

Œdema of lungs with somnolence from poison of blood with CO_2.

Sputa thin, foamy: a dynamic state: with rattling of large bubbles in chest.

Vehement palpitation with great precordial distress, followed by syncope.

Audible palpitation: great anxiety as if dying, cold sweat: invol. flow of tears: loud, difficult breathing, with trembling hands.

Angina pectoris (*Latrodect, mact.,* etc.).

Exhaustion with defective reaction.

Hysteria; symptoms simulate organic disease.

Carboneum sulph.

Kent gives *Carb. sulph.* in black type for collapse.

Frequent attacks of fainting, asphyxia.

Violent headache till mind is affected.

Sunken, staring eyes.

Expression bewildered, as if demented.

Pushed lower jaw forward, and gnashed with it against the upper.

Great thirst: great desire for beer.

Colic about umbilicus, drawing navel in (*Plumb.*).

Asphyxia from alcohol, or coal gas.

Feeling of heavy load hanging on back between scapulæ.

Sensation of vibration and trembling of whole body.

Heard voices and believed he had committed a robbery. Sensation of a hole close by, into which he was in danger of falling.

Colchicum ..

Sinking of strength, as if life will flow out from motion or exertion.

If he attempts to raise head, it falls back, mouth wide open.

Tongue heavy, stiff (? bluish, especially at base).

Bruised, sore, sensitive: *nauseated by smell or thought of food.*

Vomiting. Profuse diarrhœa and passage of blood. Stool involuntary.

Great distension of abdomen: — tympanitic.

Restlessness: cramps in legs.

Great prostration, skin cold, bedewed with sweat: cold sweat forehead (*Verat.*).

Respiration slow.

But, "without the fearfulness and dread of death of some such remedies".

Crotalus hor. ..

Rapidly becomes besotted, benumbed, putrid, semi-conscious.

Prostration almost paralytic in character.

Skin yellow, pale, bloodless with blue spots.

Rapid breaking down of blood-vessels.

SOME REMEDIES FOUND USEFUL IN SUNSTROKE
WITH INDICATIONS

Glonoinum   ..   Bad effects from being exposed inordinately to sun's
Glonoine   rays:
(Nitro-glycerine) "For over-heating in the sun, or sunstroke."

"Sudden local congestions, especially to head and
chest.

"Bursting headache, rising up from the neck.

"Great throbbing: sense of expansion, as if head would
burst.

"Cannot bear the least jar." NASH.

Undulating sensation in head:

Waves of heat, upwards.

Head feels larger.

Congestions; blood tends upwards.

Vessels (jugular, temporal) pulsate.

Temporal arteries raised, felt like whipcord.

Throbbing: constriction neck, as if blood could not
return from head.

Sensation of strangulation in throat (*Lach.*).

Whole head felt crowded with blood.

All arteries in head felt as distinct as though they had
been dissected out.

Skull too small: brain attempting to burst it.

Even nausea, followed by unconsciousness.

"*Bell.* and *Glon.* both have the fullness, pain and
throbbing, but that of *Glon.* is more intense and
sudden on onset; and subsides more rapidly when
relieved.

Bell. is better bending head back: *Glon.* worse." NASH.

Glon. has waves of pain, of blood, upwards.

Glon. has more disturbance of heart's action: *Bell.*
more intense burning of skin.

Both have very red faces (*Mel.*).

Melilotus   ..   Fearful headaches.
Sweet Clover   Confusion of thought.

Violent congestion to head.

Violent *throbbing* headache, relieved by nosebleed.

Most intense redness of face with throbbing carotids.

Belladonna ..   Also (with *Glon.*), sudden onset.

Red, flushed face: throbbing carotids: perhaps delirium, spasms, jerks and twitchings.

Eyes staring, red, bloodshot: pupils first contracted, then greatly dilated.

Skin very red and hot: "When you put your hand on a *Bell.* subject, you want to suddenly withdraw it; the heat is so intense." KENT.

Rush of blood to head: pulsation of cerebral arteries; throbbing in head.

Inflammation of base of brain and medulla from exposure to sun.

Bell. absolutely covers the text-book description of sunstroke — even at its worst: i.e. restlessness; vertigo: breathlessness; nausea and vomiting; with frequent micturition ("even if only a few drops have accumulated"). Temperature high.

Incontinence of urine and fæces.

Stertor. Pulse rapid.

Face congested: cyanosed: and (of course) convulsions.

Aconite ..   Where there is much FEAR, restlessness, and anxiety.

"Sunstroke, especially from sleeping in the sun's rays."

Head excessively hot (*Bell.*): with burning, as though brain were moved by boiling water.

Boiling and seething sensations.

High fever. Vertigo.

Face very red (*Bell., Stram., Melilotus*): feels as if it has grown much larger (*Nat. carb.*).

Tingling sensations exceedingly characteristic.

One of the remedies of apoplexy: of heat apoplexy.

Acon. is one of the remedies of sudden, violently acute, painful conditions.

Amyl nitrate ..   Heat and throbbing in head. Intense fullness in head.

Intense surging of blood to face and head (*Glon.*) as if blood would start through the skin.

Can't endure warmth: must throw off coverings and open doors and windows

Difficulty of breathing is a very prominent symptom.

Camphor   ..   Sunstroke, with restlessness and depression of spirits.

Contraction, tightness in head, *with coldness all over.*

Throbbing (head) with beats like a hammer; head hot, face red, limbs cool. (Comp. *Arn.*)

Rush of blood to head.

"The more violently the patient suffers the sooner he is cold, and when he is cold he must uncover, even in a cold room."

"Then, with a flash of heat, wants the covers on, and hot bottles." KENT.

Veratrum   ..   Sudden cerebral congestion: sunstroke.
viride

Prostration: accelerated pulse.

Head full and heavy.

Intense cerebral congestion: as if head would burst open.

Congestive apoplexy: intense headache; stupid: ringing in ears; bloodshot eyes; thick speech: *slow,* full pulse, hard as iron.

? nausea and vomiting. ? convulsions.

Worse warm drinks.

Face, cold, bluish; covered with cold sweat. Or, face flushed.

Characteristic; tongue (? white or yellow) *with a red streak down the centre.*

Cactus   ..   "Constrictions, contractions, congestions: the blood is always in the wrong place."

Vertigo from congestion: face red, bloated.

Irregularities of respiration: if he holds his breath, it seems as if his heart would fly to pieces. Increased pulsations also over body when holding breath.

Violent headaches; intense heat of head;

As if top of head would be pressed in, relieved by pressing hard on the pain.

Sounds go through the head.

Threatened apoplexy when congestion is so violent; face flushed and purple, or very red; pulsation felt in brain and all over. Choking as from a tight collar. (Comp. *Lach.*)

Cactus (cont.)   The great characteristic, constriction about heart, as if held in a vice, a wire cage; screwed tighter and tighter.

Gelsemium .. From heat of sun in summer.

Weakness and *trembling*, of any part, or the whole body.

Headache, begins in cervical spine: with bursting sensation in forehead and eyeballs. Worse from heat of sun.

Sensation of a band around head above eyes.

Great heaviness of eyelids.

Lachesis .. *Lachesis* has also a reputation for sunstroke, or effects of sunstroke.

"Paralysis depending on an apoplectic condition of brain, after extremes of heat or cold."

Face: dark red, *bluish;* bloated, as in apoplexy.

Great characteristic: worse from SLEEP.

Sleeps into an aggravation.

Dreads to go to sleep, because she wakes with such a headache.

Rush of blood to head: weight and pressure on vertex.

Great sensitiveness to touch, especially throat and abdomen.

Stramonium .. Face very red: blood rushes to face.

Congestion to head: beating of carotids.

Rushes of blood to head, with furious, loquacious delirium.

After sunstroke tormenting heat in head: pain nape of neck: very sensitive to noise, to contradiction.

NASH gives a *Stramonium* mental case, in a woman of 30, who had been over-heated in the sun, during an excursion. She was "lost, lost, lost, eternally lost," and begged minister, doctor, everybody to pray with and for her. Talked day and night about it. She would not sleep a wink, or let anybody else sleep. Said her head was as big as a bushel . . . *Glonoine, Lachesis, Natrum carb.*, etc., prescribed on the CAUSE as the basis of the prescription, were useless. But *Stramonium* covered her symptoms, and in 24 hours every vestige of that mania was gone. She had narrowly escaped the "Utica Asylum".

Arnica   ..   *Arnica* may be needed. Apoplexy; loss of consciousness.

Here the great characteristic, in any sickness, is, intense soreness and bruised feeling of body.

EVERYTHING ON WHICH HE LIES FEELS TOO HARD.

Must move, to get a new place, not yet sore.

Heat of upper part of body; coldness of lower.

Face and head alone hot: body cool (*Camph.*).

Carbo veg.   ..   Ailments from getting over-heated.

Obtuseness: vertigo: heaviness of head.

Pale greenish face, cold, with cold sweat.

Vital force nearly exhausted. Complete collapse.

Blood stagnates in capillaries: surface cold and blue.

Air hunger.

Natrum carb.   ..   Chronic effects of sunstroke.

Headache from slightest mental exertion: *from the sun,* even working under gas light.

Inability to think. Feels stupid: comprehension slow, difficult.

Head feels too large, as if it would burst (*Acon.*).

Great debility from heat of summer.

Aversion to, and worse from milk.

Natrum mur.   ..   Sunstroke. Heat in head, with red face, nausea and vomiting.

Rush of blood to head: headache as if head would burst (*Glon.,* etc.).

Heaviness occiput; draws eyes together.

Blinding of eyes: fiery zig-zags characteristic.

Worse sun: worse seaside: worse summer.

Pulsatilla   ..   Ailments from heat of sun.

Excessive vertigo. Headache with throbbing in brain.

Even apoplexy; unconscious: face purplish, bloated: violent beating of heart. Pulse collapsed.

Puls. is worse sitting; lying: better walking in open air. *Puls.* is apt to be tearful.

FATIGUE AND BRUISES

Arnica .. For bruises. Effect of falls.
For excessive physical fatigue.
"Tired heart," or dilated from exertion.
Stiffness after long riding.

Give *internally,* a few pellets, four-hourly.
Externally, two drops of tincture to the ounce of
water, saturate lint and apply, covering with cotton-
wool, or oil-silk.

(N.B.—*If the skin is broken, use Hypericum instead.*)

A FEW DROPS IN FOOT-BATH, for tired feet; or use in
the bath, for tired muscles.

SPRAINS

Rhus.   ..   Sprains.
Lumbago.
Stiff neck.
Rheumatism, where pains are worse for *first* move-
ments, agony; but relieved by continued movement
and massage.
(Bryonia is *worse for all movement*.)

         Dose. — A few pellets four-hourly.

Ruta.   ..   Also for sprains — especially of tendons.
Especially helps wrists — ankles — knees.
(N.B. — For sprained ankle, don't attempt to walk,
but stand with flexed knee and, leaning on the toes,
carefully twist and move the foot in every direction,
and so give displacements a chance to slip back into
place. Repeat this at intervals.
Compress of *Rhus,* or *Arnica* will help — 2 drops to
the oz. of water: and *Arnica* or *Rhus* internally.

BURNS AND SUPERFICIAL ULCERS

Urtica Urens (tincture of stinging-nettles.)

         Two drops to the oz. of water. Saturate gauze or lint,
and apply to burn. Cover with cotton-wool, or oil-
silk. Moisten again and again without removing
the gauze, if stuck. Quickly relieves pain, and heals.
(N.B. — Boiling water poured on stinging-nettles
will do as well as the tincture. Soak the lint in
this.)

Cantharis   ..   Or, a dose or two of *Canth.* will stop the pain.

Calendula   ..   Don't forget this remedy for burns and septic wounds.

CUTS—LACERATIONS—PUNCTURES

Hypericum .. The tincture, two drops to the ounce of water, to saturate lint or gauze, and apply. Cover with wool, or at first with oil silk and wool.

Hypericum wounds are acutely painful.

Hypericum, externally draws edges of wounds together, and promotes rapid healing.

Give *internally* also, half a dozen pellets, three doses, four-hourly.

Ledum .. For punctured wounds, wounds by rusty nails.

Insect bites.

Animal bites or scratches.

Ledum feels the COLD: yet wounded parts are cold, and are relieved by cold bathing.

(N.B. — In punctured wounds, if pains begin to shoot upwards, and tetanus threatens, go on to *Hypericum,* internally and externally.)

Apply and administer, as for *Hypericum*.

Calendula .. Cuts: rapidly heals, and prevents suppuration. Apply as above.

TETANUS

Hypericum .. Give internally, a few drops of the strong tincture, or the pellets (preferably dissolved in water), four-hourly.

Externally, *Hypericum* compress (two drops to the ounce as above) to the wound.

Strychnine .. Where the slightest touch aggravates spasm. (With *Hypericum* to wound.)

Nux .. .. Same symptoms as *Strychnine*.

Dose. — Pellets, or pellets dissolved in water, two- to four-hourly.

STINGS

Cantharis ..	Inflamed stings. Swollen, red, very bad gnat bites. Burning, biting pains: v. acute inflammation.
Ledum ..	Punctured wounds and stings. Antidotes insect, bee and animal poisons. Coldness of part, and relief from cold bathing. (Internally and externally: as *Hypericum*.)
Apis ..	Bright red, smooth swelling, with burning and stinging: worse from heat of fire.
Tarentula Cub.	Spider stings, or where stings "go septic."
Arnica ..	A drop of the strong tincture applied to a wasp sting cures it at once.

SNAKE BITES

Lachesis ..	A few pellets in half a tumbler of water, or brandy or whisky. A teaspoonful every fiteen minutes at first. Apply *Hypericum* externally, as above.

(N.B. — UNLIMITED WHISKY OR BRANDY TILL SHOCK IS PAST. In Snake bite, it fails to intoxicate.)

To antidote also, —

Carbolic Acid	Dusky face. Paleness about mouth and nose. Comatose.
Oxalic Acid ..	Violent pains in streaks, or spots. Livid, cold and numb. Trembling hands and feet.
Ammon. Carb.	Livid, weak, drowsy, aversion to cold.

BOILS AND ABSCESSES

Sulphur .. In a warm and hungry patient.

Lachesis .. For suppurations, with BLUENESS of part.

Hepar .. In the choleric patient; even to violence.
Oversensitive mentally and physically: — to a word; to contact; to pressure of dressings.

Silica .. Faint-hearted: anxious.
Confusion and want of self-confidence.
Sweats; 6 a.m., 3-5 p.m., 11 p.m.
Head sweats at night. (*Calc.*)
Boils leave indurations — to promote suppuration, and so heal. (*Calc. Sulph.*)

Calcarea .. In a chilly, sweating patient. (*Calc. Sulph.*)
Running or recurrent abscesses. Won't heal.

Pyrogen .. Great restlessness: feels bruised, sore. (*Arn.*)
Fiery-red, smooth tongue.
Very septic conditions. Pulse-rate high.

Tarentula Cub. "Lachesis — only worse." Parts bluish; burnings like *Ars.* but without the *Ars.* relief from heat.

Doses. — Four to six-hourly till relief.
Externally, compress of *Hypericum,* two drops to the oz.

CARBUNCLE

Arsenicum .. Burning like fire, with relief from hot applications.
Externally a compress of *Hypericum,* three drops to the ounce of water, or *Calendula* in potency, 30 or 200 — a few drops in water to wet compress. Cover with oil-silk and wool. Bandage very lightly.

Tarentula Cub. Like *Lachesis* with blueness of parts; (or *Crotalus*) with hæmorrhages of decomposed blood.
Burning and blueness.

(*See* BOILS above.)

Bibliography

SUGGESTED ADDITIONAL READING

Abrahamson, E. M. and Pezet, A. W. 1971. *Body, Mind and Sugar.* New York: Jove.

Adams, Ruth and Murray, Frank. 1975. *Body, Mind and the B Vitamins.* New York: Larchmont Books.

———— 1975. *Megavitamin Therapy.* New York: Larchmont Books.

Airola, Paavo. 1974. *How to Get Well.* Phoenix, Arizona: Health Plus.

Altschul, A. M. 1965. *Proteins, Their Chemistry and Politics.* New York: Basic Books.

Bailey, Herbert. 1968. *Vitamin E, Your Key to a Healthy Heart.* New York: Arc Books.

Bicknell, Franklin. 1960. *Chemicals in Food and Farm Produce: Their Harmful Effects.* London: Faber and Faber.

Bieler, Henry G. 1973. *Food Is Your Best Medicine.* New York: Random House.

Blaine, Tom R. 1974. *Mental Health through Nutrition.* New York: Citadel Press. ———— 1979. *Nutrition and Your Heart.* New Canaan, Connecticut: Keats Publishing, Inc.

Bricklin, Mark. 1976. *The Practical Encyclopedia of Natural Healing.* Emmaus, Pennsylvania: Rodale Press, Inc.

Carson, Rachel. 1978. *Silent Spring.* New York: Fawcett.

Cheraskin, E.; Ringsdorf, W. M.; and Clark, J. W. 1977. *Diet and Disease.* New Canaan, Connecticut: Keats Publishing, Inc.

Cheraskin, E.; Ringsdorf, W. M.; and Brecher, A. 1976. *Psychodietetics.* New York: Bantam Books.

Clark, Linda. 1970. *Get Well Naturally.* New York: Arco Publishing, Inc. ———— 1973. *Know Your Nutrition.* New Canaan, Connecticut: Keats Publishing, Inc.

Cleave, T. L. 1975. *The Saccharine Disease.* New Canaan, Connecticut: Keats Publishing, Inc.

Commoner, Barry. 1971. *Closing Circle.* New York: Random House. ———— 1966. *Science and Survival.* New York: Viking Press.

Davis, Adelle. 1970. *Let's Cook It Right.* New York: New American Library.

———— 1970. *Let's Eat Right to Keep Fit.* New York: New American Library.

———— 1970. *Let's Get Well.* New York: New American Library.

Fredericks, Carlton. 1975. *Eating Right for You.* New York: Grosset & Dunlap.

Fredericks, Carlton and Goodman, Herman. 1976. *Low Blood Sugar and You.* New York: Constellation International.

Fredericks, Carlton. 1976. *Psycho-Nutrition.* New York: Grosset & Dunlap.

Goodhart, Robert S. and Shils, Maurice E. 1973. *Modern Nutrition in Health and Disease,* 5th ed. Philadelphia: Lea & Febiger.

Graham, Frank. 1970. *Since Silent Spring.* Boston: Houghton Mifflin.

Heuper, Wilhelm C. and Conway, W. D. 1964. *Chemical Carcinogenesis and Cancers.* Chicago: Charles Thomas.

Hill, Howard E. 1976. *Introduction to Lecithin.* New York: Jove.

Hoffer, Abram and Osmond, Humphry. 1966. *How to Live with Schizophrenia.* New York: University Books.

Hoffer, Abram and Walker, Morton. 1978. *Orthomolecular Nutrition.* New Canaan, Connecticut: Keats Publishing, Inc.

Hunter, Beatrice Trum. 1973. *The Natural Foods Primer.* New York: Simon & Schuster.

———— Revised edition. 1980. *Additives Book.* New Canaan, Connecticut: Keats Publishing, Inc.

———— 1972. *Consumer Beware!* New York: Simon & Schuster.

———— 1978. *The Great Nutrition Robbery.* New York: Charles Scribner's Sons.

Jacobson, Michael F. 1972. *Eater's Digest.* Garden City, New York: Doubleday Anchor.

Kirban, Salem. 1979. *The Getting Back to Nature Diet.* New Canaan, Connecticut: Keats Publishing, Inc.

Kirschmann, John D., Nutrition Search, Inc. 1975. *Nutrition Almanac.* New York: McGraw-Hill.

Kugler, Hans J. 1977. *Dr. Kugler's Seven Keys to a Longer Life.* New York: Fawcett.

Lappé, Frances M. 1975. *Diet for a Small Planet.* New York: Ballantine Books.

Lewis, Howard R. 1965. *With Every Breath You Take.* New York: Simon & Schuster.

Lewis, Howard and Martha. 1970. *The Medical Offenders.* New York: Simon & Schuster.

Mintz, Morton. 1965. *The Therapeutic Nightmare.* Boston: Houghton Mifflin.

Moyer, William C. 1971. *Buying Guide for Fresh Fruits, Vegetables and Nuts,* 4th ed. Fullerton, California: Blue Goose.

Newbold, H.L. 1975. *Mega-Nutrients for Your Nerves.* New York: Berkeley.

Ochsner, Alton. 1964. *Smoking and Your Life.* New York: J. Messner.

Page, Melvin E. and Abrams, H.L. 1972. *Your Body Is Your Best Doctor.* New Canaan, Connecticut: Keats Publishing, Inc.

Passwater, Richard A. 1976. *Supernutrition.* New York: Pocket Books.
——— 1978. *Cancer and Its Nutritional Therapies.* New Canaan, Connecticut: Keats Publishing, Inc.
Pauling, Linus. 1971. *Vitamin C and the Common Cold.* New York: Bantam.
Pfeiffer, Carl C. 1975. *Mental and Elemental Nutrients.* New Canaan, Connecticut: Keats Publishing, Inc.
——— 1978. *Zinc and Other Micronutrients.* New Canaan, Connecticut: Keats Publishing, Inc.
Pinckney, Edward and Pinckney, Cathy. 1973. *The Cholesterol Controversy.* Los Angeles, California: Sherbourne Press.
Randolph, Theron G. 1962. *Human Ecology and Susceptibility to the Chemical Environment.* Chicago: Charles Thomas.
Rodale, J.I. 1975. *The Complete Book of Vitamins.* Emmaus, Pennsylvania: Rodale Press.
——— 1976. *The Complete Book of Minerals for Health.* Emmaus, Pennsylvania: Rodale Press.
Schroeder, Henry A. 1978. *The Poisons Around Us.* New Canaan, Connecticut: Keats Publishing, Inc.
——— 1973. *The Trace Elements and Man.* Old Greenwich, Connecticut: Devin-Adair.
Shute, Evan. 1977. *The Heart and Vitamin E.* New Canaan, Connecticut: Keats Publishing, Inc.
Shute, Wilfrid. 1975. *Dr. Wilfrid E. Shute's Complete, Updated Vitamin E. Book.* New Canaan, Connecticut: Keats Publishing, Inc.
Shute, Wilfrid E. and Taub, Harold J. 1972. *Vitamin E for Ailing and Healthy Hearts.* New York: Berkeley.
Stone, Irwin. 1970. *The Healing Factor: "Vitamin C" against Disease.* New York: Grosset & Dunlap.
Taylor, Reneé. 1978. *Hunza Health Secrets.* New Canaan, Connecticut: Keats Publishing, Inc.
Wade, Carlson. 1975. *Hypertension and Your Diet.* New Canaan, Connecticut: Keats Publishing, Inc.
Waldbott, G.L. 1978. *Fluoridation, The Great Dilemma.* Lawrence, Kansas: Coronado Press.
Walker, Morton. 1979. *Total Health.* New York: Everest House.
Williams, Roger J. 1973. *Nutrition against Disease.* New York: Bantam.
Williams, Roger J. and Kalita, Dwight K. 1979. *A Physician's Handbook on Orthomolecular Medicine.* New Canaan, Connecticut: Keats Publishing, Inc.
Williams, Roger J. 1978. *The Wonderful World Within You.* New York: Bantam.
Winter, Ruth. 1972. *Beware of the Food You Eat,* rev. ed. New York: New American Library.
Yudkin, John. 1972. *Sweet and Dangerous.* New York: Bantam.

List of Pharmacies and Companies in the United States and Canada that Can Supply Homeopathic Remedies

(Courtesy of the National Center for Homeopathy, Falls Church, Virginia 22042)

CALIFORNIA

City Pharmacy
1435 State Street
Santa Barbara, CA 93101

College Pharmacy
90 N. Ashwood Avenue
Ventura, CA 93003

Horton and Converse
621 West Pico Boulevard
Los Angeles, CA 90015

Mylans Homeopathic Pharmacy
222 O'Farrell Street
San Francisco, CA 94102

Nutri-Dyn
717 S. Bristol Ave.
Los Angeles, CA 90049

Santa Monica Drug
1513 Fourth Street
Santa Monica, CA 90401

Standard Homeopathic
Company
436 West 8th Avenue
Los Angeles, CA 90014

Village Drug Store
Ojai, CA 93023

ILLINOIS

Ehrhart and Karl
17 N. Wabash Ave.
Chicago, IL 60602

MARYLAND

Washington Homeopathic
Pharmacy
4914 Delray Avenue
Bethesda, MD 20014

MISSOURI

Luyties Pharmacal Company
4200 Laclede Avenue
St. Louis, MO 63108

NEW JERSEY

Humphreys Pharmacal Company
63 Meadow Road
Rutherford, NJ 07070

NEW YORK

Keihl Pharmacy, Inc.
109 Third Avenue
New York, NY 10003

Weleda, Inc.
841 South Main Street
Spring Valley, NY 10977

PENNSYLVANIA

Boericke and Tafel, Inc.
1011 Arch Street
Philadelphia, PA 19107

John A. Borneman and Sons
1208 Amosland Road
Norwood, PA 19074

VIRGINIA

Annandale Apothecary
7023 Little River Turnpike
Annandale, VA 22003.

———————————

CANADA

D. L. Thompson Homeopathic
Supplies
844 Yonge Street
Toronto 5, Ontario
Canada M4W 2H1